The Nature of Children's Well-Being

Children's Well-Being: Indicators and Research Series

Volume 9

Series Editor:

ASHER BEN-ARIEH

Paul Baerwald School of Social Work & Social Welfare, The Hebrew University of Jerusalem

Editorial Board:

J. LAWRENCE ABER
New York University, USA
JONATHAN BRADSHAW
University of York, U.K.
FERRAN CASAS
University of Girona, Spain
ICK-JOONG CHUNG
Duksung Women's University, Seoul, Korea
HOWARD DUBOWITZ
University of Maryland Baltimore, USA
IVAR FRONES
University of Oslo, Norway
FRANK FURSTENBERG
University of Pennsylvania, Philadelphia, USA
ROBBIE GILLIGAN
Trinity College, Dublin, Ireland
ROBERT M. GOERGE
University of Chicago, USA
IAN GOUGH
University of Bath, U.K.
AN-MAGRITT JENSEN
Norwegian University of Science and Technology, Trondheim, Norway
SHEILA B. KAMERMAN
Columbia University, New York, USA
JILL E. KORBIN
Case Western Reserve University, Cleveland, USA

DAGMAR KUTSAR
University of Tartu, Estonia
KEN LAND
Duke University, Durham, USA
BONG JOO LEE
Seoul National University, Seoul, Korea
JAN MASON
University of Western Sydney, Australia
KRISTIN A. MOORE
Child Trends, Washington, USA
BERNHARD NAUCK
Chemnitz University of Technology, Germany
USHA S. NAYAR
Tata Institute, Mumbai, India
WILLIAM O'HARE
Kids Counts project, Annie E. Casy Foundation, Baltimore, USA
SHELLY PHIPPS
Dalhousie University, Halifax, Nova Scotia, Canada
JACKIE SANDERS
Massey University, Palmerston North, New Zealand
GIOVANNI SGRITTA
University of Rome, Italy
THOMAS S. WEISNER
University of California, Los Angeles, USA
HELMUT WINTESBERGER
University of Vienna, Austria

This new series focuses on the subject of measurements and indicators of children's well being and their usage, within multiple domains and in diverse cultures. More specifically, the series seeks to present measures and data resources, analysis of data, exploration of theoretical issues, and information about the status of children, as well as the implementation of this information in policy and practice. By doing so it aims to explore how child indicators can be used to improve the development and the well being of children.

With an international perspective the series will provide a unique applied perspective, by bringing in a variety of analytical models, varied perspectives, and a variety of social policy regimes.

Children's Well-Being: Indicators and Research will be unique and exclusive in the field of measures and indicators of children's lives and will be a source of high quality, policy impact and rigorous scientific papers.

More information about this series at http://www.springer.com/series/8162

Alexander Bagattini • Colin Macleod
Editors

The Nature of Children's Well-Being

Theory and Practice

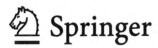

Editors
Alexander Bagattini
Department of Philosophy
University of Düsseldorf
Germany

Colin Macleod
Department of Philosophy and Faculty of Law
University of Victoria
Victoria, BC, Canada

ISSN 1879-5196 ISSN 1879-520X (electronic)
ISBN 978-94-017-9251-6 ISBN 978-94-017-9252-3 (eBook)
DOI 10.1007/978-94-017-9252-3
Springer Dordrecht Heidelberg New York London

Library of Congress Control Number: 2014948453

© Springer Science+Business Media Dordrecht 2015
This work is subject to copyright. All rights are reserved by the Publisher, whether the whole or part of the material is concerned, specifically the rights of translation, reprinting, reuse of illustrations, recitation, broadcasting, reproduction on microfilms or in any other physical way, and transmission or information storage and retrieval, electronic adaptation, computer software, or by similar or dissimilar methodology now known or hereafter developed. Exempted from this legal reservation are brief excerpts in connection with reviews or scholarly analysis or material supplied specifically for the purpose of being entered and executed on a computer system, for exclusive use by the purchaser of the work. Duplication of this publication or parts thereof is permitted only under the provisions of the Copyright Law of the Publisher's location, in its current version, and permission for use must always be obtained from Springer. Permissions for use may be obtained through RightsLink at the Copyright Clearance Center. Violations are liable to prosecution under the respective Copyright Law.
The use of general descriptive names, registered names, trademarks, service marks, etc. in this publication does not imply, even in the absence of a specific statement, that such names are exempt from the relevant protective laws and regulations and therefore free for general use.
While the advice and information in this book are believed to be true and accurate at the date of publication, neither the authors nor the editors nor the publisher can accept any legal responsibility for any errors or omissions that may be made. The publisher makes no warranty, express or implied, with respect to the material contained herein.

Printed on acid-free paper

Springer is part of Springer Science+Business Media (www.springer.com)

Contents

Part I   Children's Well-Being and Autonomy

1 **Children, Adults, Autonomy and Well-Being** 3
  David Archard

2 **Autonomy and Children's Well-Being** 15
  Paul Bou-Habib and Serena Olsaretti

3 **The 'Intrinsic Goods of Childhood' and the Just Society** 35
  Anca Gheaus

4 **Agency, Authority and the Vulnerability of Children** 53
  Colin Macleod

5 **Enhancing the Capacity for Autonomy: What Parents Owe Their Children to Make Their Lives Go Well** 65
  Monika Betzler

6 **Utilitarianism, Welfare, Children** 85
  Anthony Skelton

Part II   Children's Well-Being and Authority

7 **Paternalism in Education and the Future** 107
  Dieter Birnbacher

8 **Anti-perfectionist Childrearing** 123
  Matthew Clayton

9 **Respecting Children and Children's Dignity** 141
  Holger Baumann and Barbara Bleisch

10 **Who Decides?** 157
   James G. Dwyer

Part III Children's Well-Being and Policy

11 The Concept of Best Interests in Clinical Practice 179
Jürg C. Streuli

12 Children's Well-Being and the Family-Dilemma 191
Alexander Bagattini

13 Child Welfare and Child Protection: Medicalization and Scandalization as the New Norms in Dealing with Violence Against Children 209
Heiner Fangerau, Arno Görgen, and Maria Griemmert

14 Children's Rights, Well-Being, and Sexual Agency 227
Samantha Brennan and Jennifer Epp

15 The Grounds and Limits of Parents' Cultural Prerogatives: The Case of Circumcision.. 247
Jurgen De Wispelaere and Daniel Weinstock

Contributors

David Archard School of Politics, International Studies and Philosophy, Queen's University Belfast, Belfast, Northern Ireland, UK

Alexander Bagattini Department of Philosophy, University of Düsseldorf, Germany

Holger Baumann Centre for Ethics, University of Zürich, Zürich, Switzerland

Monika Betzler Department of Philosophy, University of Bern, Bern, Switzerland

Dieter Birnbacher Department of Philosophy, University of Düsseldorf, Düsseldorf, Germany

Barbara Bleisch Centre for Ethics, University of Zürich, Zürich, Switzerland

Paul Bou-Habib Department of Government, University of Essex, Colchester, UK

Samantha Brennan University of Western Ontario, London, ON, Canada

Matthew Clayton Department of Politics and International Studies, Social Sciences Building, The University of Warwick, Coventry, UK

Jurgen De Wispelaere Institute for Health and Social Policy, McGill University, Montreal, QC, Canada

James G. Dwyer Admission Office, William & Mary Law School, Williamsburg, VA, USA

Jennifer Epp University of Western Ontario, London, ON, Canada

Heiner Fangerau Institute for the History, Philosophy and Ethics of Medicine, University of Ulm, Ulm, Germany

Anca Gheaus Department of Philosophy, University of Sheffield, Sheffield, UK

Arno Görgen Institute for the History, Philosophy and Ethics of Medicine, University of Ulm, Ulm, Germany

Maria Griemmert Institute for the History, Philosophy and Ethics of Medicine, University of Ulm, Ulm, Germany

Colin Macleod Department of Philosophy and Faculty of Law, University of Victoria, Victoria, BC, Canada

Serena Olsaretti ICREA-Universitat Pompeu Fabra, Departament d'Humanitats, UPF, Barcelona, Spain

Anthony Skelton Department of Philosophy, University of Western Ontario, London, ON, Canada

Jürg C. Streuli University Children's Hospital Zürich, Zürich, Switzerland

Daniel Weinstock Faculty of Law, McGill University, Montreal, QC, Canada

Introduction

The concept of children's well-being or welfare is frequently invoked in public debate in a wide variety of legal, political, medical, educational and familial contexts. There is broad consensus that the well-being of children matters greatly and that it deserves special promotion and protection. Yet the very concept of child well-being is also highly contested. People often disagree about what child well-being consists in, how it is to be promoted and about its importance in relation to other goods and moral values.

Disputes about the nature of children's well-being arise in part because there are many different disciplinary perspectives from which to approach the concept. In medicine, for example, we sometimes find a narrow health-related concept of the well-being of children. Medicine, as an empirical science, tends to emphasize a conception of well-being grounded in basic physiological and psychological attributes. Well-being is treated as proper biological functioning as exhibited in the absence of disease or impairments of normal capacities. By contrast, the social sciences often focus on objective economic factors (e.g., levels of poverty), educational factors (e.g., test scores) and social factors (e.g., family structure and divorce rates) in the analysis of children's well-being. Some traditional religious communities worry that the focus on material dimensions of well-being comes at the expense of proper recognition of the spiritual well-being of children. And so on.

These diverse perspectives are not necessarily inconsistent. But a narrow focus on one perspective or one facet of well-being can generate controversies or puzzles. For example, if the well-being of children is treated primarily as a physical and psychological phenomenon, social factors that influence well-being such as family-structures or peer-pressure are easily overlooked. This in turn can result in the over medicalization of problems in which medical treatment comes to dominate efforts to promote well-being. We can see this illustrated in the alarming propensity of viewing hyperactivity in children solely as medical condition that can be remedied by prescribing powerful drugs such as Ritalin. In other cases, the concerns that some parents have for the spiritual well-being of children sometimes leads them to neglect or jeopardize their children's health. These familiar examples remind us that one general challenge in developing a satisfactory account of well-being is to determine how different facets of well-being should be integrated in a balanced and comprehensive outlook that can help guide practical decisions affecting children.

This book is intended to contribute to the project of illuminating different facets of the well-being of children and their relevance to the proper treatment of children. The specific issues addressed by the contributors are diverse as are the disciplinary perspectives and methods they employ. Together the chapters do not yield a single unified theory of the well-being of children. However, the essays are animated by a common assumption that focused attention on the character of the well-being of children is needed for at least two reasons. First, this is an understudied topic in philosophy and related academic disciplines. Second, simplistic or impoverished accounts of well-being still wield influence in various political and policy settings. The resolution of practical controversies concerning the treatment of children can be enhanced by developing more nuanced views about the nature and sources of children's well-being. Given, complexity and importance of addressing the nature of the well-being of children, there is surprisingly little academic literature that confronts the topic directly and systematically. Most philosophical treatments of well-being dwell on the well-being of adults.

Although there are, of course, commonalities between the well-being of adults and children, there are also theoretical and practically interesting differences. The essays in the volume both build upon and, in some ways, depart from general philosophical work on well-being. First, although some general dimensions of children's well-being are relatively uncontroversial, there are philosophical disagreements about the meaning and character of well-being at both the abstract and concrete level. The utilitarian tradition analyses well-being as consisting in happiness but is divided as to whether happiness should be interpreted hedonistically or whether it consists in some form of preference satisfaction. Aristotelian views, by contrast, view happiness as only one, perhaps rather small, dimension of a broader conception of eudaimonia. On these views, well-being is best seen a type of flourishing comprised of various intrinsic goods that are realized through the development and exercise of distinctively human capacities. For the most part, such expressly philosophical views have been developed with little or no attention to special features of the well-being of children. Yet children's happiness might have quite different sources and character than the happiness of adults. For instance, since children often do not understand what they want, desire satisfaction theories of happiness do not tell us much about children's happiness. Similarly, eudaimonic flourishing as a child may be quite different from flourishing as an adult. After all, at least some of the rational and affective capacities of adults that figure prominently in Aristotelian accounts of eudaimonia are not fully present in children. So in addition to determining how to address substantive philosophical disputes about the nature of well-being in general, work needs to be done on how to extend or adapt theories of adult well-being to children.

Second, interpretation of the well-being of children is complicated by the special relationships of intimacy, authority and care that obtain between adults, especially parents, and children. In most states, parents enjoy a great deal of latitude in deciding what the well-being of their children consists in and how best to promote it. Parents, for example, have wide discretion to shape their children's religious, moral and political convictions and they are permitted to make many medical, educational, dietary and lifestyle decisions (e.g., about access to media, participation in sports or music) that directly affect the well-being of children. Parental authority is often grounded in the assumption that children lack sufficient autonomy to track their interests reliably. Parents are called upon to identify and advance the well-being of their children until such time that the children become competent, independent and responsible agents. Yet parental authority over children can be exercised in ways that jeopardizes children's well-being. So parental authority to make and implement judgements about what promotes the well-being of their children is not absolute. It is always, to some important degree, limited by basic considerations of health, safety and education that are not grounded in parental judgements. Moreover, children, even before they fully mature, are not merely passive subjects. They are active and developing agents. This means facets of the independent agency they display as children are arguably relevant to the interpretation of their well-being. The well-being of children may be partly constituted by or grounded in the preferences they have and the choices they make. We may gain insight in children's well-being by being attentive to their opinions. Similarly, even when we doubt the soundness of children's judgement about their own well-being, respecting (some of) their less than ideal views, can have valuable developmental benefits and display respect for them as independent persons.

These observations give rise to practical and theoretical puzzles about how well-being should be understood in relation to parental views and what the appropriate response to potential threats to well-being is in light of the special importance of family relationships between parents and children. For example, physicians and social workers sometimes seek to protect children from their parents. Yet parents often view interventions into the private life of the family as meddlesome and destructive. In such disputes, both sides appeal to the well-being of children to justify their actions. How should such conflicts be adjudicated? How are the choices and preferences of children relevant to tracking their interests? In the face of a plurality of interpretations of child well-being, what conception of well-being should a just state employ to craft effective laws and public policies that bear upon the treatment of children? Credible answers to these and related questions depend on identifying and assessing the significance of distinct dimensions of children's well-being.

The essays in this collection contribute to that project in various ways. The book has three major parts with the essays in each part loosely organized about a common general theme. The first part focuses on issues concerning the relation between children's well-being and autonomy or agency. The second part deals with child well-being insofar as the limits of parental authority are concerned. The third part has a more applied orientation and addresses a variety of public policy controversies involving the interpretation of children's well-being.

In much literature, the concept of the child is typically defined by a purported lack of autonomy on the side of the child (Schapiro 1999) that is grounded in the cognitive, emotional and moral immaturity of children. This view emphasizes the capacities that adults normally have but that children lack: reasoning powers, time-oriented perspectives, emotional control, self-knowledge and a stable self-image (Noggle 2002). This leads some authors to view childhood as "predicament" from which children need to be helped to escape. What is valuable in a child's life is identified mainly as those activities and experiences that are instrumentally valuable in facilitating the emergence of a rational, autonomous agent (Schapiro 1999). The predicament view provides an easy basis for justifying paternalistic action against children. Children are considered to be "incompetents" (Buchanan and Brock 1990) that are incapable of reliably identifying and securing their own interests. Their well-being can only be secured through the close guidance and supervision of adults. Moreover, the orientation of paternalistic concern for children is primarily centred around preparing them for adult life and the opportunities for well-being adulthood presents. Yet, as the papers in the first part of the book demonstrate, childhood may have significance beyond its role in preparing children for adulthood. Grappling with emerging autonomy of children may be more complicated and nuanced than is often assumed.

In "Children, Adults, Autonomy and Well-Being", David Archard helps to set the stage for closer consideration of the autonomy of children and its significance by offering a subtle challenge to the widespread assumption that a sharp line can be drawn between the moral and political status of children and adults in virtue of their respective autonomy. (Adults are autonomous; children are not.) This commonly invoked "basic" view in turn underlies a liberal orthodoxy about paternalism: whereas the freedom of competent adults cannot be limited in the name of promoting their own good, promoting the well-being of children is the only consideration that matters in determining how to treat them. Archard argues that the basic view offers an unduly simplistic account of the manner in the opinions of children matter to the justification of paternalism. Children's own views about how they wish to be treated must be given weight that is sensitive both to the level of maturity and to the magnitude of the interest that is at stake when paternalism is contemplated. For Archard the point of consulting children is not solely to gather evidence about what their interests are. Instead, children's views have some weight in limiting paternalism even when they do not track their well-being perfectly.

In their paper "Autonomy and Children's Well-Being" Paul Bou-Habib and Serena Olsaretti argue for greater recognition of and respect for the distinctive autonomy of children. In their view children have a specific form of autonomy that is different from the autonomy of adults, yet it differs only in degree. Even quite young children have sufficient cognitive capacities to understand, adopt and remain committed projects and activities that they value. Securing the well-being of children, on their view, is intricately bound up in responding to the autonomy that children already display. This does not mean that children's preferences are always an authoritative guide to how they may be treated but on their account of "child-sensitive autonomy", children's reasons pose more forceful constraints on paternalism than is usually recognized. En route to developing this position, Bou-Habib and Olsaretti discuss and critique influential interpretations of the relevance of autonomy to children. They argue that many accounts of the significance of autonomy in children wrongly treat it solely as an end-state to be achieved by proper education and upbringing. Such views unduly circumscribe the capacities and authority of children in many domains to pursue their own well-being in their own way. Bou-Habib and Olsaretti also challenge Matthew Clayton's view that limits of acceptable parenting practices are set by a standard of retrospective consent. Although they are sympathetic to Clayton's opposition to the comprehensive enrollment of children into the projects of their parents, Bou-Habib and Olsaretti insist that Clayton does not adequately acknowledge the significance of children's own autonomy.

The idea that children's distinct conceptions of their own well-being need to be more fully acknowledged and respected is allied with a somewhat different theme that there are intrinsic goods of childhood. The basic suggestion is children have some special opportunities for well-being and flourishing and that value and significance of these opportunities cannot be reduced to their instrumental contribution to successful development of children into mature adults. This theme is explored in different ways in chapters by Anca Gheaus and Colin Macleod.

In her essay "The Intrinsic Goods of Childhood and the Just Society" Anca Gheaus defends the claim that there are such intrinsic goods of childhood and childhood itself has special value in virtue of the access to these goods that it affords. For example, childhood presents opportunities for carefree, spontaneous play that is fuelled by boundless imagination. Gheaus argues that proper appreciation of the value of such goods gives us reason to abandon the "predicament" view of childhood. Gheaus's proposal draws some recent research of the developmental psychologist Alison Gopnik that characterizes childhood not in terms of the absence of rationality. Rather the distinguishing feature of childhood lies in children's remarkable capacities of curiosity and their ability to learn and change in the light of new experience (Gopnik 2010). Although Gheaus acknowledges that children have more ready access to the goods of childhood, she argues adults can experience and appreciate these goods too. Indeed for Gheaus our conception of the elements of a successful adult life and the character of a just society should be revised so as to valorize and facilitate the pursuit of childhood goods by adults. On her view, at least some of the goods of childhood can and should be accessed by adults.

Although Colin Macleod also argues for the recognition of intrinsic goods of childhood, he explores the idea from a different angle. In "Agency, Authority and the Vulnerability of Children", Macleod considers how the difference between the vulnerability of adults and children is largely grounded in features of their respective agency. Adults are usually considered less vulnerable than children and this is largely because they are mature agents who have fully developed cognitive capacities in virtue they can manage important aspects of their own well-being. Children, by contrast, are juvenile agents to whom the rights to manage their own well-being are not assigned because they lack the powers of mature agency. Given our concern to reduce the vulnerability of children, one might think that we should expedite, to the greatest degree possible, the development of mature agency in children. Macleod, however, resists this suggestion because he thinks that the very absence of some features of mature agency gives children access to important sources of well-being. Macleod sees children's innocence and their capacities for imaginative play as especially valuable. Securing children access to these goods gives us a reason not to rush the development of mature agency, and this in turn affects our understanding of the rights we assign to children. Unlike Gheaus, Macleod does not think mature agents can readily access the goods of childhood. In his view, childhood has special value because it affords children more or less unique access to the goods grounded in the exercise of juvenile agency.

Monika Betzler allows that there are intrinsic goods of childhood but in her paper, "Enhancing the Capacity for Children's Autonomy: What Parents Owe Their Children to Make Their Lives Go Well", she focuses on the significance of autonomy acquisition for children's well-being. For Betzler, one of the most important duties of parents is to promote and even enforce their children in becoming autonomous persons. Betzler's basic idea is that children need to be engaged in and come to value their own projects so as to become autonomous persons. Valuing projects manifests what a person finds important, and thus satisfies an authenticity condition of autonomy. Parents have a duty to encourage their children to adopt and value significant projects. Projects are defined as norm-governed, complex action-types that are related to identity-commitments on the side of the child. By learning to pursue and value projects, children are, according to Betzler, supposed to acquire strong value-commitments that are necessary for long-term life-plans and autonomous decision-making.

Most of the essays in the first part of the volume consider how recognition and facilitation of children's autonomy or agency affects our understanding of their well-being. But the happiness of children is surely a component of well-being and it is instructive to consider how it might be understood independently of concerns about autonomy. This is challenge taken up by Anthony Skelton in his "Utilitarianism, Welfare, Children". As the title suggests, Skelton's paper draws on a broadly utilitarian perspective insofar it analyses well-being in terms of happiness. His main goal in his contribution is to overcome the general neglect of children's well-being in utilitarian ethics. Skelton reviews influential contemporary accounts of welfare in the literature and reveals its limited applicability of many views to children. He criticizes subjectivist desire accounts as ill suited to young children and objective list accounts as too exclusive. To remedy these problems, he introduces a hybrid account of well-being that embraces both subjective and objective criteria of well-being. For Skelton children's well-being should be defined by a child's subjective happiness as well by specific objective features of a child's well-being such as health. Despite its expressly utilitarian orientation, there are commonalities between Skelton's view about the characteristics of a good childhood and those endorsed by other authors in the part who do not analyze the issues from a utilitarian perspective.

Whether or to what degree the utilitarian account offered by Skelton complements the other proposals is an interesting issue.

The second part of the book picks up questions concerning the relation between children's well-being and the authority of adults to make decisions on their behalf. A standard view assigns almost complete authority to adults, and especially parents, to make judgements about children's well-being. Some degree of paternalism towards children is legitimate but there has been increasing recognition that determining the character and extent of adult authority over children is no simple matter. In his essay, "Paternalism in Education and The Future", Dieter Birnbacher addresses a puzzle about paternalism that arises in the context of education. The main question of the paper concerns the extent to which paternalism should be allowed in education. Drawing upon a line of argument due to the nineteenth-century philosopher Friedrich Schleiermacher, Birnbacher explores a special temporal dimension of paternalistic acts in education. Education is supposed to serve the long-term interests of children. However, as Schleiermacher pointed out, the realization of the expected future positive effects of paternalistic action is sometimes highly unreliable. Uncertainty about how or the degree to which educational paternalism will serve the (relatively distant) future interests of children creates an obstacle to justifying paternalism. We often have less confidence about how paternalistic intervention now will serve the interests of a person many years later. Indeed for Schleiermacher there are strict limits to the justifiability of paternalism in education. Although Birnbacher partly endorses Schleiermacher's view, he proposes a number of "tendency rules" that can help us distinguish between forms of educational paternalism that are likely to promote future interests and those that are unlikely to do so. The temporal puzzle can thereby be resolved to a reasonable degree.

Parents are widely thought to have authority not only to act paternalistically toward their children but also to secure their children's adherence to controversial conceptions of the good that they endorse but which may not be essential for securing their children's well-being. Matthew Clayton rejects this latter form of parental authority and has famously criticized the practice of what he calls "comprehensive enrollment" (Clayton 2006). Parents do not have the right to enroll their children in controversial conceptions of the good because children have a right to develop their independent worldview. In his paper, "Anti-Perfectionist Child-Rearing", Clayton defends his view against criticisms that it unduly circumscribes parental prerogatives to promote the well-being of their children. He concedes that his view does limit the manner in which parents may promote their children's well-being but he argues that these limits are justified by the considerations that parallel those that justify perfectionism by the state directed at its citizens. Just as the exercise of the state's power over citizens must satisfy criteria of political legitimacy, the exercise of parental power over children must be legitimate. However, according to Clayton the anti-perfectionist child-rearing that legitimacy requires does not gravely limit the well-being of children and is not as austere as it might seem to critics.

In their combined paper "Respecting Children and Children's Dignity", Barbara Bleisch and Holger Baumann proceed from the assumption that children are not fully autonomous agents. However, they argue that understanding children's well-being as well as what it means to respect children can be deepened through consideration of a concept of dignity. As the authors show, the concept of human dignity has remained surprisingly absent from philosophical discussions about the ethics of childhood. Drawing upon personhood accounts of human dignity, Bleisch and Baumann suggest that respecting a child's dignity involves acknowledging and appreciating the activities through which she develops and maintains an evaluative perspective of her own. Most traditional accounts of human agency highlight the concept of autonomy. On the assumption that children lack autonomy, paternalistic action against children seems easy to justify. Bleisch and Baumann's account of children's dignity does not ground dignity in autonomy but it does entail restrictions on the exercise of authority of adults over children. The proper exercise of authority over children is guided and limited by a concern to nurture and respect the activities through which a distinctive evaluative standpoint is formed. So respect for the dignity of children provides a constraint on paternalism towards them that does not depend on autonomy.

Parents are often assumed to have a kind of natural authority over children that is only limited or lost in extreme cases in which the exercise of authority by parents seriously jeopardizes the well-being of children. But in his essay, "Who Decides?", James Dwyer challenges the idea the parents enjoy ultimate authority over the lives of children. He argues that ultimate authority to determine who has custody of children and who may control important aspects of children's lives ultimately belongs to the state. On Dwyer's view, the state may delegate the authority to raise children to parents or other adults but there need be not general presumption that parents are the best custodians of children's well-being. Whether or to what degree parents should be assigned authority over children should depend on consideration by state authorities of the evidence on what arrangements are most conducive to the interests of children.

The third part of the book focuses shifts to the interpretation of children's well-being in various applied contexts in which political and policy controversies arise. As a number of papers in this part indicate, a major issue in the field is the well-being of children in the medical realm. In his paper, "The Concept of Best Interests in Clinical Practice", Jürg Streuli asks about the necessary content for a meaningful and consistent concept of best interests for use in clinical practice. He proposes a complex "constitutional matrix" that invites us to consider three kinds of discourses about children's interests and the perspectives of four stakeholders on those interests. According to Streuli, the classical analysis of best interests by Buchanan and Brock in terms of maximizing children's interests (Buchanan and Brock 1989) or the isolated consideration of the harm principle, as proposed by Diekema (2011), provide little practical guidance in complex clinical settings. An augmentation of the concept of "best interests" suitable for clinical practice requires a perspective that is sensitive to different ideologies, can determine what optimal care in a particular context is and can identify thresholds of harm. These three discourses should be informed and shaped by the views of different stakeholders: parents, clinical experts, children and future persons. So Streuli rejects a simple best interests standard as a normative principle in clinical settings. Instead he favours a more multifaceted approach that integrates and balances different perspectives on children's well-being.

In his paper "Children's Well-Being and the Family-Dilemma", Alexander Bagattini analyses a possible dilemma for physicians when they treat children as their patients: on the one hand, they have to protect children's interests and a corresponding duty to report cases where children have been maltreated. On the other hand, they have to respect parental interests in privacy of the family and parental autonomy. These duties can conflict when the physician suspects that parents have abused their child. The family-dilemma arises in legal systems that implement what David Archard calls the liberal standard: in the default case parents enjoy parental autonomy and privacy of the family. Interferences with parental autonomy are legitimate only in cases where a physician has a justified suspicion of maltreatment. This brings about the peculiar situation for the physician in which she has to decide if her evidence justifies a report to a responsible institution. Bagattini points out that the occurrence of the family-dilemma threatens the protection of vital children's interests. He shows how the values of parental autonomy and familial privacy need to be refined in order to escape the family dilemma. In the investigation of abuse, Bagattini favours shifting the burden from physicians to parents. On this approach, a physician's reasonable suspicion that a child has been abused by a parent would trigger the requirement the parent establish that he or she was not responsible for abuse.

In their combined paper, "Child Welfare and Child Protection: Medicalization and Media-Scandalization as the New Norms in Dealing with Violence Against Children", Heiner Fangerau, Maria Griemmert and Arno Görgen analyse and explore the social and political forces that influence societal norms of child protection. Their analysis gives special emphasis to the interplay of two discourses. On the one hand, various developments in medical science permitted the diagnosis of harms faced by children and introduced a vocabulary through which harms to children could be categorized and catalogued. On the other hand, discourse in the media emphasizing dramatic incidents of abuse drew public attention to the well-being of children and mobilized political support for changes to legal norms. Unlike the other papers in the volume, this essay is not expressly normative but it provides an interesting account of the evolution of norms of child protection via the interaction between medical discourse and the discourse of media-scandalization.

Samantha Brennan and Jennifer Epp observe that consideration of the sexuality of children often generates anxiety about the dangers of sexual activity for children. Children are vulnerable to harmful sexual exploitation by adults. And to the degree that they are not viewed as potential victims and are seen as engaged in voluntary sexual activity, popular discourse usually focuses on the risks for children of such activity – e.g., unwanted pregnancy or sexually transmitted diseases. Brennan and Epp acknowledge that these are legitimate concerns but in their essay, "Children's Rights, Well-Being and Sexual Agency", they argue that there has been insufficient recognition of the possibility that some forms of sexual activity may be important elements of the well-being of children. Brennan and Epp review prevailing attitudes to children's sexuality in the literature and identify ways in which it has failed to grapple adequately with children as emerging sexual agents. In some respects, their analysis is provisional: they seek to prepare the ground for more sustained and reflective investigation of this controversial topic. However, they do insist that children, even before they are fully autonomous, can meaningfully consent to some kinds of lower risk sexual activity (with other children). Moreover, they endorse "sex positive" programs of sex education that teach children not only about the risks of sexual activity but also its potential contribution to well-being.

Finally, in "The Grounds and Limit of Parents' Cultural Prerogatives: The Case of Circumcision", Jurgen De Wispelaere and Daniel Weinstock discuss the degree to which parents should be permitted to require children to participate in religious or cultural rituals to which children cannot consent. Their analysis focuses on controversies surrounding the legitimacy of circumcision that is not medically necessary but that is viewed, by some parents, as having great religious or cultural significance. De Wispaelaere and Weinstock offer a qualified defense of the permissibility of circumcision that is safely performed and does not impair normal sexual functioning. Their rationale is located in the way in which permitting circumcision can contribute to the well-being of parents and children by facilitating intimate relationships that are grounded in joint participation in cultural traditions. This does not mean that all cultural or religious practices that facilitate "intimacy goods" are permissible. Protecting children from excessive harm remains a paramount concern. However, De Wispaelaere and Weinstock maintain that the risks of circumcision fall below the threshold of serious harm. So, in this case, there is not a troubling trade-off between realizing intimacy goods and protecting the basic well-being of children.

We think that the papers in this volume reveal the richness of the topic of the well-being of children. Of course, we hope that they have yielded some substantive insights about the components of children's well-being as well as their rights and moral claims in relation to adults. However, the essays in this volume are not the final word on the subject. Instead, they are an invitation for further exploration that we hope others will take up.

Düsseldorf, Germany   Alexander Bagattini
Victoria, BC, Canada   Colin Macleod

References

Buchanan, A., & Brock, D. (1989). *Deciding for others. The ethics of surrogate decision making*. Cambridge: Cambridge University Press.
Buchanan, A., & Brock, D. (1990). *Deciding for others*. Cambridge: Cambridge University Press.
Clayton, M. (2006). *Justice and legitimacy in upbringing*. Oxford: Oxford University Press.
Diekema, D. (2011). Revisiting the best interest standard: Uses and misuses. *Journal of Clinical Ethics, 22*(2), 128–133.
Gopnik, A. (2010). *The philosophical baby*. New York: Picador.
Noggle, R. (2002). Special agents: Children's autonomy and parental authority. In D. Archard & C. Macleod (Eds.), *The moral and political status of children*. Oxford: Oxford University Press.
Schapiro, T. (1999). What is a child? *Ethics, 109*(4), 715–738.

Part I
Children's Well-Being and Autonomy

Chapter 1
Children, Adults, Autonomy and Well-Being

David Archard

1.1 Introduction

Here is a simple and brief summary of a view that should nevertheless be readily recognisable. I will entitle it the 'basic view'. Children and adults enjoy a different moral and political status. The well-being, or interests, of both adults and children matter. Indeed, they matter equally to the extent that we should not think that age makes any difference to how we weight the interests of an individual adult and an individual child. In the famous words attributed to Jeremy Bentham by John Stuart Mill, 'Everybody to count for one and nobody to count for more than one' (Mill 1969: 257). All human beings are equal and are so in respect of their shared humanity. Nevertheless, there is this difference between adults and children. Adults can and should be permitted to make choices as to how they lead their lives. By contrast, children cannot and should not be permitted to make such choices. Thus adults have fundamental liberty rights, whereas children, if they do have any rights, only have basic welfare rights.

This view is of course crudely stated. Much has been written, especially in recent years, on the moral and political status of children (Archard and Macleod 2002: Part 1). The sharply drawn contrast between adulthood and childhood has been challenged. Proper acknowledgement of what is specific and peculiar to childhood, and what follows morally as a result, has been demanded. The extent to which children lack any rights or any acknowledged capacity to make decisions has also been critically discussed. Nevertheless, the 'basic view' exercises considerable influence. It does so not just within the domain of philosophy, but also in law and social policy. Children and adults, on this 'basic view', are very different from one another, and

D. Archard (✉)
School of Politics, International Studies and Philosophy, Queen's University Belfast,
University Road, Belfast BT7 1NN, Northern Ireland, UK
e-mail: d.archard@qub.ac.uk

© Springer Science+Business Media Dordrecht 2015
A. Bagattini, C. Macleod (eds.), *The Nature of Children's Well-Being*,
Children's Well-Being: Indicators and Research 9,
DOI 10.1007/978-94-017-9252-3_1

this fact should make a big and real difference to how they are treated socially, legally and politically. Since it serves well to illustrate some of the issues I will be treating, consider the case of biomedicine. Adults cannot be subjected to any medical procedure or to participation in any medical research without their informed consent. Children, by contrast, have no such status. When it comes to the question of whether or not children should undergo a medical procedure what matters is what is in their best interests.

In what follows I shall not attempt any fresh review of the 'basic view'. Rather I shall explore what it implies for how, in the context of the distinction between adults and children, we think about the relationship between autonomy and welfare, and in particular, in consequence, for how we evaluate paternalism.

1.2 The Nature and Value of Autonomy

Let me start then by outlining another familiar view, one about the nature and value of adult autonomy. Adult human beings are autonomous or self-governing creatures. This capacity for self-rule marks humans out from other animals and is of great value. It merits the ascription to adult human beings of a certain moral status, one that is possessed equally. What further follows is that adults should be permitted, subject to certain qualifications, to make their own decisions about matters affecting only their own interests. Although it is acknowledged that adults differ in their abilities to make independent choices, and to make sensible or prudent choices, nevertheless inasmuch as all adults do have a basic capacity to choose how to lead their own lives they should be allowed the freedom to do so.

Let me now spell out what this view claims in a little more detail, and say something about how I shall understand autonomy. The ideal of autonomy here being appealed to is often attributed to Kant. Or at least Kant is cited as a key source of this ideal. However, Kantians, such as Onora O'Neill, are quick to distinguish a properly Kantian ideal of moral autonomy – the capacity of human beings to regulate their decisions in conformity with the moral law vouchsafed to them by their possession of reason – from that of personal autonomy – which is a general capacity to think about and subsequently act upon one's own desires and beliefs (O'Neill 2002). In what follows it is the ideal of personal autonomy that is in question.

Some feminists have criticised what they regard as the individualist or atomist presuppositions of the ideal of personal autonomy. To that end they have favoured what is termed 'relational autonomy' and stressed the importance of an individual's social and personal relations (Nedelsky 1989; Mackenzie and Stoljar 2000). It is unclear whether the criticism is that such relations are important as a necessary context for the acquisition and exercise of personal autonomy, or whether it is that autonomy just is to have and live within those relations. In what follows I ignore such controversy and endorse no particular view of what autonomy is or requires.

Personal autonomy is a capacity whose value lies in its exercise. The capacity is roughly one of being able in the right kind of way to think about and to revise one's beliefs and desires. What matters, then, is that humans are able to exercise that capacity in the leading of their lives. 'By exercising such a capacity, persons define their nature, give meaning and coherence to their lives, and take responsibility for the kind of person they are' (Dworkin 1988: 20). Of the capacity in question much more can be said, and there has been extensive discussion of what exactly it involves. It suffices to indicate here that, broadly, there are two kinds of capacity, one having to do with the ability of the individual to choose independently of others, and one having to do with the ability of the individual to choose in the light of what are genuinely her own desires and beliefs.

Why exactly is autonomy valuable and just how valuable is it? Ascribing moral and political significance to the capacity of humans to make their own choices is a product of modernity and of the Enlightenment. At bottom the idea is that individuals owe nothing to others simply in virtue of their inherited or acquired social position, and that for each of us no course of life is indicated in advance as required or predetermined. We can be, and should strive to be, the authors of our own lives.

It is contentious just how valuable autonomy is and, again, much has been written on the subject. Let me roughly sketch three possible ways in which the value of autonomy might be expressed. On the first, which we might call a transcendental valuation, the exercise of autonomy is essential or necessary if anything else is to be of value in a life. Autonomy is a precondition of individual well-being. We have reason to enhance and to develop everybody's autonomy just insofar as doing so thereby necessarily serves to increase their overall well-being (Haworth 1984). On this view a non-autonomous life will always be worse than one led autonomously. Expressed in another and very influential manner an endorsement constraint operates upon the value of any life. This holds that, 'No life goes better by being led from the outside according to values the person does not endorse' (Kymlicka 1990: 203). This amounts to the first view inasmuch as such endorsement must be autonomous if the constraint is to be credible.

On a second view the exercise of autonomy is instrumentally valuable. Insofar as individuals choose autonomously they choose well and what is for their own good. This is because individuals know better than others what makes their life go well. Mill appeared to endorse this view when he claimed in *On Liberty* that, respecting their own interests, the 'ordinary man or woman has means of knowledge immeasurably surpassing those that can be possessed by anyone else' (Mill 1989: Chapter 3, Paragraph 4). Nevertheless, it is implausible to think that each and every exercise of autonomy by each and every 'ordinary' person is always for the best. To that extent autonomy only has contingent value.

On the third view autonomy is intrinsically valuable. Choice has value independently of the value of what is chosen (Dworkin 1972: 76). Autonomy is a part of what makes life go well. A life led autonomously goes better in consequence of being led autonomously. However, it goes well in other regards as well. This leaves open the possibility that in some overall estimation of a life the value of autonomy might be balanced against other considerations. A non-autonomous life might not be worse than one led autonomously – if those other considerations are of such value as to outweigh the loss of autonomy. Now, of course, it is consistent with this third view to regard autonomy as being of such value that no outweighing of this kind is possible. However valuable those elements of a life, apart from autonomy, might be, they can never, even in aggregate, amount to more than autonomy. There are, thus, stronger and weaker versions of the third view.

I note that talk of weighing in this context is congenial to a consequentialist account of value. Non-consequentialist approaches might baulk at such talk and view the honouring of personal autonomy as a side-constraint upon any treatment of individuals. Again, I sidestep such issues. I want only to allow that autonomy may be viewed either as so important that we ought always to strive to be autonomous or such that it would be all right sometimes to be non-autonomous. I will talk later of weighing autonomy against other considerations in the estimation of a life because it is a useful way of representing the problem of how to evaluate autonomy in the overall context of the life well led. Moreover, such talk fits with the concerns of this volume.

J.S. Mill's work, especially his *On Liberty*, is an important source of the ideal of personal autonomy. Mill himself never uses the phrase 'personal autonomy'. His ideal of 'individuality' is nevertheless a close approximation. Now, Mill is notoriously ambiguous as to why he thinks autonomy is valuable. As noted, he seems to endorse an instrumental valuation of autonomy. However, he also entitles the third chapter of his essay, 'Of Individuality, as *One* of the Elements of Well-Being' (emphasis added), suggesting that he subscribes to a version of the third view. In his explication of the harm principle in the 'Introductory' chapter – that the 'sole' purpose for which the freedom of any individual might be limited is to prevent harm to others – Mill writes that a person's 'own good, either physical or moral, is not a sufficient warrant' for any interference with her liberty (Mill 1989: Chapter 1, Paragraph 8). This suggests that he believes that the prevention of harms a person might cause herself can never be of such weight as to trump the exercise of her own choices, however imprudent these might be. Mill, thus, might subscribe to a strong version of the third view adumbrated above, or to some version of the first or second views.

1.3 The Liberal Orthodoxy

This is not the place systematically to evaluate any of these views. However, what I will term the 'liberal orthodoxy' holds with Mill that individuals should be permitted to make decisions concerning their own good and that a limitation of a person's freedom is never justified, whatever the gains to that person in terms of harms thereby avoided or good thereby promoted. The orthodoxy rests ultimately upon a strong valuation of personal autonomy. In recent years there has been a growth of scepticism about the orthodoxy (Arneson 2005; De Marneffe 2006, 2010; Grille 2009; Conly 2013). The sceptics doubt that there are never sufficient reasons to supplant an individual's autonomous choice of her own good. I shall not assess the arguments. I shall make three comments.

First, I note that the orthodoxy and associated strong valuation of autonomy draw strength from a conflation of two ways in which we can understand the exercise of autonomy. These are 'occurrent' and 'global' (Young 1980). An occurrent exercise of autonomy is one in respect of some particular decision; autonomy is exercised globally in respect of a life. Now, it makes much more sense to think that an autonomous life is the more valuable for being autonomous than it does to think that each and every autonomous choice is all things considered better for the individual. A life that is autonomous may be *on the whole* better for being autonomous; it is less clear that a life that is *wholly* autonomous – autonomous in respect of every choice made – is always better than one in which some decisions are non-autonomous.

Similarly, it is fair to comment that the endorsement constraint makes evident sense in respect of some choices – the example of freely endorsed religious worship is frequently cited – but not of all. And that the constraint may derive much of its plausibility from the generalisation of those cases in which it works best across a lifetime (Wall 1998).

Second, an ascription to individuals of a right or authority or warranted freedom to make decisions about self-regarding matters, those that affect the interests of the individual alone, makes most sense when autonomy is construed as instrumentally valuable. Inasmuch as individuals know better than others what is in their own interests it makes little or no moral sense to deny them the right to act in what they autonomously decide is best for themselves.

Of course it will be said that adults but not children have such a right or authority precisely because adults but not children are able to know what is in their interests. However, the problem addressed in this piece is the warrant for the basic view that sharply distinguishes between adult and children. Thus, third, in the context of the present discussion the orthodoxy – anti-paternalism and the ascribed authority of individuals to make self-regarding choices – is yoked to the basic view. An absolute and clear distinction between the moral and political status of adults and children informs the scope of the orthodoxy. Put as simply as possible, an adult's own good is never a sufficient warrant for a limitation of her freedom, whereas in respect of children the child's best interest is the only consideration in the making of decisions that determine what shall be done to or for her. Adults should always be allowed to make self-regarding decisions, children never.

The essential burden of this piece is that the basic view gives us further reasons to be sceptical of the orthodoxy. Moreover, seeing more clearly how and why adults and children are regarded as separate sheds important light on the relation between autonomy and well-being in the cases of both categories of human being. It is important next to say more about the line that is drawn between them.

1.4 Drawing Lines

Of any capacity that is exercised it may be said that it is possessed, and exercised by those who do possess it, to different degrees. This is true of personal autonomy. Adult human beings are not autonomous to the same extent. Some can be more independent than others of human influences upon them; just as some are able to identify more authentically with what are their own views and values. Why then should we attribute such importance to a capacity that is far from being equally possessed and displayed?

The answer given by many is that the capacity for autonomy has a 'significant threshold'. What matters is that we can sensibly view a class of persons as having such a capacity above that threshold. Further, nothing of moral import follows from the fact that those above the threshold differ in their possession and exercise of the capacity in question (Dworkin 1988: 31–2). Put in terms of the distinction between adults and children the thought is this. Adults have enough autonomy; children do not. The fact that adults have and display autonomy to varying degrees is not important; all that matters is that they have enough autonomy and children do not.

This claim is deeply problematic. The criticisms of it extend to any attempt to mark equality of status within one group by means of the possession of features that vary both across members of the group in question and within those outside the group. This is a version of what Richard Arneson terms the 'Singer problem', arising from the failure, in Singer's eyes, to mark a morally significant and defensible distinction between humans and non-humans (Arneson 1999). To understand the problem some simple notation may help in the first instance. Call 's' the feature in respect of which status is conferred and allow that individuals who are candidates for the ascription of that status vary in their possession of s. Call 't' the 'significant threshold' at which enough s is possessed for individuals to acquire the status in question. Then, those who fall below t – call them 'C' – have less of s than those who are above t – call them 'A'.

Let me now identify two problems. The first is the 'threshold problem' and is that of being able to identify and defend a non-arbitrary point at which possession of sufficient s justifiably marks the difference in status of C and A. The second problem is the 'gradation problem'. Members of A differ in their possession of s, just as members of A differ in their possession of s from members of C. Why, then, shouldn't status be accorded in a gradated form both to those below t and those above it? In other words, why shouldn't status be proportionate to one's possession of s *wherever* an individual falls on the scale of s possessed?

Even if the threshold problem is addressed and resolved, the gradation problem remains for those above t. The problem is that members of A differ from members of C in their possession of s such that it is appropriate to mark that difference by the attribution of a different status. Nevertheless, members of A still differ amongst themselves in respect of just that feature, s, that marks them off from members of C. Why, then, shouldn't members of A be accorded more or less status depending upon their possessed degree of s?

Rendered back in the terms of adults, children and autonomy the problems are these. The threshold problem is why adults differ so significantly in their possession and exercise of personal autonomy from children that a certain status is accorded to the former but denied to the latter. The gradation problem is that of why adults who differ in their possession and exercise of autonomy shouldn't be granted a liberty to choose autonomously that is the greater (or lesser) the more (or less) of the capacity to be autonomous they have.

Lest this discussion seem all too abstract let me couch the problems in the form of a familiar type of decision-making. Imagine a simple, risk-free medical procedure that is necessary to relieve an individual of a debilitating, painful and possibly life-threatening condition. The basic view combined with orthodox anti-paternalism yields the following ways in which to proceed. A child's expressed wish not to undergo the procedure is heard but not treated as morally equivalent to a refusal of consent since the child lacks the capacity for autonomous decision-making and is not granted a power of agreeing to or refusing a medical procedure. In the child's case the decision taken will be one that is in the child's best interests. In the case of an adult – one who is not judged incompetent to make a decision in virtue of some determinate mental failing and who is sufficiently informed about matters – refusal of the procedure is sufficient moral (and legal) reason not to proceed, indeed for doctors proceeding in the face of such a refusal to be guilty of assault. Adult incompetence can be defined, as does the 2005 English Mental Capacity Act, in the following way: ' a person lacks capacity in relation to a matter if at the material time he is unable to make a decision for himself because of an impairment of, or disturbance in the functioning of, the mind or brain,' and that 'it does not matter whether the impairment or disturbance is permanent or temporary' (Mental Capacity Act 2005).

A capable adult's refusal of the simple life-saving treatment must be respected even if it is judged by reasonable persons to be grossly imprudent and to be clearly contrary to the adult's best interests. So long as the adult is above a certain 'significant threshold' of competence, the standing presumption being that all adults are above this threshold, then his refusal to have the medical procedure is determinative of what shall happen.

But why – in the terms of the gradation problem – should we not think that adults are capable of making autonomous decisions to varying degrees? Some are more influenced than others by what doctors or those close to them would wish. Some are less able critically to review their own beliefs and wishes about the procedure, to understand and appreciate the procedures and its outcomes. Some are less capable of revising their outlook after such inspection. In short, adults differ in their degrees of decision-making independence and authenticity. So why wouldn't we conclude that the refusal of a competent adult to an eminently sensible medical procedure does not have decisive weight? Why not instead think that it should be given *some* weight, but one that is proportionate to the degree of autonomy displayed? That refusal may be sufficient to discount the judgment that it is not in the individual's interests. But it need not be. For some individuals, those whose refusal to have the procedure manifests very little capacity for autonomous decision-making, it would be appropriate, and permitted, to go ahead with the medical procedure in the face of the refusal.

Before I show how the gradation problem is compounded by a complication in the basic view, let me first say something briefly about the 'threshold problem'.

1.5 The Threshold Problem

There are in fact two threshold problems. The first is why some particular threshold is fixed; the second is that of whether it is appropriate to have any threshold. Here, once again, is the essential difficulty. Individuals vary in their possession of some relevant feature. Yet they are divided into at least two status classes by means of a 'significant threshold' in the possession of that feature. This is such that those above the threshold have the status denied to those below it. Children and adults differ according to the basic view in their moral and political status. The difference between children and adults is, in the first instance, one of age so the significant threshold is a particular age. Hence, the first problem is whether it is right to have that age be 18 or 16, or whatever age is in fact set by law or social convention. The second problem is whether or not age should serve as the marker of a difference in status.

Of course, it is not age as such that makes the difference but the correlation of age with a difference in capacities. That correlation is not perfect and without exceptions. However, it can be argued to hold in general. Thus, it be will be said that most children lack those capacities that most adults have. Moreover, a generalisation of this kind can be defended in such a way that it makes sense to argue for one age threshold as opposed to another.

A comparison helps. Legal systems will determine that it shall be a crime to drive whilst under the influence of alcohol, and they will do so because drunk driving is properly regarded as an action that significantly risks harm to others. What is fixed upon as the significant threshold of alcohol consumption will vary from jurisdiction to jurisdiction. It varies from zero tolerance (0 mg of alcohol per 100 ml of blood) in some countries to 80 mg in the United Kingdom and the United States. However, it will reflect an informed belief as to what constitutes a level of consumption that occasions a significant enough subversion of the possibility of safe driving. The threshold generalises across driving capacities. Some drivers may be able to drive safely above the threshold; others may be incapable of safe driving below the threshold. The point is that a defensible generalisation that is not without exceptions underpins the determination of the appropriate threshold.

In this manner the use of some particular threshold can be shown to be warranted and the threshold problem is to that extent disarmed. The problem of thresholds also needs to be set in the context of feasible alternatives. Where a threshold is argued not to be sufficiently sensitive to relevant differences between individuals who may, contrary to the generalization that fixes it, fall above or below it, the following is possible. We may simply test each and every individual to determine whether or not she does have or display what is needed to qualify for the award of the status in question. Thus, we might, for instance, see if any particular child has the capacity for independent and authentic choice-making that would merit regarding her as an autonomous adult entitled to make her own decisions.

Now, the construction and operation of any such test would bring in its wake enormous problems: How would it be devised? Who would use it? Would everyone be tested? How could we revise the test? How would we ensure that is fairly applied?

Seen in the light of such problems a simple threshold procedure that rests on a generally reliable generalization is preferable. Moreover, we could still regard the use of any significant threshold as open to forms of appeal. Thus, the English law 'Gillick' test of competence regards children, those below the significant age threshold, as able in principle to show that they do have (in the famous words of Lord Scarman) 'sufficient understanding and intelligence to understand fully what is proposed' (Gillick 1985). In this manner the presumption of childish incompetence is defeasible.

For what follows it is important to note that something like a Gillick test of competence can be employed in conjunction with a threshold that distinguishes children from adults. The test allows that some below the age threshold may be able to demonstrate that they have the capacity which is presumed to be possessed only by those above it. Nevertheless, the use of the test complements rather than replaces the presumption of a threshold. Moreover, it is distinct from the idea of weighting which I shall now discuss.

1.6 A Child's Voice

The basic view is complicated by an understanding of why and how we should attend to the wishes of the child. The claim that we should listen to children is most notably expressed by Article 12 of the United Nations Convention on the Rights of the Child: 'States Parties shall assure to the child who is capable of forming his or her own views the right to express those views freely in all matters affecting the child, the views of the child being given due weight in accordance with the age and maturity of the child' (UNCR 1989).

This right comprises two entitlements. One is that the child should be listened to; the other is that views expressed should be given a weight proportionate to the child's maturity. Two questions can be asked of the right. One is why the child does have such a right; the second is what it means to accord the views of the child 'due weight'. In answer to the first question, I differ from those, such as Harry Brighouse, who see the point of hearing the child in consultative terms (Brighouse 2003). On such an account, adults can learn from the expression of a child's views what is, in fact and all things considered, best for the child. On my own view the child has a right to be heard just because and insofar as the child is an independent source of opinions about matters affecting its own interests (Archard and Skivenes 2009a, b). This is not to deny that attending to the views of a child may not reveal what is in a child's interests. It is to deny that this is the *only* reason to listen to a child capable of expressing her views. Doing so is also to recognise that such a child has her views on what is in her interests and a voice to express what these are.

Notwithstanding these differences, there is the further question of what it means to weight the views of the child 'in accordance with' the child's age and maturity. The problem of doing so is not one of thinking how the weight of views might be proportionate to the child's maturity. The problem is that of understanding how a greater or lesser weight for those views might make a difference to an outcome. Consider again the example of the medical procedure. The child refuses to have it. Doctors and parents are agreed that it is in the child's best interests. How is the child's refusal given 'due weight' and how would we know that it had been given due weight? Presumably there is and has to be a tipping point at which the child's maturity is such that her view, in this instance the refusal of the procedure, outweighs the contrary judgment. In short, her refusal counts and the medical procedure is not done.

Importantly, this approach is distinct from that exemplified by the use of something like 'Gillick competence'. On that approach, one is either mature enough for one's views to be determinative of the decision taken, or one is not. Age serves in the first instance as the marker of the threshold of sufficient maturity. However, someone below the threshold age can demonstrate sufficient maturity in respect of some particular decision. It is not that those below the threshold age have their maturity assessed and given 'due weight'. They are either mature enough or they are not.

We should note that the views of a child are weighed against considerations of the child's interests. Thus, when determining if a child's views are weighty enough to be determinative of the outcome, we should take account not simply of how mature the child is (and in respect of the matter under review) but also of how significant, and weighty, are her interests in this matter. Thus, for instance, a child refuses to have a simple and relatively risk free life-saving operation. Should her refusal count? We need to estimate two things: first, how well does she understand what is involved in this refusal; second, how momentous are the consequences of her refusal. She is choosing to die. Does she know and appreciate what this means? Is her continued life of such value that acting to preserve it trumps her refusal even when this is given its 'due weight'?

We can now see an interesting asymmetry in the use of any weighting approach. Above the critical threshold are adults whose refusal is determinative of matters. They have enough maturity for their decision to count decisively. Below the threshold are children whose refusal will be given a 'due weight' proportionate to their maturity and weighed against the outcome to be decided upon. But, once again, the question posed by the 'gradation problem' presses. Why shouldn't the wishes and views of adults, just like those of children, also be given 'due weight'? Why should we have and make use of a threshold that separates adults from children, rather than employ a scalar weighting of maturity against decision outcomes? In short, the important qualification to a simple threshold approach made by a weighting one (such as is represented by Article 12 of the CRC) throws into sharp relief the shortcomings of the basic view when it underpins orthodox anti-paternalism.

1.7 Complications

The unhelpful role of the basic view is compounded by a number of factors. First, the more broadly and loosely autonomy (as a minimally defined capacity) is construed so as to include all but incapacitated adults, the less obviously it sharply distinguishes adults from children. In other words, to the extent that all adults can be gathered as a group beyond a threshold, that threshold begins to look less 'significant' and appears to mark less of a clear, bright dividing line between adults and children.

Second, childhood and adulthood are understood in mutually exclusive terms and as sharply divided from one another. This is achieved in a number of ways. Thus, childhood is standardly understood *privatively*, as that which is simply not adulthood. To be a child is simply and solely to lack that which defines adulthood. This misrepresents both the extent to which children exhibit features and characteristics that are distinctive of childhood, and the extent to which children are in many regards very close to adults. Again, childhood is often understood *teleologically* as a preparation for adulthood. To be a child is to be on the way to being, but to not yet be an adult. Again, this misrepresents by omission and understatement what childhood amounts to. Finally, such privative and teleological conceptions of childhood presume that adulthood is normatively superior to childhood. By comparison with the achieved state of adulthood, childhood is not a loss, rather it is only a necessary albeit inferior, preliminary stage on the way to better things. St Paul's famous words are a perfect illustration of this outlook: 'When I was a child, I spake as a child, I understood as a child, I thought as a child: but when I became a man, I put away childish things' (The Holy Bible 1986, 1 Corinthians 13:11).

1.8 Conclusion

The basic view that sharply distinguishes the normative status of adulthood from that of childhood is yoked to an orthodox anti-paternalism that gives personal autonomy priority over welfare to yield this simple account: adults can and should decide how to lead their lives; children cannot and should not be given that liberty. Understanding how the line is drawn between adulthood and childhood gives grounds for being sceptical of orthodox anti-paternalism. The asymmetrical favouring of an adult's right to make choices over the absence of any such right on the part of a child is unjustified. Making better sense of how the basic view and orthodox anti-paternalism are combined shows more clearly why, and how, both are deeply problematic positions.

References

Archard, D., & Macleod, C. (Eds.). (2002). *The moral and political status of children*. Oxford: Oxford University Press.

Archard, D., & Skivenes, M. (2009a). Hearing the child. *Child & Family Social Work, 14*(4), 391–399.

Archard, D., & Skivenes, M. (2009b). Balancing a child's best interest and a child's views. *The International Journal of Children's Rights, 17*(1), 1–21.

Arneson, R. (1999). What if anything renders all humans equal? In D. Jamieson (Ed.), *Singer and his critics* (pp. 103–128). Oxford: Blackwell.
Arneson, R. (2005). Joel Feinberg and the justification of hard paternalism. *Legal Theory, 11*(3), 259–284.
Brighouse, H. (2003). How should children be heard? *Arizona Law Review, 45*(Fall), 691–711.
Conly, S. (2013). *Against autonomy, justifying coercive paternalism.* Cambridge: Cambridge University Press.
De Marneffe, P. (2006). Avoiding paternalism. *Philosophy and Public Affairs, 43*(1), 68–94.
De Marneffe, P. (2010). *Liberalism and prostitution.* Oxford: Oxford University Press.
Dworkin, G. (1972). Paternalism. *The Monist, 56,* 64–84.
Dworkin, G. (1988). *The theory and practice of autonomy.* Cambridge: Cambridge University Press.
Gillick v West Norfolk and Wisbech Area Health Authority [1985] *3 All ER* 402.
Grille, K. (2009) *Anti-paternalism and Public Health Policy.* Doctoral thesis in Philosophy, Stockholm, Sweden.
Haworth, L. (1984). Autonomy and utility. *Ethics, 95,* 5–19.
Kymlicka, W. (1990). *Contemporary political philosophy.* Oxford: Oxford University Press.
Mackenzie, C., & Stoljar, N. (Eds.). (2000). *Relational autonomy: Feminist perspectives on autonomy, agency, and the social self.* New York: Oxford University Press.
Mental Capacity Act. (2005). http://www.legislation.gov.uk/ukpga/2005/9/section/2. Last accessed July 2013.
Mill, J. S. (1969). Utilitarianism [1861]. In J. M. Robson (Ed.), *The collected works of John Stuart Mill, Vol. X, essays on ethics, religion and society.* Toronto: University of Toronto Press and Routledge & Kegan Paul.
Mill, J. S. (1989). On liberty [1859]. In S. Collini (Ed.), *On liberty' and other writings* (Cambridge texts in the history of political thought). Cambridge: Cambridge University Press.
Nedelsky, J. (1989). Reconceiving autonomy: Sources, thoughts, and possibilities. *Yale Journal of Law and Feminism, 1*(1), 7–36.
O'Neill, O. (2002). *Autonomy and trust in bioethics.* Cambridge: Cambridge University Press.
The Holy Bible. [1611] (1986). Cambridge: Cambridge University Press.
UNCR (United Nations Convention on the Rights of the Child). (1989). http://www2.ohchr.org/english/law/crc.htm. Last accessed July 2013.
Wall, S. (1998). *Liberalism, perfectionism and restraint.* Cambridge: Cambridge University Press.
Young, R. (1980). Autonomy and socialisation. *Mind* 89m, pp. 565–576.

Chapter 2
Autonomy and Children's Well-Being

Paul Bou-Habib and Serena Olsaretti

2.1 Introduction

There is little controversy over some of the preconditions for a good childhood. Consider, for example, a few of the indicators of children's well-being in a recent report by UNICEF (2007) comparing children's well-being across 21 developed countries: 'material well-being', 'health and safety', and 'family and peer relationships'.[1] Most would agree that a child's well-being is most likely undermined, or under threat of being so, if the child lives in poverty, is in poor health, or has no close relationships with her parents or friends. If policy makers, parents and carers were able to secure or facilitate high scores for children across all of these indicators, most would agree that they would have made substantial progress in ensuring that children enjoy a good childhood.

There are other aspects of a good childhood that are more controversial than those identified by the three above indicators. Consider, for example, the question of how great an emphasis parents should place, in rearing their children, on preparing them for adulthood. Does there come a point – and if so, where should that be drawn? – at which the 'concerted cultivation' of skills and aptitudes in children

---

[1] UNICEF, 'Child poverty in perspective: An overview of child well-being in rich countries, *Innocenti Report Card* 7', (Innocenti Research Centre, Florence, 2007).

P. Bou-Habib (✉)
Department of Government, University of Essex, Wivenhoe Park, Colchester CO4 3SQ, UK
e-mail: pbou@essex.ac.uk

S. Olsaretti
ICREA-Universitat Pompeu Fabra, Departament d'Humanitats, UPF, c/Ramon Trias Fargas, 25-27, 08005 Barcelona, Spain
e-mail: serena.olsaretti@upf.edu

begins to undermine the goodness of a childhood?² Should we insist, if not at the level of public policy, then at the level of the norms that surround parenting, that childhood be less regimented and less heavily focused on its being a transitional phase onto adulthood? Another controversial question concerns what Matthew Clayton has termed the practice of 'comprehensive enrolment', which is the practice by (some) parents of enlisting their children into their religious ways of life or other commitments that are premised on their comprehensive conceptions of the good life (Clayton 2006: 87). If parents wish to secure a good childhood for their children, should they abstain from seeking to enrol their children into their comprehensive conceptions of the good life, at least assuming that they do or should recognise that there is reasonable disagreement over the truth of such conceptions?

Our aim in this paper is to make a case for taking into account, when settling such controversial questions, the importance of the autonomy of children *as children* – that is, the limited autonomy they enjoy during their childhood. In particular, we argue that the autonomy of children places constraints on how they may be reared by their parents and treated by the wider community, and that it prohibits parents from enrolling them into their particular religious and other comprehensive views. In holding this view, we give support to Clayton's position against comprehensive enrolment, but give it a different basis from the one he offers.

2.2 Children's Claims and the Agency Assumption

As a starting point for our discussion, it is helpful to examine a proposal by Colin Macleod that we dispense with what he calls the "agency assumption" in seeking to identify the kinds of goods and treatment to which children have claims. Macleod makes this proposal after observing that leading approaches to social justice identify persons' claims of justice in ways that fail to adequately capture the claims of children.[3] Consider the Rawlsian standard for identifying the claims of persons. Rawls argues that we should identify those claims in terms of a set of 'primary goods'. He includes within that set goods that facilitate our exercise of two fundamental capacities: our capacity for justice, which consists of our capacity to identify and act from principles of political justice, and our capacity to have, pursue and revise a conception of the good. The primary goods that facilitate our exercise of these powers include: (1) basic rights and liberties such as freedom of thought and liberty of conscience; (2) freedom of movement and free choice of occupation; (3) powers and prerogatives of offices and positions of authority and responsibility; (4) income and wealth and (5) the social bases of self-respect (Rawls 2001: 58–9).

---

[2] The term 'concerted cultivation' comes from Annette Lareau's fine study of class-based parenting styles Lareau (2003).

[3] See Macleod (2010). Macleod's criticism seems applicable also to other theories of social justice, including Ronald Dworkin's theory of 'equality of resources'.

To illustrate the inapplicability of this list of primary goods to children, Macleod asks us to consider two children who have an equal share of Rawls's primary goods (Macleod 2010: 180).

> One child has a secure and loving family and is exposed to a rich range of opportunities for imaginative play, adventure, and aesthetic exploration and experience. The other child leads a safe but dull childhood with little or no access to goods readily available to the first child. Suppose, moreover, that the expectations of primary goods of these children over the course of a complete life are equal. On the index of primary goods there is no justice-salient advantage enjoyed by the first child that the second child lacks. Yet this conclusion seems implausible.

Macleod is clearly correct, in our view, in maintaining that this conclusion is implausible.

Macleod argues that the reason Rawlsian justice is inapplicable to children is that it rests on what he calls an *agency assumption*. Rawls assumes that: (a) persons have and can exercise the two moral powers, (b) they must assume responsibility for their ends, and (c) they are able and expected to interact with others in ways that respect the agency of fellow participants in social cooperation. All three parts of that assumption are questionable in the case of children. That is the reason, so Macleod suggests, why the list of primary goods that is informed by the agency-assumption is inapplicable to children.

It is important to distinguish two lessons one might draw from Macleod's analysis of Rawlsian justice. The first is that we must substitute or supplement primary goods with other goods as the relevant ones for assessing the claims of children. This lesson strikes us as true and important. The second lesson is that 'the agency assumption that dominates Rawls's theory provides an unsatisfactory basis for constructing a metric of individual advantage' in the case of children (Macleod 2010: 183). We are worried that drawing this lesson in these terms may be misleading. It is certainly true that the agency assumption *as Rawls conceives of it* does not (and was not intended) to apply to children. But that doesn't mean that the agency of children, on a conception of it that is appropriate to their capacities, should not play a central role in how we identify the kinds of treatment that children have a claim to receive (and to avoid). It may be the case that children are able to *some extent* to do all of (a), (b) and (c) in the previous paragraph. The correction needed is not, therefore, to drop the agency assumption as a basis for identifying the claims of children but to revise it, along with the list of facilitating goods it entails, in a manner that more accurately reflects their capacities.

That these two lessons come apart can be seen if we recall Macleod's helpful example, quoted earlier, comparing a child who is exposed to 'a rich range of opportunities for imaginative play, adventure, and aesthetic exploration and experience' with a child who leads a 'safe but dull childhood'. We share Macleod's reaction that this difference in childhoods matters a great deal, and we agree that the fact that this difference matters discredits the use of Rawlsian primary goods in the case of children. But we also believe that the example resonates with the proposal that children's claims of justice centrally involve their agency. The deficiency experienced in the second child's childhood is a deficiency from the point of view of his agency (and it may be a deficiency in other respects, too). An important part of what is regrettable about his childhood is the limited range of values he has opportunity to explore and appreciate. It is therefore possible to reject Rawlsian primary goods as the goods to which children have claims of justice, while retaining the fundamental idea that the agency of children should play a central role in our account of the goods and treatment they have a claim to receive.

In this paper, we argue that children's claims must make reference to their autonomy *as children*. The view we defend is compatible with different accounts of why we should respect a person's, and a child's, autonomy. On some views, respect for a person's autonomy matters, in part or wholly, because of the impact that doing so has on that person's well-being. Different connections might be made between respect for a person's autonomy and her well-being, which vary in accordance with whether we hold that a person's either autonomously choosing or at least endorsing a certain good or treatment is either often or always necessary for that good or treatment to either positively contribute to her well-being, or for it to avoid diminishing her well-being. It is also possible to hold, either alongside the view just sketched, or instead of it, a different account of why we should respect a person's autonomy, on which respecting a person's autonomy matters for its own sake, independently of, and perhaps sometimes in spite of, the impact of our doing so on her well-being.

In this paper we do not take a stance on which of these views of autonomy's value we should adopt; instead, our main aim is to examine how a concern with the autonomy of children should constrain the kinds of treatment they receive from others. (The three accounts we examine of the relevance of children's autonomy for how they ought to be treated are, we believe, compatible with either of the two views of autonomy's value briefly sketched above.) In Sect. 2.2, we examine Joel Feinberg's well-known view that the future autonomy of children – the autonomy of the adults the children will become – should constrain their treatment during childhood. In Sect. 2.3, we examine Clayton's proposal that our treatment of children should be constrained not only by their future autonomy, but also by a particular component of their autonomy, namely, their *independence* (we explain the notion of independence in more detail below). Clayton's proposal has the merit, in our opinion, that it does not, unlike Feinberg's, restrict the basis of the autonomy-claims of children purely to the future autonomy they will enjoy as adults. However, we do not believe that the concern with independence adequately captures the autonomy claims of children. In Sect. 2.4, we give an alternative account of how the autonomy of children *as children* constrains the goods and treatment they have a claim to receive from others.

2.3 The Right to an Open Future

If children lacked autonomy, would this mean that considerations about autonomy have no role to play when determining what may and should be done for children? Matthew Clayton discusses this question at length in his *Justice and Legitimacy in*

Upbringing, where he identifies two views that answer it in the negative and affirm that the autonomy that children will and should have *as adults* constrains what may be done to them as children. The first view, which Clayton attributes to Feinberg and developed in Feinberg's classic defence of a child's right to an open future, conceives of autonomy as an 'end-state' or as an 'achievement' (Feinberg 1994). On this argument, Clayton suggests, the importance of autonomy inheres in the achievement of a self-determined life, a life in which a person deliberates rationally about which goals to pursue and is able to pursue them. Autonomy is violated, according to the achievement view, when others deprive a person of an environment that presents her with sufficiently varied goals to choose from, or undermines her deliberative faculties, or prevents her from pursuing the goals she has settled upon.

How exactly the achievement argument might justify constraints on childrearing needs to be spelt out a little. After all, if we claim that children lack the deliberative faculties necessary for achievement, then it is not clear why, so far as achievement is concerned, their autonomy generates constraints on how parents may rear them. One way to spell out the achievement argument is to specify that it is the *future* achievement of children – i.e. the achievement they will be able to realize *as adults* – that requires that parents abstain from rearing them in certain ways *during their childhood*. As Feinberg puts it, it is the child's 'right to an open future' that constrains what may be done to him or her now, while she is a child. For example, parents may not so insulate their children from other ways of life that their children are unable, later, at the start of their adulthood, to pursue goals other than those that are part of their parents' way of life. The rearing of children must be constrained in such a way that it does not undermine the child-as-adult's capacity for autonomy.

The argument that children must be reared in a way that ensures they enjoy a capacity for autonomy as adults can be used in order to justify state intervention in communities that withhold their children from exposure to a diversity of ways of life. In the US Supreme Court case, *Wisconsin* v. *Yoder* (1972),[4] for example, Amish parents asked for an exemption from a compulsory school attendance law which required attendance until the age of 16. Although Justice White ultimately supported the Court's endorsement of that exemption, he was keen to set limits to the extent to which children may be deprived of education. In justifying such limits, he gave an eloquent expression of the end-state argument:

> It is possible that most Amish children will wish to continue living the rural life of their parents…Others, however, may wish to become nuclear physicists, ballet dancers, computer programmers, or historians, and for these occupations, formal training will be necessary…A state has a legitimate interest…in seeking to prepare them for the life style that they may later choose, or at least to provide them with an option other than the life they have led in the past.[5]

Consider now some unsuccessful objections to the end-state argument.

---

[4] *Wisconsin v. Yoder* 406 U.S. 205 (1972).

[5] See *Wisconsin v. Yoder* (White, J., concurring). White ultimately supported the court's majority opinion in favor of the Amish parents on the grounds that the Amish request to reduce their children's education by 2 years would only make a slight difference to their qualifications.

First, it might be argued that if parents heeded the demands of the end-state argument, this would actually threaten their children's autonomy. It might be said that the end-state conception requires that parents must take their children through a bewildering tour of lifestyle options during the course of their childhoods. They must expose their children to the great variety of world religions, take them to career fairs from an early age, and survey the costs and benefits of all the different marital arrangements they might consider entering into during their adulthood. The adult that would emerge from this process would be a disorientated, paralyzed mess. Similarly, it might be thought that the end-state conception requires that parents ensure that their children are not tied to any goals before they reach adulthood, so that they may be able to identify with and pursue goals of their choosing at that point; but by abstaining from encouraging children's loyalty to goals or projects, parents would fail to instil in children a capacity to commit themselves to goals, or to have more than a shallow view of such commitments, thereby actually hindering their children's future autonomy.[6] This sort of objection fails. The end-state conception is not self-defeating. If promoting children's future autonomy requires that parents expose them to only a manageable range of goods, and encourage loyalty to them, then the end-state conception will recommend precisely these courses of action. Saying this, however, is not the same as permitting parents to insulate their children from exposure to other ways of life. (Indeed, that a child be exposed to the possibility of her endorsing other goals may be necessary in order for her to properly learn what it means to remain committed to the goal she currently identifies with).

The objection we want to raise to the end-state argument is different from the objections we have just considered. We believe the argument fails to fully capture the autonomy claims of children. Even if parents rear their children in a way that ensures that their child's capacity for autonomy upon reaching adulthood is robust, it is still possible that the manner in which they have reared them does not respect their autonomy. Consider two illustrations of this objection. First, suppose that a child's natural tendency is to be diffident and inward-looking. The child prefers not to expose himself to new activities, or to form new relationships. His parents are anxious about this. They are worried that if this tendency is left unchecked, the range of goals their child will be able to genuinely consider as worthy of pursuit, upon his entering adulthood, will be narrow and impoverished. They thus resolve to change his character. They insist, against much protest from their child, that he try new activities and socialize more energetically with peers. After little sign of progress, the parents decide that bolder action is needed: they send their child off to a boarding school known for producing socially confident and adventuresome young men and women. Let us assume that their child emerges from this experience with a greater capacity to explore and pursue goals than he would have had, had his parents left him to develop more in line with his natural tendencies. The end-state view would seem to applaud this example of childrearing; indeed, it would require it in the name of the child's autonomy. In our view, however, this example of childrearing comes at the expense

---

[6] A version of this objection is raised by Mills (2003).

of *at least some part* of the child's autonomy. It is not true that the rearing of this child is an entirely happy story from the point of view of his autonomy.

Consider, next, the following very bizarre illustration. Suppose parents with rather specific views about the good life discover a magical pill that ensures that the person who ingests it attains a robust capacity for autonomy. They resolve to force their young child to practice their view of the good life: he must engage in certain personal eating and dress habits informed by that view, he must attend regular lessons on weekends that lead him to hold the core beliefs associated with that view and he must restrict his socializing to children whose parents hold the same view of the good life. While celebrating his eighteenth birthday, the parents then slip the magical pill into their child's drink, so that he can move forward into adulthood with a robust capacity for autonomy. If the end-state view fully captured the autonomy claims of the child, there would be nothing regrettable in this bizarre story, at least from the point of view of the child's autonomy. But we think there is something regrettable. The end-state argument thus misses an important dimension of the autonomy of the child.

2.4 Autonomy as Independence

Our proposal is that we need to take seriously the autonomy of children as children in identifying the constraints on the kind of treatment others may give them. Before we turn to that proposal, we now consider an alternative attempt to capture the autonomy claims of children put forward by Matthew Clayton. Like the end-state argument, this argument assumes that children lack capacities for autonomy, but insists that their autonomy, understood in a particular way, can still be violated while they are children, independently of whether their *future capacity* for autonomy is compromised.[7] According to Clayton's independence view, achievement, though immensely important, is not the only thing that matters for autonomy. A person's autonomy imposes constraints on others even if that person is not currently capable of achievement, for example, because she currently lacks the deliberative faculties that are necessary for setting goals for herself. As Clayton explains (2011: 361):

> …violation of the independence of an individual who is incapable of choice is a real possibility, because others can determine which goals she pursues when she is unable rationally to decide for herself…Independence renders it impermissible to set someone else's ends, including the ends she pursues for only a period of her life, even when she is incapable of setting ends for herself.[8]

---

[7] At one point in the argument, however, Clayton suggests that the demands of autonomy as he understands them can be defended, among other reasons, on the grounds of their having instrumental value for a person's future capacity for autonomy. See Clayton (2006: 105–9).

[8] In this article, Clayton restates and develops the argument of *Justice and Legitimacy in Upbringing* in the face of objections raised by Cameron (2011).

According to Clayton, the demands of independence, when a person lacks the capacities necessary to set goals for herself, can be cashed out using the idea of retrospective consent: when a person lacks those capacities, any interference with her should be one we are confident she will retrospectively consent to.[9] This, as Clayton suggests, seems plausible in those cases where an adult is temporarily incapacitated, as when someone lies unconscious after having an accident and a doctor must decide whether to operate on her. In such cases, the doctor should ask whether the operation he can carry out on his patient is one the patient would retrospectively consent to. The test seems to be passed, for example, by an operation aimed at saving the patient's life, but not by a further intervention aimed at fixing a fertility problem the doctor discovers in his patient while carrying out the life-saving operation. We should, Clayton suggests, apply the same test to the case of children.

Clayton holds that the commitment to autonomy as independence, and the retrospective consent test that he thinks expresses that ideal, justify a constraint that prevents parents from setting ends for their children. The kinds of childrearing that are excluded by that constraint include, in particular, comprehensive enrolment, or, the enrolment of children into their parents' comprehensive conceptions of the good life, such as, for example, any religiously-informed doctrines. (Children are 'enrolled' into such doctrines when they are encouraged to regard them as true and as worthy of pursuit prior to having the capacity to properly scrutinize them.) The autonomy of the child demands that a parent hold back in that way because:

> To do otherwise would be to treat the person as a mere means, as an individual whose goals and activities are chosen by others who are more powerful. She would, thereby, become like a tool, which is used by others in fulfilling their chosen projects (even if their project is her perfection according to their conception of the good) (Clayton 2006: 104).

The retrospective consent test confirms this conclusion: assuming that parents recognise that adults, including the adults their children will become, could reasonably disagree with the comprehensive conception which they, the parents, hold, parents cannot be confident that their enrolling their children into that conception will elicit their children's retrospective consent.[10] Comprehensive enrolment therefore fails to pass the retrospective consent test.

---

[9] As Clayton writes (2011: 361): 'the independence view of autonomy asserts that the comprehensive enrolment of children is morally wrong, because…it is an instance of others deciding one's characteristics or goals without one's consent or in the absence of confidence of eliciting one's retrospective consent.'

[10] As we understand the independence argument and the retrospective consent test, they specify necessary but not sufficient conditions for meeting the demands of autonomy. It is in principle possible to respect someone's independence, and not set goals for him, but to fail to provide him with the opportunities that are required for him to become autonomous. So we understand Clayton to hold that parents are under the demands of *both* the achievement and the independence view. Similarly, thinking that retrospective consent is sufficient may license 'self-justifying paternalism': this might permit parents to instil in their children the very preferences and character that lead the children to retrospectively consent to the ways in which their parents reared them. But this would not guarantee that the child's autonomy has been respected. It would seem necessary that

Although we are in broad agreement with Clayton's conclusions, we do not think he fully succeeds in providing a rationale for them. In particular, we agree with Clayton's claim that the comprehensive enrolment of children is unjustified, but have three main qualms about his argument.

Our first qualm concerns the distinction between the independence and the achievement conceptions of autonomy as Clayton draws it, and the role that distinction can play in Clayton's argument. That distinction, we think, actually collapses into two different ones: there is, first, a distinction between views on which there is value in the sheer possession of the capacity for autonomy, regardless of whether it is exercised, and views on which the exercise of that capacity, by contrast, is what has value (the latter views could be characterised as emphasising the value of achievement). This distinction between opportunity and achievement conceptions of autonomy is different from the distinction between self-determination and independence. On views of autonomy as self-determination, autonomy consists in either having the opportunity or actually setting goals for oneself; this contrasts with the view of the value of independence, which insists that there is value in not having goals set by others, value that is irreducible to, and independent of, the value of self-determination. It is in principle possible for people to be independent while failing to be self-determined (a fickle person in the grip of her changing whims is an illustration), and in any event, so the defender of independence would insist, even when a person achieves independence *through* being self-determined, the fact that one is independent adds further, and distinct, value.

Now, the fact that there are here two different distinctions at play – that between capacity and achievement, and that between self-determination and independence – is relevant for the following reason. We can agree with Clayton that, from the point of view of autonomy, more matters than just that people actually set themselves goals, or exercise their capacity for self-determination. We could also agree, specifically, that there is distinct value in others not setting goals for oneself, regardless of whether one achieves the good of self-determination. But just as we hold that self-determination has value only if someone has the capacity to be self-determining, we could believe the same about independence: we could think that, unless someone has the capacity to be self-determining, or to set goals for oneself, then there is no value in respecting her independence. So insisting on the importance of the value of autonomy as independence, rather than, or additionally to, the value of self-determination, does not help establish a case for the value of independence when the capacity for self-determination has not yet been formed.[11]

---

the retrospective consent that the child-as-adult gives to ways in which she was reared as a child not owe itself solely to the manner in which her parents reared her. It is thus more plausible to hold that retrospective consent is only a necessary condition for respecting the child's autonomy, and not a sufficient condition. For an illuminating discussion of self-justifying paternalism, see Archard (1993).

[11] The point we are raising here is similar to, but different from, Cameron's objection to Clayton. Cameron believes that there can be no objection to comprehensive enrolment from autonomy-as-*achievement* when a child lacks the capacity for autonomy: 'I fail to see how whether or not another person chooses for you at a time when you cannot choose for yourself can be relevant to

Our second qualm about Clayton's argument concerns the suggestion that comprehensive enrolment can be said to be generally impermissible because religious parents who enrol their children in their comprehensive conceptions of the good life, and do so deliberately, treat their children as 'mere means' or 'tools' in the pursuit of their own projects. That description of what parents do would be true, we submit, if what motivated the parents in enrolling their children into their comprehensive doctrines were the achievement of a goal in which only they, the parents, had an interest. This would be true if, for example, parents enrolled their children into their religious views only so that they, the parents, can duly observe their religion. But most religious parents engage in the comprehensive enrolment of their children *for the sake of their children*. It is true that the parents rely on their own conceptions of the good in order to identify what exactly is in their children's interest, but that does not make it any less true that they are acting for the sake of their children, or with the children's interests at heart.

In response, one might deny that acting for the sake of one's children precludes the possibility of using them as a means. Suppose, for example, a parent wants his daughter to be an Olympic gymnast. He forces her to train every day and keeps her to a diet that ensures that her body is in optimal shape for gymnastics. Suppose also that this parent sincerely does this for the sake of his child. It seems reasonable to say that he is using his child as a means: he is taking her, as she currently is, and shaping her into a Olympic gymnast, not unlike the way a sculpturer might take a rough piece of marble and shape it into a beautiful sculpture. One can be said to be using someone as a means, so it might be argued, just insofar as one shapes her into an ideal one has set for her, even if one acts for her sake.

We are sympathetic to this suggestion, but we would insist that one needs to appeal to the child's autonomy as a child in order to vindicate the charge that it is wrong to use one's child as a means in this way. Recall that we are assuming that the child's right to an open future is respected – if the above-mentioned father's plan to make her daughter into a gymnast compromised her future capacity to set goals for herself, then that plan would be condemned by the requirement to maintain and promote the child's future capacity for autonomy, as explained by the achievement conception. Clayton's suggestion is that he is identifying a *further* constraint on the parent's conduct. We are questioning that he can do this by appealing to the wrongness of setting goals for the child, unless we assume that the child's autonomy matters. It is not wrong, after all, to shape a rough piece of marble into something else, or to train an untrained dog into a well-behaved dog. That is because a piece of marble and a dog lack autonomy. The reason it is wrong to try and shape a child into an Olympic gymnast in the way just described is that the child, as a child, has autonomy. So it is only by taking seriously the child's capacity for autonomy that we can explain why comprehensive enrolment, even when it respects the child's right to an open future, is wrong.

---

the autonomy of your life as a whole.' Cameron (2011: 347). Our objection is that it is unclear that there can be an objection to comprehensive enrolment from autonomy-as-*independence* when a child lacks the capacity for autonomy.

Thirdly, we do not think that the idea of retrospective consent establishes the conclusions Clayton supports: the retrospective consent test does not clearly condemn comprehensive enrolment. To see this, note that when we ask whether children, as adults, retrospectively consent to the upbringing they received as children, we should disambiguate between two importantly different things which could inform whether consent will be given: (a) whether parents showed dispositions of love, affection and concern, which animated what they did for the children, or (b) whether the particular ways in which parents manifested those dispositions reflect comprehensive conceptions of the good which are shared by the child-as-adult. These two things come apart: it is perfectly possible for a child-as-adult to disagree with his parents' conception of the good, but still retrospectively consent to his upbringing because he recognises that that upbringing exhibited the dispositions of love and care a parent should be moved by. It may well be that children-as-adults will come to appreciate the dispositions of love, affection and concern that they see their parents showed them during their childhood, even if some of the ways those dispositions manifested themselves consisted of the parents' raising the child in a religious doctrine which the children, as adults, reject. True, sometimes the nature of the particular manifestation of parental concern can be such that it affects whether a child-as-adult will retrospectively approve of what his parents did to and for him; this is likely to be so if the upbringing was especially stifling in some important ways, perhaps to the extent that it makes a child-as-adult entertain doubts about whether his parents really were animated by caring dispositions.[12] But this is not the standard case, nor the case that we are supposed to consider: recall once again that the retrospective consent test is applied to cases in which we are assured that a child's right to an open future was not violated by the parent. In such cases, it seems to us that (a) above, rather than (b), is what *will and should* be relevant and decisive for settling the question of whether a child retrospectively consents to the upbringing she received. We think that this fact reflects two important distinctive aspects of the upbringing of children, which make this case relevantly different from other cases (involving a doctor's decisions of how to treat unconscious patients) that Clayton applies the retrospective consent test to.[13]

First, children, at least up to a certain age, and unlike adults who lose consciousness (whether temporarily or permanently), do not have a conception of the good prior to parental interference. Secondly, parents have an all-round responsibility for their children's well-being as children, rather than a narrowly circumscribed responsibility to restore an adult to a certain physical condition. Because of these two facts, whether or not the conception of the good which guided the parent is one the child-as-adult agrees with, seems relatively unimportant for determining whether the child will and should consent to the upbringing he received. A doctor who must decide what sort of operation to perform on you

---

[12] The case of genetic enhancement, which Clayton thinks stands condemned by the value of independence, can be explained in this light. See Clayton (2011: 361).

[13] See Clayton (2011: 357–61).

while you are unconscious, if she guided herself by a conception of the good she knows you may disagree with, would be replacing a judgement you *would make* if only you were conscious, and would be riding roughshod over that judgement, exploiting your inability to express that judgement. This goes against the doctor's responsibility which is, insofar as that is possible, to act *in line* with that judgement – a judgement which expresses the convictions and comprehensive views you already have and which you have guided you life by so far. This is not so with children. There *is as yet* no conception of the good that the parent is going against. That there will be *in the future* a conception of the good, and that it may be different from the one that guides the parent, seems less relevant for assessing the parent's actions: unless we assume that children already have some autonomy, there is, in the case of children, no distortion or bending of the child's view of the good.

Similarly, disagreement on the comprehensive conception that guides parents seems less damning than disagreement in the case of a doctor and her patient, because parents have an all-round responsibility to care for their children and look after their children's well-being. The fact that they have such responsibility means two things. First, it means that parents cannot and should not prescind from considerations about what is good for their children when bringing them up, and that, since such considerations must be wide-ranging – parents are in charge of the physical, emotional, cognitive well-being of their children, both as children as future adults – there is ample room for disagreement, between different adults, concerning the particular conception of the good that moves different parents. Secondly, because it is parents' special and distinctive responsibility to care for their children, and to provide them with love and attention, and because of the important role that love and affection have for the child's and the future adult's well-being, it seems that these aspects of the parental upbringing role are most salient when the child-as-adult asks whether she retrospectively consents to her upbringing. It matters a great deal that my parents displayed love and attention towards me. The nature of the dispositions that move the surgeon who performs a life-saving operation on me, by contrast, seem important mostly instrumentally, that is, insofar as they impact on whether the surgeon does what is in my best health interests by my lights.

So, we think that the special character of the parenting role explains well why the retrospective consent test will and should primarily be sensitive to the dispositions that move parents, and relatively insensitive to whether the child-as-adult agrees with the conception of the good that moved the parent. The retrospective consent test, then, does not seem to condemn comprehensive enrolment. We add that we do believe that parents wrong their children when they enrol them into their comprehensive doctrines even as they thereby manifest dispositions of love and affection towards their children. We just do not think that the wrong that parents thereby do to their children is to be explained by reference to the absence of the retrospective consent of their children-as-adults. The trouble with comprehensive enrolment lies elsewhere.

2.5 Child-Sensitive Autonomy

Our aim so far has been to cast doubt on the adequacy of arguments that aim to capture the autonomy claims of children in terms of either their future autonomy as adults or their independence. We believe the concern these arguments fail to express is best expressed by an argument that takes the autonomy of children *as children* seriously. In this section, we explain the sense in which we think it is true that children have a capacity for autonomy and we attempt to show the constraints on childrearing that this limited capacity for autonomy justifies.

Our starting point in formulating the idea that we should take seriously the idea of children as autonomous are the concluding remarks in Feinberg's discussion of children's rights to an open future, and it is worth quoting those at length (Feinberg 1994: 95):

> There is no sharp line between the two stages of human life; they are really only useful abstractions from a continuous process of development, every phase of which differs only in degree from that preceding it.(...) Any 'mere child' beyond the stage of infancy is only a child in some respects, and already an adult in others. In the continuous development of the relative-adult out of the relative-child there is no point before which the child himself has no part in his own shaping, and after which he is the sole responsible maker of his own character and life plan.

These remarks, which seem unexceptionable, are not denied outright by writers in this area, but we think that their significance is neglected. Even Feinberg himself raises the points just made with a view to solving what he thinks are only apparent paradoxes concerning the possibility of *adult* autonomy: Feinberg aims to show that there is no paradox in the idea that adults can achieve self-determination and self-fulfilment, because adults are not fully the product of external inputs; rather, he notes, they are also, and increasingly, the product of their earlier selves.

What we would like to focus on instead is the following: persons develop the various intrapersonal capacities for autonomy gradually, and accordingly, they hold those capacities to increasing degrees.[14] Children, even fairly young children, may then be said to possess some degree of autonomy, understood as the effective ability to act in line with one's commitments, and that fact has some significance for how they may be treated. It is useful here to distinguish three intrapersonal factors that are necessary for people to have the capacity for autonomy. First, there are some cognitive abilities: a person must have the ability to reason, such as, for example, the ability to undertake means-ends reasoning; she must be able to understand relations between ideas and to make inductive and deductive inferences. Second, a person must have the ability to appreciate value or, more generally, must be able to

---

[14] For people to enjoy autonomy, either across a life and overall or at specific times and in particular domains, they must have both certain intrapersonal and certain environmental capacities. Our claims concern intrapersonal capacities, since it is these that children are thought to lack. Moreover, we are talking here about children having 'local autonomy', or autonomy with regard to particular actions.

have commitments. Thirdly, a person must have a sufficient strength of will to act in line with her judgement of what she should do, or so as to strive at what she cares about. These different factors can be held in different degrees and what the autonomy of children demands will thus vary correspondingly. As Amy Mullin has argued, even children in the 3-to-8 year old group may be said to display these capacities to some degree and to enjoy some local autonomy, and as they increasingly improve on such capacities, they acquire a gradually greater capacity for autonomy (Mullin 2007).

The fact that children after infancy and early childhood have some capacity for autonomy, we believe, has two different sorts of implications, which can be roughly categorised as concerning, respectively, the actions children may be made to perform, and the beliefs they may be expected to form.

Consider, first, the way in which the fact that children are autonomous to some degree should constrain the actions they may be made to perform, and the way in which they may be made to perform them. Children's preferences about what to do, their propensities and inclinations, are clearly not always authoritative, even if we accept that children enjoy some degree of autonomy. There are clearly cases in which parents must override a child's choices, and this is not only compatible with, but arguably required by, a concern with the child's autonomy. The most straightforward cases are those in which children lack the reasoning ability required for making a particular choice. For example, it is plainly not possible for 5-year olds to decide whether or not they need to visit a doctor, which doctor to visit, and the extent to which they should follow the doctor's orders. It is then not an exercise of their capacity for autonomy for them to chose one way or another in that particular matter. In that case, when a parent insists against a child's wishes that the child must be taken to the doctor or that she must take foul-tasting medicine that the doctor has prescribed, the parent is not impeding the child's exercise of her autonomy.

Another class of cases in which childrearing can override a child's preferences without undermining the child's autonomy, and indeed in line with respecting the child's autonomy, involve insufficient strength of will on the part of the child. A child may lack the strength of will needed to adhere to a conclusion about what she must do that she has been able to properly reason herself to. For example, an old enough child may be able to understand that brushing her teeth every evening before bedtime is necessary for her to avoid having to undergo painful treatment at the dentist and yet she may be still young enough to stubbornly refuse to brush her teeth before going to bed. Assuming that her refusal is due to weakness of will, requiring her to brush her teeth is not an interference with her exercise of autonomy.[15]

Much unobjectionable and everyday childrearing consists of parents overriding children's preferences for their own good in ways that make up shortfalls in the

---

[15] A related class of cases in which parents may override a child's wishes in line with her autonomy are those in which the parent thereby teaches the child the discipline of adherence to her own chosen projects. We would insist, however, that the projects the parent may require the child adhere to must be the child's *own* projects, not projects the parent has chosen for her. For a discussion of the relevance of adherence to the autonomy of children, see Callan (2002).

child's reasoning capacities or strength of will. The claim that children have a limited capacity for autonomy that needs to be respected does not conflict with this large portion of childrearing.

There are other cases, however, in which respect for a child's autonomy seems to require abstaining from making her do certain things. Children can give good reasons for why they do not wish to pursue certain activities. Take the example of an 8-year old who finds playing the piano boring and pointless. Assume that she has been exposed to the possibility of learning the piano for a while and that she never voluntarily plays the piano but does so only after being offered rewards or being threatened with punishment. Insisting that she continue learning to play the piano would be disrespectful of her autonomy. Alternatively, a child may develop a passion for a particular activity that the parents find utterly devoid of value. A 7-year old's obsessions with building robots out of cans, or collecting bugs, might cause her parents a great deal of annoyance. Yet, while her parents might reasonably attempt to entice her into doing something they regard as more valuable, it would be disrespectful of her autonomy for them to prevent her from engaging in these harmless activities.

It is worth pausing to reflect on why it is acceptable to override a child's initial resistance to playing the piano and to insist that she at least try playing the piano for a while, whereas it is obviously unacceptable to do the same in the case of an adult. Why does a child's lack of endorsement of a given activity count as a weaker constraint on how others treat her with respect to that activity than an adult's lack of endorsement?

Here it is helpful to recall the distinction between two reasons for why respecting a person's autonomy ultimately matters, namely, her well-being and the intrinsic importance of respecting her autonomy. Both reasons can be invoked to explain why the endorsement constraint is weaker in the case of children. In reasoning from well-being, one can point out that the preferences and dispositions of adults are settled to a much greater degree than those of children and that an adult's initial judgement that a particular activity will not be worthwhile for her is thus more likely to be accurate than the initial judgement of a child. The intrinsic importance of respecting another person's autonomy also justifies a stronger endorsement constraint in the case of adults. An adult has a greater capacity to appreciate value than does a child, and thus to decide what activities are worthwhile. Insisting that it is good for an adult to play the piano is thus more likely to override a judgement she is perfectly able to make for herself, where this is not necessarily the case with respect to a child.

With regard to the question of what kind of actions children may or may not be made to engage in, then, the requirement that we respect the autonomy of children as children complies in large measure with commonsense views about childrearing. However, we think that the implications of the requirement to respect the autonomy of children are more controversial where the issue at stake concerns what beliefs children may be expected to form. In particular, we think that in this domain respecting the autonomy of children has the following two implications for the conduct of parents (and other carers as well). First, parents should, wherever possible, provide children with the information and the explanations which children are capable of understanding and appreciating. Insofar as a child already has the capacity to understand x, it is wrong to deceive him about the facts and mislead him about x. For example, once a child is capable of having at least a rudimentary understanding of the causes of rainfall, it is wrong to tell him that rainfall is caused by angels' shedding tears. Telling him that would disrespect his capacity to reason.

Second, parents should not aim to induce their children to hold beliefs about matters that children are incapable of understanding the evidence or reasons for. This second requirement is different from the first, although both could be subsumed under the broad requirement of striving for a fit between children's held beliefs and their capacities to form and assess beliefs. The second requirement applies where what is in question is the parent's decision to expose his child to the acquisition of beliefs the child cannot be given reasons or evidence for, *either because of her still immature cognitive abilities*, or *because of the nature of the belief at hand*. On this view, the enrolment of children into comprehensive doctrines – doctrines which reasonable people can disagree about – is wrong insofar as it is a special case of the more general category of conduct aimed at making children come to hold, through non-rational means, beliefs which they cannot assess or understand the reasons for. It disrespects the child's autonomy to make him hold beliefs which he is incapable of understanding or assessing the reasons for, such as a complex mathematical theorem, or a belief that there exist such places as Heaven and Hell.[16]

To be sure, it is permissible to tell children that there are such things as complex mathematical theorems, which some people study, understand fully and set out to prove. But it would be wrong to resort to manipulation or deception (as one would have to do, as the child could not get to understand the theorem by reasoning her way to it) so as to get the child to actually believe the theorem, or to affirm it as something she knows. Similarly, it is fine for parents to explain to their children, for example, that many people believe in certain religious propositions – for example, that Jesus was the son of God, or that there exists such places as Heaven and Hell. But parents disrespect their children's autonomy when they aim to make their children believe those propositions at a time when their children are not yet able to grasp or scrutinize the reasons for them. This implies that parents should not take their children to churches or religious institutions with the intention of getting their children to adopt their religion and also that they refrain from urging religious beliefs on their children at home.

Eamonn Callan reports an example of childrearing that we regard as violating the requirements we have identified. The example is Nicholas Wolsterstorff's induction, as a child, into the tradition of the Dutch Reformed Church. Wolsterstorff describes

---

[16]With the latter sort of beliefs, unlike with the former, it is true that even adults cannot come to hold it by reasoning their way through it. Our view does not commit us, however, to suggesting that it is somehow wrong for adults to choose themselves to embrace such beliefs; what is wrong is to make autonomous *others*, even partially autonomous children, believe such things.

that induction in an autobiographical essay, from which Callan quotes, as follows (Callan 2002: 128):

> My induction into the tradition, through words and silences, ritual and architecture, implanted in me an interpretation of reality – a fundamental hermeneutic. Nobody offered 'evidences' for the truth of the Christian Gospel; nobody offered 'proofs' for the inspiration of the Scriptures; nobody suggested that Christianity was the best explanation for one thing or another…The scheme of sin, salvation, and gratitude was set before us, the details were explained, and we were exhorted to live this truth.[17]

Callan uses this example as part of an insightful explanation of how Wolsterstorff's religious upbringing did not eventually undermine his capacity for autonomy as an adult. But Callan does not consider the possibility we are highlighting here: that this kind of childrearing undermines the child's autonomy during his childhood. Whatever the long-run effects on the child-as-adult's autonomy, we believe adults disrespect the child-as-child's autonomy when they exhort him to comply with a scheme of sin, salvation and gratitude without offering him a justification for why he should do that.

Before concluding, we would like to consider two objections to the view we have just sketched.

A first objection to our claim that respect for the autonomy of children requires that parents abstain from enrolling their children into their own religious views is that it appears to be in tension with our earlier claims. For example, we said earlier that parents do not disrespect their children's autonomy when they insist, against their child's wishes, that she go to the doctor. The reason we gave for this was that she does not have the capacity to decide whether or not to go to the doctor. Her autonomy is therefore not being thwarted when her parents make that choice on her behalf. Exactly the same, so it might be objected, can be said in defence of permitting parents to enrol their children into their religious views. Young children do not have the capacity to decide whether or not to believe that Jesus is the son of God, or that there are such places as Heaven and Hell. We should therefore conclude, in parallel, that the child's autonomy is not thwarted when her parents make her adopt those religious beliefs.

However, we believe there is an asymmetry between making a child act in a particular way and making a child hold a particular belief. Consider how parents usually make a young child act in a particular way, such as, say, going to the doctor, or taking foul-tasting medicine. They do so by offering rewards ('an ice cream!') or by threatening punishment ('no ice cream all week!'). In short, they alter the pay offs of her options so that the particular option they want her to exercise becomes the most attractive one for her, either because of the reward they attach to it, or because of the penalty they attach to alternatives to it. Parents cannot make their children hold beliefs in the same way – that is, by altering pay offs. The process of belief-formation does not respond to reward and punishment. The route through which they make their children believe something is the route of authority, such as for example the 'silences, ritual and architecture' that Wolsterstorff mentions in the above passage.

---

[17] The original source of the Wolsterstorff passage is Wolsterstorff (1997).

That difference is important. A child's capacity to reason is preserved intact when a parent makes her go to the doctor by altering her pay-offs. If she goes because she will get an ice-cream, she goes for a reason that she herself is able to appreciate. But to get a child to believe something on authority is quite different. It circumvents her capacity to reason. To this, it might be responded that when a child believes on authority she believes for a reason, the reason being the authority, or the 'ritual and architecture' that surrounds the conclusion – here, a religious belief – she is being made to adopt. But our autonomy, including the autonomy of children, requires that the reasons for which we believe something not include authority. Once we are made to believe on authority, our autonomy is undermined, either by ourselves, if we are old enough to know better, or, if we are too young, by those who made us believe on authority.

A second objection is that the claim that children should not believe on authority is too strong. Surely there are many instances in which parents make their children believe something on authority that are entirely unobjectionable. Is it really wrong to make a 4-year believe in Santa Claus or the Tooth Fairy? If not, then why single out the practice of comprehensive enrolment in religious belief for criticism?

The reply here is that it matters what the beliefs that we make children believe are about. Religious beliefs are full of 'do's and don'ts' and involve some of the biggest questions we can ask about the meaning of our lives. The belief in Santa Claus is about much less. Santa has a big white beard, is pulled along by reindeer and delivers presents at Christmas time. Now if parents made children believe a much more comprehensive Santa Claus story – imagine parents who justified all manner of 'do's and don'ts' to their children and all manner of beliefs about our lives and the world in which we live by appealing in some way to Santa Claus – then that would indeed be wrong.

So, we think that the case for taking seriously the autonomy of children as children can be defended. We think that competing accounts of how the demands of autonomy constrain parental conduct either do not capture fully the autonomy claims of children (as with the end-state account) or do not seem defensible unless it is assumed that children as children have autonomy (as with the independence account). This does not mean that these accounts should be discarded altogether, but that we do not do justice to children's interests unless we also recognise that their gradually increasing capacity for autonomy has implications for what may be done to and for them.

References

Archard, D. (1993). Self-justifying paternalism. *The Journal of Value Inquiry, 27*, 341–352.
Callan, E. (2002). Autonomy, child rearing, and good lives. In C. Macleod & D. Archard (Eds.), *The moral and political status of children* (pp. 118–141). Oxford: Oxford University Press.
Cameron, C. (2011). Debate: Clayton on comprehensive enrolment. *The Journal of Political Philosophy, 20*(3), 341–352.
Clayton, M. (2006). *Justice and legitimacy in upbringing*. Oxford: Oxford University Press.

Clayton, M. (2011). Debate: The case against the comprehensive enrolment of children. *The Journal of Political Philosophy, 20*(3), 353–364.
Feinberg, J. (1994). The child's right to an open future. In J. Feinberg (Ed.), *Freedom and fulfillment*. Princeton: Princeton University Press.
Lareau, A. (2003). *Unequal childhoods: Class, race, and family life*. Berkeley: University of California Press.
Macleod, C. (2010). Primary goods, capabilities, and children. In H. Brighouse & I. Robeyns (Eds.), *Measuring justice: Primary goods and capabilities*. Cambridge: Cambridge University Press.
Mills, C. (2003). The child's right to an open future? *Journal of Social Philosophy, 34*(4), 499–509.
Mullin, A. (2007). Children, autonomy, and care. *Journal of Social Philosophy, 38*, 536–553.
Rawls, J. (2001). *Justice as fairness: A restatement*. Cambridge: Harvard University Press.
UNICEF. (2007). *Child poverty in perspective: An overview of child well-being in rich countries, Innocenti Report Card 7'*. Florence: Innocenti Research Centre.
Wolsterstorff, N. (1997). The grace that shaped my life. In K. J. Clark (Ed.), *Philosophers who believe* (pp. 259–275). Downers Grove: Intervarsity Press.

Chapter 3
The 'Intrinsic Goods of Childhood' and the Just Society

Anca Gheaus

3.1 'Intrinsic Goods of Childhood'

Philosophers' interest has recently turned to the issue of the so-called intrinsic goods of childhood; the existence and identity of such goods are likely to carry important implications for what is a good childhood and for what adults collectively owe to children. The concern with the intrinsic goods of childhood, as it has been expressed by philosophers such as Samantha Brennan (forthcoming), Colin Macleod (2010) and Harry Brighouse and Adam Swift (forthcoming, 2014), covers several interconnected questions. At least three different issues are being addressed under the heading of the intrinsic goods of childhood:

(a) Is childhood itself intrinsically valuable?

The first, and fundamental, issue is whether childhood itself is an intrinsic good – that is, a stage of life that is intrinsically good, rather than valuable only instrumentally, in preparation for adulthood.[1] Is it worthwhile to have had a childhood? If we had the choice to skip childhood and come into the world as fully formed adults,[2]

I am grateful to Monika Betzler, Matthew Clayton, Jurgen De Wispelaere, Tim Fowler, Colin Macleod, Thomas Parr, Lindsey Porter, Norvin Richards, Adam Swift and Patrick Tomlin for helpful comments on earlier drafts. While writing the last version of this paper I have benefited from a De Velling Willis Fellow at the University of Sheffield.

[1] This is the focus of Brennan's paper, who also raises the second question but engages with it to a lesser extent.

[2] 'Possible' both metaphysically and practically. Some will think it is a metaphysical impossibility to 'skip' childhood, since the identity of adults is constituted, in part, by memories and experiences that presuppose childhood.

A. Gheaus (✉)
Department of Philosophy, University of Sheffield, 45 Victoria Street, Sheffield S3 7QB, UK
e-mail: a.gheaus@sheffield.ac.uk

would it be rational to do so? If childhood is intrinsically good, then some of childhood's own goods – that is, things that are necessary for a good childhood – also have intrinsic value, rather than being merely instrumental for subsequent stages of life. In different words, if it is desirable that we start life as children, then it is important that we enjoy the things that make for a good childhood even if not all these things will also be conductive to a good adulthood – indeed, even if enjoying the goods of childhood was to jeopardise some of the goods of adulthood.

For example, suppose that having significant economic responsibilities as a child makes one's childhood overall worse, and one's adulthood overall better. If childhood was valuable only as preparation for adulthood, little would speak against assigning significant economic responsibilities to children. But if childhood has intrinsic value, the question is how much, if any, economic responsibility should be attributed to children in order to secure the best trade-off across individuals' different life stages.

In this paper, I take the position that childhood is indeed intrinsically good; by 'the intrinsic goods of childhood' I refer to those goods that, first, make an important and direct contribution[3] to a good childhood, and that are, therefore, intrinsically important for a well-lived human life; and, second, have some developmental value for children. To illustrate, play is an intrinsic good of childhood and therefore, on the view of childhood that I adopt, play is valuable beyond its usefulness to a good adulthood. (That is, above and beyond the fact that it helps children acquire information and skills that will be useful to them later on). Instead, childhood play is an intrinsic good of a human life. In contrast, fulfilling sexual relationships, for instance, are an intrinsic good of a human life, but not of childhood.

(b) Are the intrinsic goods of childhood only valuable for children?

The second issue at stake is whether some of the intrinsic goods of childhood are also *special* goods of childhood – that is, whether they are valuable, or particularly valuable, for children, and not valuable for adults.[4] Is it true that (a subset of) the intrinsic goods of childhood cannot also directly contribute to good adulthoods? Unstructured time and play, a sense of being carefree, and sexual innocence are among the suggested examples of things that are good for children, but not, or much less so, for adults. The focus of this paper is on exploring what it means for childhood goods to be special, and whether it is plausible that there are any special goods of childhood.

I shall argue that the intrinsic goods of childhood discussed so far in the philosophical literature are not likely to be special: they are also good for adults. In the case of children, however, I assume that many of these goods also play an important developmental role. For this reason, individuals who had been deprived of them in childhood cannot simply be compensated for the loss by being allowed to enjoy

---

[3] I cast my argument, and its terminology, in terms of goods that make an important contribution to a good childhood rather than goods that are *necessary* for a good childhood, in an attempt to minimise the contentious nature of the claims I make.

[4] This seems to be the main concern of Brighouse and Swift (forthcoming 2014).

these goods later in life. On this account, play – for instance – is good for adults as well as for children; but it benefits children both *qua* children and *qua* future adults, because it is necessary in order to foster, in children, the acquisition of knowledge and skills that are essential for a good adulthood.

(c) What goods are owed to children?

The third issue, very closely related to the second, is whether just treatment of children requires that they be provided with goods that are different in nature from the goods owed to adults: this is the question of an appropriate metric of justice towards children.[5]

Is Childhood Itself Intrinsically Valuable?, Are the Intrinsic Goods of Childhood Only Valuable for Children? and What Goods Are Owed to Children? are independent questions. The first two need not be dependent on each other: It is possible that childhood has intrinsic value, and hence some goods of childhood are intrinsically valuable, but that these goods are not specific to childhood. If so, then all the things that are good for children are also, at least potentially, good for adults. (This is the position for which I argue). It is also possible that childhood and its goods are intrinsically valuable and, at the same time, that some things, such as play, are only valuable during childhood. The other two combinations are possible as well: perhaps only adulthood has intrinsic value, but the things that make for a good childhood also make for a good adulthood; and they are intrinsically valuable only when enjoyed during adulthood. That would be to say – to keep with the same example – that childhood play is merely instrumentally valuable, while playing as an adult is intrinsically valuable. (A somewhat odd, but not incoherent, view). Finally, it is possible to believe that childhood is only instrumentally valuable and that some of its intrinsic goods loose their value once we reach adulthood. The intrinsic goods of childhood, on this view, will contribute only indirectly to a good human life. Indeed, this is the position identified as the conventional view by Brennan.

There is one obvious[6] line of resistance to the claim that these two questions are independent: if those goods that make childhood good are indeed good for and available to adults as well, if therefore they are available throughout a person's life, then why would it be irrational to skip childhood? Can childhood have special value if its goods can be realised in adulthood? I do not deny the force of this challenge; but I work with the assumption, which I find plausible, that the intrinsic goods of childhood – at least those I discuss here – are, for a variety of reasons, *more easily* available to children though also realisable in adulthood. Loosing yourself in unstructured play, for instance, may come a lot easier if you are a child than if you are an adult, and yet be a good and feasible thing to do in both cases. The intrinsic goods of childhood may be sufficiently valuable for us to think that a good live should have plenty of them. In this case it would be irrational to skip childhood, given how difficult they are to come by in adulthood.

---

[5] And has been discussed by Macleod (2010).
[6] And I am grateful to several readers of previous drafts, who brought it to my attention.

The last two questions – of whether the intrinsic goods of childhood are only good for children, and of what children are owed – bear more on each other, but the relation is unidirectional. A positive answer to the former implies a positive answer to the latter: if some of the intrinsic goods of childhood are different in kind from adulthood goods, this means that some of the goods owed to children are of a different kind than those owed to adults. A negative answer to the former question may seem to imply a negative answer to the latter question, but it does not. The relationship between the two issues is complicated by the different kinds of authoritative relationships between, on the one hand, states and its citizens, and, on the one hand, between states, adults and children.

In liberal societies, adults are supposed to be autonomous, to stand in relationships of equality to each other, and hence to be governed by states that are neutral with respect to citizens' conceptions of the good. For this reason, it is plausible to think that justice requires states to watch over the redistribution of only a limited number of goods – say, income and wealth, and possibly other basic goods. Adult recipients of these goods are then free to pursue their own plans and preferred lifestyles. There is no complaint of justice that many other kinds of goods, that can be essential to leading good human lives (such as music lessons), are left out of state redistribution. Adults should be free to pursue these goods, if they wish to, but there is no injustice if they are not being provided with these goods – and, of course, they should never be *forced* to pursue them.

By contrast, children stand in relationships of authority with both the adults who rear them and the state: the latter kinds of agents are allowed – and often required – to be paternalistic towards children. It is contentious whether parents or states should have the final say with respect to what goods should be provided to children. But the legitimacy of paternalism in relationships with children is rarely disputed; it entails that children ought, as a matter of justice, to be provided with the kinds of goods that are important for their well-being *qua* children and *qua* future adults and, possibly, that they should be compelled to accept these goods.

Therefore, even if one could draft a plausible list of intrinsic adulthood goods, this list would not necessarily have a direct consequence for the metric of justice towards adults: adults should be allowed to choose whether to pursue or not things that are good for them. In contrast, the existence of childhood goods does have direct consequences for the metric of justice towards children. Moreover – and this is an additional point – some things that are good for both children and adults may be too scarce to be available, or equally available, to all members of the society and there may be reasons of justice to give priority to children when we distribute them.

This means that the position I adopt here – that the intrinsic goods of childhood are not specific to childhood – is compatible with the belief that children and adults are not owed the same goods. To illustrate, it is possible to think that unstructured time is equally good for children and for adults but it is owed, as a matter of justice, only to the former.

The focus on this paper is on the question of whether the intrinsic goods of childhood are only valuable for children; I provide a very sketchy defence of a positive answer to the question of whether childhood is intrinsically valuable in the next section,[7] and then I move on to defend a view according to which the intrinsic goods of childhood are also valuable to adults in the third section. The short narrative intermezzo in the fourth section invites readers to examine their own beliefs concerning the relationship between childhood goods and adulthood goods. I engage only tangentially with question "What Goods Are Owed to Children?", of the adequate metric of justice for children. In the last section I draw a tentative conclusion about the social implications of childhood goods.

3.2 Childhood's Intrinsic Value

According to an influential view, childhood is a predicament, a stage of life to be overcome in order to enter adulthood, the truly valuable state of life.[8] One important duty that child-rearers have towards children is to help them grow up psychologically and morally, that is to overcome the state of childhood, because 'were one condemned … to remain a child throughout one's existence…it would be a personal misfortune of the utmost gravity.' (Lomasky 1987: 202)

Does this necessarily mean that childhood is a harmful, or otherwise regrettable state? I take the position that it is not. A belief that childhood is in no way intrinsically harmful is compatible with the existence of a duty to help children grow out of childhood and become adults. Here is a plausible explanation of this duty: in order to have an even minimally good life, children need adults' care. But since adults become frail, and die, they are unable to provide care endlessly. Therefore, if they are to avoid being harmed, children have to eventually grow out of their childhood state. This is to say that childhood is not, as such, a harmful state but rather that it can become one under certain conditions that, indeed, apply in the real world.

On the predicament view of childhood, childhood is valuable only because it leads to adulthood; it does not have intrinsic value: the child's present good is a function of its status as a prospective project pursuer' (Lomasky 1987: 202) – that is, an adult. How plausible is it to believe that childhood is to be gotten over with as soon as possible and, if possible, skipped altogether? That it would be good for individuals to forego their own childhood?[9] Samantha Brennan suggested the following thought experiment as a test for whether one believes that childhood has any intrinsic value: if a pill existed that could turn newborns into adults instantaneously would it be rational to take it? I cannot do full justice to this question here.[10]

---

[7] I address this question more fully in paper 'Unfinished adults and defective children' (work in progress).

[8] A classical text in analytical philosophy that can be interpreted as advancing this view is Tamar Schapiro (1999).

[9] Brennan raises these questions in her forthcoming paper.

[10] A variation on this question qualifies it: if individuals are given adulthood-time instead of childhood-time, would this make it rational to skip childhood? To show that it wouldn't, one would

But, since the argument I propose in this paper is strengthened by a negative answer to this question, I start by indicating how implausible the view of childhood-as-mere-predicament is.

Many will perhaps find it unnecessary to argue that the above view of childhood is implausible; childhood nostalgia is common, and childhood is often represented as the golden age of one's life. Even adults who do not judge their own childhoods as good, are often longing for the sense of freshness, limitless possibilities, excitement and relative freedom from social expectations they had as children. But at least some of these attractive features of childhood are, presumably, the bonus of being at the beginning of one's life rather than that of a particular age. Of course, we all start life as children, and therefore, in the world as it is, these are typical advantages of being a child. However, this does not necessarily mean that one *has* to be a child in order to enjoy them. Possibly, if the instant-adulthood pill from Brennan's thought experiment existed, the instant adults would enjoy the same sense of freshness, limitless possibilities and excitement that children enjoy in the real world. Many of the good things about being a child may in fact derive from being at the beginning of one's life rather than from being a child. (Assuming, that is, that 'being at the beginning of one's life' is not an sufficient feature of being a child).

The place to look for the intrinsic value of childhood then is in the essential feature(s) of childhood, that is the feature(s) that necessarily separate children from adults. Philosophers have traditionally identified children's temporary lack of rationality and autonomy – which, in turn, were said to make even older children less than full agents – as the distinctive characteristic of childhood.[11] And children's defective agency made some doubt that childhood can be an intrinsically valuable life stage; therefore, this conception of childhood is also responsible for qualifying childhood as a predicament to be overcome.

This view may come in a stronger or a weaker version. One may think, quite extremely, that since children lack rationality, they also lack personhood and hence they are less morally worthy than adults. Or one may, less extremely, hold that in spite of their diminished rationality children are persons, hence proper objects of moral concern, but that children's irrationality justifies paternalistic attitudes towards them – that is, the denial of freedom considered basic in the case of adults.[12] The belief that childhood has intrinsic value may be compatible with paternalism, but not with the stronger version of childhood-as-predicament.

---

have to explain not only why childhood has intrinsic value, but why it has a value that is of a different kind than that of adulthood, such that skipping childhood would impoverish one's life in a way that cannot be made up for with the extra years of adulthood. Indeed, this seems to be the more interesting and difficult issue, since few people would think it rational to just skip childhood. Here I gesture towards such an explanation, which I discuss at length in 'Unfinished adults and defective children'.

[11] Or, at least, the characteristic that matters morally and legally; thus, adult human beings lacking sufficient rationality and autonomy have traditionally been deemed on a par – morally and legally – to children.

[12] Amongst contemporary philosophers, Schapiro herself holds this Kantian view.

The normative belief that rationality is *the* source of personhood and hence of (full) moral status, combined with a descriptive belief that children are insufficiently rational, yields the conclusion that childhood is a predicament. If both the descriptive and the normative elements of this view on childhood are correct, then children's moral status is indeed derivative from the expectation that they will reach adulthood. In this case, there would still exist childhood goods: things that make childhoods go well. But if childhood was merely instrumentally valuable, then things that prepare children for a good adulthood should be considered the most important childhood goods, since a childhood could not be considered overall good if it failed to prepare you for adulthood. Similarly, the view that childhood has merely instrumental value and contains merely instrumental goods implies that what is owed to children *qua* future adults should always have priority over what it is owed to them *qua* children. On this view, a successful adulthood can easily redeem, for example, a tedious or stressful childhood, if the same things that caused misery during childhood brought about success during adulthood.

Here I assume – with very little argument – that the descriptive element of the above argument is false. In this age and time, nobody would probably want to uphold a sharp contrast between children's utter irrationality and adults' rationality. Not only is rationality a matter of degree, but, more importantly, children's ability to reason in general, and, in particular, to understand and give consideration to other people's interests, has arguably been underestimated. Developmental psychologists seem increasingly confident of toddlers' ability to use reasoning, imagination and empathy within the constraints of their lack of experience, that is information about the world (Gopnik 2009) . In Alison Gopnik's words:

> we used to think that babies and young children were irrational, egocentric, and amoral. Their thinking and experience were concrete, immediate and limited. In fact, psychologists and neuroscientists have discovered that babies not only learn more, but imagine more, care more, and experience more than we would ever have thought possible. In some ways, young children are actually smarter, more imaginative, more caring and even more conscious than adults are. (Gopnik 2009: 5)

According to this newly emerging understanding of childhood, 'children aren't just defective adults, primitive grown-ups gradually attaining our perfection and complexity. Instead, children and adults are different forms of *Homo Sapiens*.' (Gopnik 2009: 9). The real distinguishing mark of childhood is children's superior ability to learn and change in the light of experience. and their exceptional mental flexibility, that allows them to imagine how things could be – as opposed from how they actually are – better than adults. On this view, children have, to a higher degree than adults, a distinctive and particularly precious human feature: the ability to conceive of change. Adulthood, by contrast, is the age when we are best suited to bring about the changes that we can only envisage thanks to our child-like abilities. So children, like adults, are rational beings; the difference between them is that children are better at imagining things while adults – who have the benefit of experience and enhanced self-control – are better at turning imagination into reality.

As I discuss in more detail in the next section, Gopnik compares children with small scientists or social reformers, a comparison that makes sense if we think that scientists and social reformers need child-like qualities. We of course often think this – and we also think that artists or philosophers exhibit to a high degree child-like qualities like curiosity and the ability to see the world with a fresh eye, that other adults have lost in the transition to adulthood. This means that, at the very least, childhood is a mixed state with respect to the constitutive features of rational and moral agency. Childhood contains elements that are intrinsically – and especially! – valuable and others that are less valuable, such as lack of experience or a relative low ability to control the expression of one's emotions and their impact on one's behaviour.

Much detail is still missing from this picture of childhood and adulthood. But its core – the discovery that babies not older than a few months and young children have a very active mental life that includes logical thinking – makes it plausible that children in general are above the threshold of rationality necessary to give them equal moral worth to that of adults. Thus, if developmental psychologists are right, even if rationality was indeed the source of full moral status, children from very young ages onwards would be likely to qualify.

The normative element of the childhood-as predicament view is also contentious. It is very contentious that rationality is the unique, or even supreme, source of moral status. Sentience, and the capacity for empathy – and with it, an ability to relate to others emotionally – are important contenders for moral status, and they obviously characterise children. Not that it has never been contested that (very young) children possess sentience or empathy: It is interesting to note that in the late nineteenth, and early twentieth, century newborns were deemed incapable of pain – to the extent of having medical procedures including surgery done on them without anaesthesia[13] – a theory fully disproved nowadays. Similarly, one twentieth century school of childrearing seems to deny much of babies' emotions and interprets their signs of distress as attempts to manipulate their adult caregivers. The denial of emotional relatedness, however, is only possible by postulating a form of instrumental – in this case, manipulative – rationality. There seems to be no way of consistently denying to children *qua* children *all* grounds for moral status on any minimally plausible view.

Childhood, I will assume for the remaining of this paper, has intrinsic worth. Taking a pill that makes one skip childhood and plunge straight into adult life would be irrational, because it would deprive the pill taker of a part of her life during which she can exist as an individual whose life has intrinsic value. Some things, hereby called 'the intrinsic goods of childhood', will be necessary or at least conductive to good lives for children.

---

[13] Fortunately, in the beginning of the twentieth century scientific experiments started to be made to test – and refute – this belief. One of the earliest such experiments is reported in M.G. Blanton (1917). For more on this, see D. B. Chamberlain (1991).

3.3 The Intrinsic Goods of Childhood in Adulthood

The next question is whether the intrinsic goods of childhood necessarily lose their value once individuals have grown up. I suggest not: it is implausible that the intrinsic goods of childhood are also *special* goods of childhood – in other words, that they cannot also be adulthood goods. Of course, different adults have different ideas of what represents a good life, and therefore few things are likely to be considered universally good. But the things that have been recently suggested as likely intrinsic goods of childhood *are* considered important goods by many adults. One of them is play, as I will soon illustrate. Moreover, there is nothing about the intrinsic goods of childhood that is necessarily inimical to good adulthoods, even allowing for the vast diversity of reasonable conceptions of the good held by different adults.

The truth of this claim obviously depends on what it could mean that some goods are specific to childhood. I distinguish between several likely interpretations:

(1) First, if one has in mind valuable dispositions and abilities, one may want to say that we can only enjoy these goods as children, and not as adults, because as adults we had most probably lost them. Possible examples include the ability to learn very quickly, the disposition to react with wonder to new persons, objects or events or the ability to take a lot of joy from one's imagination and from unstructured play. It would be difficult to deny that the above abilities and dispositions characterise children, and not adults, *in general*. But this is a merely descriptive interpretation of the claim 'there are intrinsic goods of childhood'; I will turn to the exploration of its normative import below.

(2) More interesting is a second possible claim, that some dispositions or states of mind are good for us only when we are children, and once we have reached adulthood they turn bad, or at most indifferent. Examples may include sexual innocence or a sense of being care-free, as suggested by Harry Brighouse and Adam Swift: 'innocence about sexuality, for example, is good in childhood, even though for most people it would not be valuable for their adulthood. A certain steady sense of being carefree is also valuable in childhood but is a flaw in most adults.' (Brighouse and Swift forthcoming, Chap. 4). Certain dispositions may be childhood-specific goods because they advance the well-being of children, but not that of adults – as it seems to be the case with sexual innocence. Other dispositions seem to be morally significant: virtues if they characterise children and are vices, or perhaps morally neutral, if they characterise adults. This would be the case with a disposition of being care-free.

(3) A third sense in which some things could be special goods of childhood concerns the goods at which we can hope to have access at different stages of life. It is perhaps reasonable to expect to enjoy certain goods during childhood, but not after we had become adults. An example is the unstructured time that is necessary if children are to use the capacities mentioned in (1): to learn, play, discover the world at their pace. In this interpretation, the intrinsic goods of childhood are those that would have value for adults but to which adults could not reasonably aspire because it would be too impractical to structure society

such that adults have access to them. This interpretation of what it is for something to be a special good of childhood is, of course, not independent from the issue of what goods are being owed to children, respectively to adults: even if it was indeed impractical to ensure that adults have access to some goods given the current social organisation, these goods may still be owed to adults and – at least above a certain threshold of affluence – considerations of justice trump considerations of efficiency.

So how plausible is it that there are any intrinsic goods of childhood on any of the above interpretations? With respect to the abilities and dispositions listed in the first category, it is likely that they would be good for adults if adults could keep them, just as they are good for children; it is *regrettable* when adults loose them. In fact, many adults *do* retain curiosity, the ability to be excited by novelty, imagination and the ability to learn and to enjoy play – to varying degrees. Perhaps it is possible to ensure the retention of these abilities and dispositions in most adults. And some adults who attain excellence in fields such as science, arts, or philosophy[14] possess some of these abilities and dispositions to a very high degree. That we admire these people and the accomplishments made possible by their child-like abilities and dispositions indicates that the loss of child-like abilities and dispositions is regrettable. (I cannot go into a lengthy discussion of whether the loss is regrettable all things considered or only in some way; curiosity – for instance – may get you into trouble in some circumstances, and it is thinkable that such circumstances pertain more to adult life than to children's lives). A possible implication is that adults should be helped and encouraged to retain as much as possible the valuable abilities and dispositions that children display spontaneously; they are not childhood specific goods in a normative sense – they are not indifferent or bad for adults.

I assume that adults can, within limits, influence the extent to which they can enjoy the capacities mentioned in (1). This can be achieved for instance through particular educational practices (based perhaps on Montessori-like pedagogical principles) and, as adults, through the creation of a society conductive to their exercise. The pursuit of art, science or philosophy as a hobby, easy access to popularised science and learned societies, arts, sports and dancing clubs and, crucially, sufficient leisure time, are examples of social features that can make a difference to adults' ability to remain curious, fun-loving and adventurous, if they wish to.

Similarly, the dispositions from the second group seem, at least sometimes, capable to benefit, or to count as virtues in, adults. Occasionally, the ability to forget that they are sexual beings,[15] and to behave as if they were not, will allow adults to better

---

[14] Gopnik repeatedly uses the image of children as experimental scientists in order to convey the typical mental abilities of babies and small children, which is another way of saying that scientists and children share a high level of curiosity and imagination. Imagination has also been closely connected to artistic creativity. And Plato and Aristotle famously claimed that wonder is the distinctive reaction of philosophers to the world: philosophy begins in wonder (see, for instance, Aristotle, *Metaphysics*, Book 1,2: 982b.)

[15] Note that on a moral view, once very widespread, according to which sex is evil, sexual innocence could be good for both children and adults.

attain valuable goals such as pursuing friendships or allow themselves to enjoy activities that are more enjoyable when one is unselfconscious of one's sexual nature (such as a pillow fight, or a visit to a nudist beach).[16] A sense of being care-free may be enjoyable, attractive, and morally unobjectionable in adults as well as in children, as long as it does not result in irresponsible behaviour. If it leads to irresponsible behaviour, it ceases to be admirable in children as well as in adults.

But perhaps the real concern behind the emerging discussion of childhood specific goods is that some of the good things in life – which many adults are able to enjoy, although perhaps not quite as much as children – cannot be afforded, or at least cannot be guaranteed to, adults. Most adults *cannot afford* to follow their imagination, sense of curiosity and wonder, to exercise their capacity to enjoy new things, people and ideas and to have a care-free attitude. One may think this is for good reason: adults should collectively bear the responsibility of providing for themselves and for their young. On this view, if individuals and society are to survive and thrive, adults have to give up these kinds of leisure and devote themselves to productive and reproductive pursuits. But different social organisations of work and child-rearing will be more or less compatible with adults' enjoyment of these capacities.[17] A worker who works 30 h per week will have more time to play, learn and explore new interests that are not relevant to her job than a worker who works 50 h per week. A parent who is not the only one responsible for her children's access to adequate nutrition, health care and educational opportunities (because, for instance, much of childcare is provided in social contexts such as institutions or less formal communities, and/or socially subsidised) can afford to cultivate a general sense of being care-free that good parents who are alone responsible for these things cannot. Generally, the practicality of adults continuing to enjoy childhood goods is not a given; it depends on how societies are set up.

Let me illustrate the claim that the intrinsic goods of childhood are not specific to childhood, either in the sense that only children *can* enjoy them, or in the sense that only children *should* enjoy them, or in the sense that it is *unreasonable* for adults to expect them. Norvin Richards, a philosopher who believes that children ought to be allowed to enjoy some unstructured time whether or not this advances children's good *qua* future adults, notes that talented children trained for stardom have childhoods too much like adulthood in the sense that their work is virtually all there is to their lives. Such children, according to Richards, miss out on the only

---

[16] It is not easy to see, in the first place, why sexual innocence is a childhood good. A plausible interpretation may be to see sexual awareness as either a body of knowledge or a disposition that may, but need not, afford more benefits than burdens. Since an active sexual life does not benefit children, they have no need of sexual awareness, which would therefore be a net burden to them. But the same is true about full knowledge of the traffic code: we do not need this knowledge as children because as children we are not supposed to drive cars, so it would be an unnecessary burden. Yet, it would be odd to suggest that ignorance of the traffic code is a specific good of childhood.

[17] And, if Bertrand Russell (1935) in his *In Praise of Idleness* was right, we have since long reached the technological development to afford the leisure necessary for the enjoyment of childhood goods.

time in their lives when they could explore the world freely, enjoy the pleasures of aimlessness and the chance to discover and cultivate other capacities they have.[18] But, of course, adulthood is not *necessarily* a time of life when work is virtually all there is to one's life[19] (in addition, perhaps, to enjoying those parts of family relationships and friendships that are not work). Such an exclusive focus on work is merely one among several conceptions of a good adulthood. The childhood goods discussed by Richards seem capable of being good for adults as well: adults can explore the world freely, enjoy aimlessness and cultivate capacities that are not directly relevant to their work. Doing these things can obviously be valuable for adults, and they seem admirable things to do. Finally, it is up to us collectively to make ample space for such activities in adults' lives – albeit not without sacrificing to some extent other valuable things.

It is therefore far from obvious that the intrinsic goods of childhood discussed in this paper are specific to childhood. How appealing would it be to shape society such that a majority of adults can continue to enjoy the intrinsic goods of childhood? The highly stylised stories in the next section are three variations on a short episode in the life of children and adults. They are meant to tease your intuitions with respect to the desirability of some the above-discussed childhood goods for adults.

3.4 Three Stories

One
It has been snowing the entire weekend, and the public transportation stopped working. Schools closed, and children are happily playing in the snow for hours. Adults struggle to get to work and to carry on with business as usual. This is an urban image that I remember from my own childhood, as I assume many other readers will. It is a world of Care-free Childhood and Serious Adulthood, where children and adults lead partially separate lives and enjoy partly different goods.

Two
It has been snowing the entire weekend, and the public transportation stopped working. Schools closed, and children, who have to stay at home, received additional homework by email. They concentrate on independent study and try to make sure they don't fall behind with it. Adults struggle to get to work and to carry on with business as usual. Twenty years later, the children in world Two will be slightly better off as adults than the children in world One; they will have a slightly better work ethics, and as a result will be slightly more prosperous. If they ever meet, most

---

[18] See the discussion in Richards (2010), at page 156.

[19] Nor does Richards claim that it is; his argument is an argument about what children are owed in the world as it is, given contingent social expectations.

One-people will say they would never trade their wonderful childhood for a slightly better adulthood. But Two-people may not understand what One-people mean by their wonderful childhood and its memories, and perhaps nobody will be able to arbiter who is, overall, better off. This is an urban image that one can occasionally see these days. It is a world of Serious Childhood and Serious Adulthood, one in which children and adults lead more similar lives than in world One because children do not have access to some goods which are plausibly intrinsic to a good childhood.

Three

It has been snowing the entire weekend, and the public transportation stopped working. Schools closed, and children are happily playing in the snow for hours. The government grants a national holiday to everybody, but all adults and children have to take turns in cleaning the roads and providing emergency services according to their ability. (Organisation gets occasionally messy). Adults join in the play, and in the evening everybody eats reheated leftovers from the previous days. Nobody worries too much about damages to the economy, which do not affect basic necessities, and everybody is ready to share equally the losses. In the middle of snow fun, adults often forget they are mature, sexual beings and play with each other just like the kids. This is a world that I have not really experienced,[20] but perhaps others have and I can easily imagine it. It is a world of mostly Care-free Childhood[21] and relatively Care-free Adulthood, one in which children and adults lead more similar lives than in world One because the intrinsic goods of childhood are also amply available to adults.

In which of these worlds would you like to live as an adult? Which of these worlds would you choose for your children? Together, these questions can help us evaluate the comparative worth of the three worlds above.

3.5 Minimal Trade-Offs and the Just Society

I expect that different adults will answer the first question differently – some would go for fun, others for more work and the additional rewards that more work can bring. Children may incline for world Three because here we assume that they value fun over maximal prosperity, and world Three contains the greatest amount of fun over the course of one's life. But we would not typically put the first question to children, because we would not know what to do with their answer: what if their opinion about how they would like to live diverges from ours? Paternalism in

---

[20] At times, however, the world of my own childhood was similar to the world in Three.

[21] Children here do a bit more work – such as shovelling snow – than in the first world; I assume the added 'care' is however very small, since adults, not children, bear the ultimate responsibility for getting things done.

relationship with children, I assume, is legitimate, and so it is ultimately adults' responsibility to decide what is good for children both *qua* children and *qua* future adults.

Any adult preference for one of the three worlds falls within the range of reasonable comprehensive conceptions of the good. So is there anything that can guide a principled choice between the three worlds[22]? In this section I explain why there is a case in favour of world Three, if indeed childhood is intrinsically valuable, as argued in the second section, and if the intrinsic goods of childhood are not special goods of childhood, as argued in the third section.

Preference for more fun versus more prosperity will determine one' preference for one of the three worlds. Those who prefer more fun and less prosperity would be happy to live in world Three. But adults who would prefer the additional benefits of more work – and hence a Serious Adulthood – will hesitate between One and Two. One source of hesitation is the lack of a general consensus about how to weight a good childhood against a good adulthood. If Two-people have better adulthoods, but worse childhoods than One-people, whose life is better overall? As Brennan notices, there is a widespread tendency to evaluate practices or policies aimed at children in the light of the long-term good they are likely to produce for the future adults.[23]

One consideration that can help to narrow down the choice is the premise that childhood is an intrinsically valuable stage of life, and hence that a miserable childhood cannot be compensated for by a good adulthood. Here I assume – possibly controversially – that adults collectively know what a good childhood is. A good childhood should include significant amounts of free time, unstructured play, opportunities for joyful and experimental social interaction, and a sense of being carefree.[24] These features of the good childhood are the same as those identified by Brennan and by Brighouse and Swift as plausible intrinsic goods of childhood. (They are of course not all, or the most important, things that children need: protection from violence and cruelty; freedom from hunger; clean water and air; shelter; loving and caring adults – all these seem basic to a good childhood. But the focus here is on those intrinsic goods of childhood that are threatened by attempts to weigh good childhoods against good adulthoods, and that may be sacrificed for the sake of the latter). If childhood is intrinsically valuable, then children are owed good childhoods; hence, adults should choose the Care-free Childhood worlds One or Three.

---

[22] There are several complications in these comparisons that I would like to leave on the side. A main complication is that perhaps One-people and Two-people will participate in common competitive quests as adults, and that Two-people will then have a competitive advantage over One-people. To avoid this additional complication, let us assume that they will never meet in competitive contexts. Another complication for comparisons that I shall not consider at this stage is that adults' sharing play with children can impact on the evaluation of both childhood and adulthood.

[23] She writes: 'When we enquire whether a particular practice or policy is good for children our usual entry into that problem is in terms of its long term effects.'

[24] This belief is encoded in article 31 of the United Nations Convention on the Rights of the Child (1989), which stipulates a 'right of the child to rest and leisure, to engage in play and recreational activities appropriate to the age of the child and to participate freely in cultural life and the arts.'

3 The 'Intrinsic Goods of Childhood' and the Just Society

The second consideration that can guide the subsequent evaluation of worlds One and Three is the belief that the intrinsic goods of childhood such as play, fun and unstructured time are not specific to childhood. If the intrinsic goods of childhood are also capable to directly contribute to a good adulthood, there is a case for ranking Three as the best of the above worlds. Depending on the relative weight that the intrinsic goods of childhood have in an adult life, Three may appear to be the better world because in Three adults as well as children have access to the intrinsic goods of childhood whereas in One they do not. (The qualification is explained by the possibility that childhood goods are good, but extremely trivial, for adults).

But, given that adults in Three cannot choose to give up the opportunity to enjoy intrinsic goods of childhood in exchange for more work-and-prosperity, is Three also the more just world? Many of the conditions necessary if most adults are to retain and enjoy as much as possible their capacities to learn and play are public, rather than private, goods: labour market regulations to allow people to have decently paid jobs without long hours, a level of general prosperity and equality that makes it possible for individuals to enjoy leisure, clubs and societies accessible to all. In practice, it may take a high level of redistribution to create such a society. Moreover, additional services such as social security, public provision of healthcare and education may be necessary to ensure individuals against the vagaries of markets, and allow them to lead the relatively care-free lives that are necessary for the enjoyment of most of the intrinsic goods of childhood. Redistribution and the creation of these public goods at everybody's expense *for the sake of adults' enjoyment of particular goods* may be objected to on grounds of state neutrality: the enjoyment of the capacities to learn or play do not figure in every adult's conception of the good. Do the individuals who would prefer a Serious Adulthood, and who live in world Three, have reasons to complain that they cannot pursue their idea of a good life – that is, less fun, more work and more prosperity?

I am not sure about the answer to this question. But here comes a *pro tanto* reason why something like world Three is more likely to be desirable on grounds of justice than world One: because world One is more likely to antagonise good childhoods and good adulthoods. As noted above, the tendency to evaluate childrearing practices mostly in light of how well they serve the interests of children *qua* future adults may indicate that we discount the intrinsic goods of childhood. But it *need* not indicate such discounting. Instead, it may indicate adults' worry that there will be a time when they no longer can protect the children for whom they are responsible – and in whose future they take legitimate interest. Such adults may feel morally obliged to ensure, as far as they can, and perhaps as quickly as they can, that children become able to take care of themselves. Therefore, a source of hesitation between world Two and world One[25] is that world Two, of hard work and little play, seems to provide individual children with the best safeguards against a life of adult

---

[25] Even adults who wholeheartedly prefer world Three may experience this hesitation, if there is not enough prosperity in world Three. To avoid complicating the examples too much, I assume that conditions in world Three are such that everybody can enjoy a decent living standard even if adults as well as children play occasionally.

deprivation. In world Two children are rushed through childhood and likely to become self-standing quicker than in the other two worlds.

Few people, I assume, are willing to risk that their children will have a deprived adulthood for the sake of a good childhood. Of course, the degree to which such worries are warranted depends on the degree to which particular social arrangements provide safety nets to their members. If safety nets are not available, or if they are not reliable or sufficiently robust, parents will have good reasons to worry in case their children are left at the mercy of the society. Not providing adequate safety nets is therefore a way in which social organisation can antagonise good of childhoods and good adulthoods. Another way is extreme competitiveness in the acquisition of material goods and social prestige. In a very competitive economy, that rewards individuals strictly according to their market contribution, parents and teachers will know that, in order to fare well as adults, children should learn to be goal-oriented, hard working and efficient very early in life; it may then be rational for parents and teachers to sacrifice unstructured time – and maybe other intrinsic goods of childhood – for the sake of a safer adulthood.

If there is an obligation to give children good childhoods, this obligation narrows the choice down to One or Three. However, as long as there is a real possibility that their children will live in over-competitive societies lacking safety nets, parents have reasonable incentives to shape the worlds of their children to resemble more world Two. Individual parents have reason to push their children towards a Serious Childhood, in order to make sure that they will not end up deprived in a world of Serious, and very competitive, Adulthood. Assuming that world One, rather than world Three, is more likely to exhibit high competitiveness and lack of safety nets, then world One is less stable in the protection it gives to children's enjoyment of the intrinsic goods of childhood.[26] In world Three, by contrast, children can safely enjoy the goods of childhood.

If children are owed the intrinsic goods of childhood, then world Three seems better suited to protect justice for children. Given that it is rational to seek to minimise the trade-offs between the long-term and the short-term interests of one and the same person, world Three also appears more rationally organised: in world Three children can enjoy the intrinsic goods of childhood without worry that this will impair their future ability to compete in the adult world of work, and hence their chances to a good adulthood. Would-be workaholics who live in world Three can be told that limitations on the hours they can work serve the purpose of protecting justice for children.

This is not sufficient to argue that structural limitations on adults' use of time, of the type present in World Three, are necessarily just. To settle this question one would need to address other questions: Is it possible to secure justice for children without putting constraints on the combination of work and leisure that adults can choose? (That is, is a hybrid of worlds One and Three possible?) And if not – if

---

[26] I assume the antecedent of this conditional is true in the real world, but I cannot argue for this belief here.

practical conflicts between the demands of justice towards children and the demands justice towards adults are unavoidable – which should be given priority? These questions are beyond the scope of my paper.

3.6 Conclusion

Philosophical interest in the intrinsic goods of childhood is being fuelled by a sense that it is wrong to make children's lives more adult-like – that is, to move closer to something like World Two. Here I argued that, in fact, there are two alternatives to this development, both of which can acknowledge the intrinsic value of childhood: one emphasises the differences between childhood and adulthood and to tries to avoid putting pressure on children to live like adults. The other one makes space for more childish adulthoods and thus moves closer to World Three. I hope to have shown that there are good reasons in favour of the latter option.

This is not to deny that childhood and adulthood are different stages of life and that the precise content of our duties to children differ from what is owed to adults. Even so, it is possible that the same kinds of goods contribute to a good childhood and to a good adulthood; the difference may be one of degree. Even if we strived to preserve forever some of the features that make childhood valuable – such as the capacity to learn or to derive pleasure from play – we would probably not be able to enjoy them, as adults, to the same degree as we had enjoyed them as children. And even if we were able to hold on to child-like capacities for learning and for play, the legitimate burdens of adulthood might prevent us from enjoying these capacities as much as we would like to. Nonetheless, as a society we do have a considerable level of freedom to determine exactly how much the lives of children and those of adults *can* have in common – and, in fact, in different times and places childhood and adulthood have been more or less similar to each other. Some philosophers who pay close attention to childhood deplore that recently, in at least some social environments, too much of adults' goals and time structuring are being imposed on children. I share these worries, while at the same time believing it would be wise to resist this trend without overemphasising the difference between the two stages of life. Instead, I argued, we should aim to make the lives of children and adults more alike by making more space for childhood goods in the lives of adults. Adults can, and should, have the freedom to cultivate and enjoy capacities to learn and play a lot more than they are typically able to in highly competitive and efficiency-driven societies. Making room for more child-like adulthoods would be conductive to a desirable society by accomplishing three important goals: first, it would make it easier to live up to the requirements of justice towards children; second, it could improve the lives of adults; and third, it would minimise the (possibly unavoidable) trade-offs between childhood and adulthood goods. The first two are moral requirements; the third, a rational desiderata – provided we give enough weight to children's interests *qua* children.

References

Blanton, M. G. (1917). The behavior of the human infant in the first 30 days of life. *Psychological Review, 24*(6), 456–483.

Brennan, S. (forthcoming). The goods of childhood, children's rights, and the role of parents as advocates and interpreters. In F. Baylis & C. McLeod (Eds.), *Family-making: Contemporary ethical challenges.* Oxford: Oxford University Press.

Brighouse, H. & Swift, A. (forthcoming 2014). *Family values.* Princeton University Press.

Chamberlain, D. B. (1991). *Babies don't feel pain: A century of denial in medicine.* International symposium on circumcision. Online at http://www.nocirc.org/symposia/second/chamberlain.html. Accessed 10 Nov 2012.

Gopnik, A. (2009). *The philosophical baby.* New York: Farrar, Straus and Giroux.

Lomasky, L. (1987). *Persons, rights and the moral community.* Oxford: Oxford University Press.

Macleod, C. (2010). Primary goods, capabilities and children. In H. Brighouse & I. Robeyns (Eds.), *Measuring justice: Primary goods and capabilities.* Cambridge: Cambridge University Press.

Richards, N. (2010). *The ethics of parenthood.* Oxford: Oxford University Press.

Russell, B. (1935). *In praise of idleness.* Available online at http://www.zpub.com/notes/idle.html

Schapiro, T. (1999). What is a child? *Ethics, 109,* 715–738.

United Nations General Assembly (1989). *United Nations Convention on the Rights of the Child.*

Chapter 4
Agency, Authority and the Vulnerability of Children

Colin Macleod

> When I was a child, I talked like a child, I thought like a child, I reasoned like a child. When I became a man, I put childish ways behind me.
>
> *1 Corinthians 13:11*

In the Shel Silverstein song 'A Boy Named Sue' that was immortalized by Johnny Cash, the protagonist explains the consequences of having been named Sue by the father who abandoned him as a child. He says: "Well, I grew up quick and I grew up mean, My fist got hard and my wits got keen". When, as an adult, Sue confronts his father, his father says:

> Son, this world is rough
> And if a man's gonna make it, he's gotta be tough
> And I knew I wouldn't be there to help ya along.
> So I give ya that name and I said goodbye
> I knew you'd have to get tough or die
> And it's the name that helped to make you strong (Silverstein 1969).

The song lyrics and their otherwise odd juxtaposition with the line from Corinthians illustrate some themes of this paper. First, there is the contrast between the vulnerability of children and adults. Children are viewed as especially vulnerable and need more help in securing their basic interests than adults. The well-being of children seems fragile when compared to the well-being of adults. Yet despite this general vulnerability, children can display remarkable resiliency: they have, or can rapidly acquire, capacities that permit them to deal with adversity in a mature and

---

For helpful feedback on this paper I would like to thank Alex Bagattini, Anca Gheaus, Christine Straehle and audiences at the meetings of the American Philosophical Association and the Canadian Philosophical Association.

C. Macleod (✉)
Department of Philosophy and Faculty of Law, University of Victoria,
PO BOX 1700 STN CSC, Victoria, BC V8W 2Y2, Canada
e-mail: cmacleod@uvic.ca

successful fashion. Growing up 'quick', as Sue did, involves acquiring some of the skills and capacities characteristic of adults. Becoming this kind of mature agent renders the child less vulnerable and more able to track his or her own well-being than the person who 'reasons as a child'. This brings into focus a common assumption about the relationship between agency and vulnerability, namely that the development of mature agency reduces vulnerability. However, I will suggest that this relationship is more complex than we often assume. Second, despite the apparent advantages, in terms of vulnerability, of becoming an adult, losing one's childhood *too* quickly seems to involve a significant loss of value. Although there is a time to put 'childish ways' behind us, there seems to be a place within a good human life for a period in which 'childish ways' should hold sway. Even if growing up 'quick' renders a child less vulnerable to many familiar threats to well-being than one who remains a child longer, there seems reason to regret a truncated childhood. There are, I believe, intrinsic goods of childhood[1] and an adequate account of the well-being of children should pay attention to them.

The suggestion I wish to explore in this essay is that facets of children's well-being are tied to such intrinsic goods and realization of these goods depends on the *absence* of mature agency. Appreciation of this feature of some childhood goods complicates our understanding of the value of mature agency and the relationship of agency to the attribution of rights and responsibilities to persons. We often think that children should not be assigned certain rights and responsibilities because they lack the capacities requisite to meaningful or competent exercise of some rights and duties (Griffin 2002: 2008).[2] However, I will suggest that facilitating some goods of childhood may justify not assigning certain rights and responsibilities to children even though they have (or could be raised to have) the agential capacities associated with recognition of rights and responsibilities in adults. Moral authority to make certain decisions and moral liability for the consequences of those decisions is often taken to be a straightforward function of agency: mature agents (adults) have both full authority and liability and immature agents (children) lack full authority and liability. I will try to show that the relationship between agency and authority is more complex. To some degree, our understanding of the moral rights and responsibilities of children should be shaped by attention to the importance of securing the goods of childhood and not simply by the degree to which children have or can acquire the powers of mature agency.

---

[1] Elsewhere I have discussed the significance of such goods to the debates about distributive between advocates of Rawls's theory of primary good and the advocates (Macleod 2010). For other recent discussions of the intrinsic goods of childhood see (Brennan 2014; Gheaus 2014).

[2] I do not share Griffin's general skepticism about the attribution of moral rights to children because I reject the idea that genuine moral rights can be attributed only to autonomous moral agents. In my view, some moral rights protect fundamental dimensions of well-being. Children's well-being is of sufficient moral importance to assign rights to them that are aimed at protecting their well-being. The view I develop below holds that the particular scheme of rights we assign to children should be sensitive to the importance of facilitating intrinsic goods of children. For discussions of issues concerning the attribution of rights to children see (Brennan and Noggle 1997; Brennan 2002; Brighouse 2002; Liao 2006; Macleod 2003; Schrag 1980).

The rest of the paper is organized in the following way. First, I will explain why reflection on the relation between agency and vulnerability requires us to refine the way in which we view children as comprehensively more vulnerable than adults. Second, I will sketch some ways in which the moral status that typically accompanies mature agency can be corrosive to some goods of childhood and explain why this should give us pause about assigning rights of moral authority to children at too young an age. Third, I will offer some illustrations of the implications of the analysis for the rights and responsibilities of children.

4.1 Agency and Vulnerability

Vulnerability involves some kind of susceptibility to harm. The sense in which a person is or is not vulnerable will depend both on the specific content of their interests and the ways and degree to which these interests are protected from threats. People vary in their interests and thus how they can be injured. They also vary in the protections they have against threats to their interests. So people will vary, potentially considerably, in the vulnerabilities they have. For example, a physically strong but gullible person may be relatively invulnerable to assault but very vulnerable to exploitation. The opposite will be true of a weak but canny person. Whether a person is vulnerable to a particular threat will depend both on the person's particular traits (e.g., intelligence, strength, immune system, sense of self) and features of the social and material conditions of the person (e.g., wealth, political environment, attitudes of other people toward the person). Together this means that there is a good deal of fluidity to the concept of vulnerability as it applies to persons or groups of persons. For instance, in a sexist society, women are vulnerable to discrimination but since sexist attitudes that generate this vulnerability are socially contingent, we cannot say that women are vulnerable to discrimination per se.

Despite this fluidity, we frequently characterize whole classes of persons (e.g., infants, the elderly, the poor) as vulnerable in a general or systematic way. Moreover, this kind of systematic vulnerability often triggers distinctive moral claims to attention, care and protection. Thus because we recognize the general vulnerability of young children we monitor their lives closely, regulate their behaviour and provide them with goods that they cannot procure for themselves.

As Schapiro observes: "Our basic concept of a child is that of a person who in some fundamental way is not yet developed, but who is in the process of developing. It is in virtue of children's undeveloped condition that we feel we have special obligations to them, obligations which are of a more paternalistic nature than are our obligations to other adults. These special obligations to children include duties to protect, nurture, discipline, and educate them. They are paternalistic in nature because we feel bound to fulfill them regardless of whether the children in question consent to be protected, nurtured, disciplined, and educated" (Schapiro 1999: 716). Young children are physically weaker than most adults and that fact plays a role in explaining their vulnerability. But it's tempting to locate a significant dimension of the general vulnerability of children in their limited powers of agency. Schapiro, for instance, goes on to characterize childhood as a 'predicament' that is rooted in the fact that children lack the full powers of agency (Schapiro 1999: 716). On this kind of "deficit conception of childhood" (Matthews 2008: 27) raising children properly is entirely oriented to facilitating the development of mature agency. Once freed from the wanton state of childhood, a mature adult can reason effectively about her own good and how best to pursue it.

Just what constitutes full or mature agency is, of course, a complex and controversial matter and I do not propose a specific account here. However, we can identify some salient features of mature agency that young children and to a lesser degree adolescents typically lack. First, a certain threshold of realized cognitive capacity seems important to mature agency. Mature agents can employ their cognitive powers to understand and reason about the world. Some degree of instrumental rationality is important here: mature agents can employ practical reason to set and pursue complex goals and projects successfully. Second, mature agents have a reasonably reliable and broad understanding of salient features of their social and natural surroundings. They have knowledge, for instance, about basic goods that contribute to well-being and about common threats in their natural and social environment. Third, mature agents have a sophisticated array of affective and integrated psychological traits. This kind of psychological maturity is characterized, in part, by a reasonably stable sense of self, marked by an ongoing and self-aware commitment to values and projects that the agent recognizes as hers. To some degree, this involves a coherent integration of such commitments and a capacity to locate their current preferences and values in relation to their future selves (Noggle 2002). These three facets of mature agency – viz., advanced cognitive skills, wide practical knowledge, and stable psychological unity – are, I suspect, interdependent. A person with severe cognitive deficits will be unable to understand her surroundings or achieve a coherent integration of commitments that is reasonably stable over time.

But beyond this broad depiction of some its constitutive elements, I take no position on how the concept of mature agency is best developed or what additional traits figure in a complete picture of it. What matters for our purposes is that young children and even adolescents usually fall short, along one or more, of thresholds of cognitive powers, understanding and psychological integration of the self that comprise mature agency. Children, even young children, do of course have preferences and remarkable cognitive capacities.[3] They can meaningfully set and pursue some ends. Similarly, some of their preferences and choices merit moral recognition and respect. Moreover, children bear some moral responsibility for their actions. They are, consequently, capable of action and not mere behaviour. So it is appropriate to consider them to have a form of agency that I will label juvenile agency.

---

[3] In some respects, it is arguable that the cognitive capacities of young children exceed those of adults. For example, children can more readily acquire new languages than adults Matthews (2008: 28). Alison Gopnik (2010) provides a valuable account of recent research into the remarkable capacities of young human minds. Gopnik's findings do not, however, challenge the idea children are not mature agents.

It's difficult to say precisely when children graduate from juvenile agency and reach the developmental thresholds that constitute mature agency. (The transition is gradual and its progression can vary between different children.) But however the transition is understood in detail, there are two points concerning the emergence of mature agency that are relevant to subsequent analysis. First, children are viewed as especially vulnerable because they have not reached the relevant developmental thresholds associated with mature agency. Second, the way children are treated can have a bearing on how quickly they acquire the relevant capacities. In other words, onset of mature agency is, to some degree, sensitive the way children are reared.

The idea that children are especially vulnerable in virtue of their immature agency is to some extent reasonable. However, we should avoid exaggerating the significance of agency because its relation to vulnerability is surprisingly complex. On the one hand, agency confers protection from harm to agents. There seem be at least two dimensions to the protective facet of agency. First, recall that agency depends on the acquisition of cognitive powers that permit agents to understand and reflectively reason about their natural and social environment. Call this *cognitive competence*. In virtue of cognitive competence, agents can identify and pursue goods and can detect threats to well-being and act so as to avoid or minimize them. They can reflectively consider both long and short-term objectives and they can assess the significance of risk to practical deliberation.[4] Second, mature agency confers a special kind of moral status on persons. Mature agents have special authority to organize and direct their own lives. Call this *agential authority*. Agents can exercise this authority in ways that decrease their vulnerability to some kinds of harm. For instance, most adults have the authority to enter into valuable relationships with others (e.g., friendships) that facilitate their well-being and afford protection against threats to their interests (e.g., insurance contracts).

On the other hand, the same facets of agency that are protective can also be a source of vulnerability. Cognitive competence can generate vulnerability in two ways. First, it can lead to knowledge that generates risks. Thus it facilitates the discovery and creation of dangerous technologies (e.g., weapons) that pose threats to well-being. Second, it can alter the character of caring relations between persons and thereby diminish attentiveness to the well-being of agents. For instance, because we assume that adults have the kind of knowledge and practical wisdom that allows them to cross roads safely, we are less inclined to monitor and assist them as they navigate traffic as pedestrians. By contrast, we are much more attentive to the dangers children face as pedestrians. Agential authority can generate vulnerability since agents have the authority to enter into relationships or to engage in activities that put them at greater risk of harm. Whereas we allow adults to act in ways that we know are harmful to them, we frequently prevent children from exposing themselves to parallel harms.

---

[4]This is not to say, of course, that mature agents always exercise their cognitive capacities effectively.

These observations are not inconsistent with the widely held view that children have distinct moral claims to attention and protection that are grounded in their vulnerability. But they do show, I think, that the acquisition of mature agency does not uniformly diminish vulnerability. That fact influences our understanding of the well-being of children in relation to their gradual development of mature agency. If the development of agency in children were an unqualified benefit to them then we would have strong reasons to facilitate the rapid acquisition of agency in children. We would think that the sooner children could be assigned agential authority the better it would be for them. There are, of course, biological limits to accelerating the (usual) age that children can acquire the cognitive skills, knowledge and affective psychological trains requisite to competent agency. No process of enhanced early childhood education and intense socialization can transform infants into agents. However, with older children and adolescents there does seem to be variation in the age at which persons can function as competent agents. To some degree, the age of agency acquisition is malleable.

Indeed, it appears that one way to accelerate the acquisition of agency is to assign relatively young children demanding 'adult' tasks, roles and responsibilities. In other words, treating children as though they already have the competencies of mature agents contributes to the developmental processes through which they actually become mature agents. Children who 'grow up quick' are often children who are expected at a young age to assume significant responsibilities for managing their own welfare and the welfare of others. They can acquire practical knowledge that will help them to negotiate the social world as agents. Relatively young children can learn how to cook, clean, work and generally take care of themselves and others. They can comprehend rich and detailed knowledge about the so-called adult world of politics, law, commerce, sex, death and etc. so that they can deliberate and make decisions about how to act in an informed and responsible fashion. Such children become, as the phrase goes, wise beyond their years.

The degree to which the acquisition of agency is socially constructed in this way and thus capable of being expedited is unclear. Perhaps there is little room to rush the development of agency. But suppose, for the sake of argument, that by assigning responsibilities to children at an early age and by furnishing them with knowledge about 'worldly matters', we could significantly reduce the age at which most children become mature agents. Should we welcome adoption an approach to child rearing that facilitates the development of mature agency at the earliest possible age? If the acquisition of agency was an unqualified benefit to a person by rendering her systematically less vulnerable to harm and better able to secure her own well-being, then concern for the promotion of human well-being would seem to favour such a child rearing approach. However, as we have seen mature agency does not diminish vulnerability across the board. Nonetheless, even if agency brings with it some exposure to harm, it might typically confer a net gain in well-being on persons and there would be strong welfarist reasons to facilitate early agency. Similarly, if achieving the moral status of a mature agent has moral significance in its own right then there will be an additional reason to orchestrate the acquisition of agency as soon as possible. To the degree that we locate the distinct value of human life in being a mature agent and exercising the powers of agency then expediting the onset of mature agency would have great moral urgency. These observations push us towards a rather bleak but common vision of childhood. It is a vision in which the juvenile agency of childhood is intrinsically inferior to the mature agency of adulthood. Childhood assumes, at best, instrumental value: its principal significance lies in preparing a person for mature agency. As Michael Slote puts it: "what happens in childhood principally affects our view of total lives through the effects that childhood success or failure are supposed to have on mature individuals" (Slote 1983: 15). Similarly, Schapiro's characterization of childhood as a 'predicament' from which children need to helped to escape depicts childhood as a normatively limited and regrettable state.

4.2 Agency and Goods of Childhood: Against Rushing Mature Agency

This is a vision of childhood that I wish to reject. By way of challenging it, I shall identify two good components of a human life to which children as juvenile agents have privileged and perhaps unique access. I hasten to add that children's access to these goods can be blocked or disrupted by various kinds of social and material deprivation. In our unjust world, not all children enjoy these goods fully or adequately but I think they are amongst the goods that can be a source of intrinsic value in the lives of children. Moreover, in my view, they are important goods that contribute significantly to making a person's life go well overall. Their normative importance should not be discounted because they are fleeting and only readily accessible during childhood.

4.3 Innocence

First, childhood is characterized by a type of innocence that contributes distinctive value to the activities and relationships of children. Children, especially young children, are receptive to very diverse activities, experiences and relationships. They can be amused, engaged, scared, and puzzled by things that strike adults as banal or familiar. Innocence permits various childhood choices and new discoveries to be accompanied by a sense of wonderment and joy. As innocents children are untroubled by disturbing and troubling dimensions of the adult world. Similarly, childhood innocence seems to facilitate a kind of unmediated trust and intimacy between children and those who love and care for them. The intense caring relationships and emotional states that are unmediated by reflection or analysis that one can experience via the innocence of childhood seem good in their own right. Although preservation of such innocence throughout a full human life would stand in the way of experiencing other valuable emotions and relationships, we have reason to regret that some children are denied access to the goods of innocence. But notice that innocence of this sort involves a kind of ignorance of or unfamiliarity with the workings of the world. In adults innocence can be an obstacle to agency precisely because it involves epistemic errors that bear on prudent and successful planning. As cognitively competent mature agents we know how to scrutinize the motives and intentions of others and this very scrutiny, though it serves a protective function, mediates and alters the character of our love and trust of others. Innocent adults are naïve and they are less able to set and pursue their ends rationally. But the innocence of children does not seem like an encumbrance to meaningful childhood activities and relationships at least when viewed on its own terms. As we mature, the character and extent of our innocence diminishes and we can no longer experience activities and relationships from the distinctive vantage of the innocent. Of course, the gradual transition from innocence to a more worldly perspective has its own rewards and benefits. Indeed, experiencing that transition is arguably itself a component of human flourishing. Although the loss of innocence at a suitable age is not itself regrettable, denying children an opportunity to experience innocence would be regrettable.

4.4 Imagination

Second, juvenile agency is characterized by remarkable and distinctive imaginative powers. Children can imaginatively transform ordinary household items into the elements of a complex make-believe world. Similarly, they can ascribe personality and agency to inanimate toys and include these imaginatively animated creatures in wonderful adventures and narratives. These imaginative capacities seem to be sources of rich and intense emotional experiences from giddy excitement and the reckless abandon of many childhood games to the peculiar delight of entering the scary world of monsters. From the perspective of mature agency, many of these exercises of imagination present themselves as defects – a failure to see and appreciate the world as it really is. For adults to enter into such imaginary worlds, even partially, they must summon 'the willing suspension of disbelief'. By contrast, children's entry seems spontaneous and unselfconscious. However, it seems clear that the lives of children are enriched by their imaginative participation in make-believe worlds and, at a suitable age and stage, it does not seem regrettable that children make choices and embark on projects that are predicated on false or distorted views of the world. Moreover, even if the playful exercise of imagination contributes crucially to the development of mature agency,[5] I do not think its normative significance should be viewed entirely in developmental terms. Similarly, play has value as an expression of juvenile agency independently of its hedonic value. Of course, a child who 'chooses' to be a dragon slaying knight has fun but the creative expression of juvenile agency involved in play has, I believe, significance in its own right.

---

[5] Schapiro plausibly suggests that imaginative play is important to the development of agency that helps children to "become themselves" Schapiro (1999: 732).

4 Agency, Authority and the Vulnerability of Children

I hope the foregoing remarks provide credible motivation for the idea that there are some intrinsic goods of childhood. As with many claims about sources of value in a human life, it is difficult to provide proof of them beyond that provided via the resonance of some examples with our reflective judgements of value. So I hope the examples have resonance for readers. However, for the purposes of the rest of the analysis, it is important to emphasize a couple of features of these goods. First, they should not be interpreted as inferior to or as pale, simplified, versions of the goods accessible to mature agents. On my view, they goods in their own right and constitute independent and important elements of an overall account of human flourishing. It is good to be a child for part of one's life and it is valuable to have access to the distinctive goods of childhood. We should not, consequently, deprive or unduly circumscribe the access that persons have to the goods of childhood even if limiting their access had no regrettable developmental effects and we could instead secure them access to goods of mature agency.

Second, there is an important sense in which realization of these goods for children is undermined by acquisition of the cluster of attributes that confer mature agency on persons. Reaching a threshold of cognitive maturity and acquiring true beliefs about the world involves a loss of innocence and irrevocably changes our capacity for carefree imaginative play. I assume that the normal progression of cognitive and psychological development of children imposes some limits on what kinds of reasoning capacities they can normally have at given ages and consequently what kinds of knowledge of the world they can have (and grasp its significance). Very young children, for instance, cannot understand and reliably negotiate various dangers that the world may present and they cannot tend to their basic needs by themselves. However, as children grow older and approach adolescence, it seems possible to equip them with skills and knowledge that allow them to secure for themselves many of their basic interests and to protect themselves from harm. And this returns us to the issue posed above as to whether we have reasons connected with our concern for the vulnerability of children to expedite, as much as possible, the process of acquiring mature agency. Recognition of the goods of childhood provides reasons to resist such a suggestion.

We can see this via reflection on the hypothetical case of Sue with which we began. Sue, and real children like him, who have demanding responsibilities thrust upon them at a young age, mature very rapidly and function effectively as mature agents. The early assignment to children of responsibilities to care for themselves and others seems to facilitate the rapid development of mature agency. Children come to understand the real challenges they must address in order to meet their own needs and the needs others. Because their powers of instrumental rationality are regularly deployed to solve practical problems, they develop rapidly. It also seems plausible that, perhaps out of necessity, they develop a coherent sense of and become capable of the kind of temporal extension characteristic of mature agency. Along many dimensions they are less vulnerable to harm than their less mature counterparts. Yet in such children's lives there is little room for innocence and imagination and it is their very competency as mature agents that cuts them off from such goods. If this is plausible then there is a sense in which the development of mature agency *too quickly* generates harm by frustrating realization of the goods of childhood. Of course, it is tricky to determine what exactly the appropriate rate at which mature agency should be acquired. Similarly, an excessive prolongation of childhood that might be achieved by infantilizing older children and adolescents is not desirable either. However, I think we should conclude that the interests of children are not uniformly advanced by the development of mature agency. Indeed, because mature agents cannot readily access the goods of childhood, there is an important sense in which the acquisition of mature agency is a source of vulnerability for children. Rapid onset of mature agency in children undermines their well-being by diminishing their opportunity to realize the distinctive goods of childhood.

4.5 Rights, Responsibilities and Agency

By way of conclusion, I want to briefly speculate on the way in which the foregoing analysis may complicate our understanding of the attribution of rights and responsibilities to children. We often assume that there is a special connection between agency, responsibilities and rights. Although adults and children have some moral rights in common, we assign some rights to adults that we deny to children and the standard rationale for doing so is grounded in claims about the agential capacities of adults and children respectively. Consider, for instance, examples of rights associated with what I called agential authority. Adults have the right to make wide-ranging choices about how the kinds of risks and harms to which they wish to expose themselves. To a much greater extent than children, they have the authority to regulate their own vulnerability. Hence paternalism towards adults requires special justification. Similarly, adults, in virtue of their mature agency, are held responsible for their conduct in distinctive ways. Adults are expected, in many contexts, to take much greater responsibility for seeing to their own interests and needs than children. Adults also have special responsibilities to attend to the interests of others while children typically have fewer and less demanding responsibilities. Similarly, adults are subject to more extensive censure and punishment than children when they flout moral or social norms.

On one standard account, the attribution of characteristically adult rights and responsibilities to persons tracks agency in a straightforward way: rights and responsibilities are assigned to persons in relation to the agential capacities they have. On this view, children do not qualify for 'adult' rights and responsibilities because they lack the capacities constitutive of agency that are requisite to such moral claims. They acquire rights and responsibilities as they acquire the relevant capacities of agency.

In light of this it is tempting to suppose that children are denied rights to make a wide variety of self-regarding choices about their own lives (and hence regulate their own vulnerability) *solely* because they lack relevant agential capacities. But given the malleability of the onset of mature agency, children can acquire agential capacities requisite to rights and responsibilities at younger ages than they are typically assigned some moral rights and responsibilities. And this might seem to justify attributing at least 'adult' rights and responsibilities to older children and adolescents as soon as it is developmentally feasible. Suppose, for instance, that most 12 year old can – through suitable processes of education and socialization – acquire the cognitive capacities, knowledge and psychological traits that permit them to track their own interests and to manage their lives in an independent and successful fashion. Such children would have the cognitive competence and agential authority required to regulate their own vulnerability. On the standard view, it would seem that we should assign adult rights – e.g., rights to make wide ranging self-regarding decisions, rights to work and vote along with corresponding responsibilities and liabilities – to such children and we should welcome the processes that facilitate the early acquisition of adult rights. But once we recognize the importance of childhood goods, the standard model looks too simple.

The account I have sketched about the relationship between mature agency and the intrinsic goods of childhood suggests a different, more nuanced, understanding of the relation between rights and agency. It allows for the possibility that some rights can be predicated on the value of juvenile agency itself and the intrinsic goods it can generate. So rather than viewing rights as oriented *solely* towards the facilitation and protection of mature agency, we can say that rights can also arise in relation to the protection and facilitation of juvenile agency. The right of children to play and to be free consequently of various demanding adult responsibilities may, on this approach, turn out to be an important moral right even though it is not grounded in mature agency. More needs to be said, of course, about how these kinds of rights are to be tempered if they conflict with claims children have to the facilitation of mature agency. I will not address that matter here. The main point is simply to suggest that an overall account of children's rights needs to be sensitive to the value of the goods of childhood. If I am right then some, arguably premature, ways of developing the mature agency of children may violate their rights as juvenile agents.

4.6 Conclusion

We care about the special vulnerability of children and we seek, consequently, to protect them from the various threats to their well-being that they cannot negotiate themselves. One way to diminish their vulnerability is to equip them as quickly as possible with the capacities of mature agency. But the very features of juvenile agency that render children vulnerable also give them access to important human goods. This means that we often have reason to be ambivalent about reducing children's vulnerability by getting them to abandon 'childish ways'.

References

Brennan, S. (2002). Children's choices or children's interests: Which do their rights protect? In D. Archard & C. Macleod (Eds.), *The moral and political status of children* (pp. 53–69). Oxford: Oxford University Press.

Brennan, S. (2014). The goods of childhood, children's rights, and the role of parents as advocates and interpreters. In: F. Baylis & C. McLeod (Eds.), *Family-making: Contemporary ethical challenges* (pp. 29–48). Oxford University Press.

Brennan, S., & Noggle, R. (1997). The moral status of children: Children's rights, parents' rights, and family justice. *Social Theory and Practice, 23*, 1–26.

Brighouse, H. (2002). What rights (if any) do children have? In D. Archard & C. Macleod (Eds.), *The moral and political status of children: New essays* (pp. 31–52). Oxford: Oxford University Press.

Gheaus, A. (2014). The 'intrinsic goods of childhood' and the just society. In *The nature of children's well-being: Theory and practice* (pp. xx–xx). Dordrecht: Springer.

Gopnik, A. (2010). *The philosophical baby*. New York: Picador.

Griffin, J. (2002). Do children have rights? In D. Archard & C. Macleod (Eds.), *The moral and political status of children: New essays* (pp. 19–30). Oxford: Oxford University Press.

Griffin, J. (2008). *On human rights*. Oxford: Oxford University Press.

Liao, S. M. (2006). The right of children to be loved. *The Journal of Political Philosophy, 14*(4), 420–440.

Macleod, C. (2003). Shaping children's convictions. *Theory and Research in Education, 1*(3), 315–330.

Macleod, C. (2010). Primary goods, capabilities and children. In H. Brighouse & I. Robeyns (Eds.), *Measuring justice: Primary goods and capabilities*. Cambridge: Cambridge University Press.

Matthews, G. (2008). Getting beyond the deficit conception of childhood: Thinking philosophically with children. In M. Hand & C. Win Stanley (Eds.), *Philosophy in schools* (pp. 27–40). London: Continuum.

Noggle, R. (2002). Special agents: Children's autonomy and parental authority. In D. Archard & C. Macleod (Eds.), *The moral and political status of children* (pp. 97–117). Oxford: Oxford University Press.

Schapiro, T. (1999). What is a child? *Ethics, 109*, 715–738.

Schrag, F. (1980). Children: Their rights and needs. In W. Aiken & H. LaFollette (Eds.), *Whose child? Parental rights, parental authority and state power* (pp. 237–253). Totowa: Littlefield, Adams, and Co.

Silverstein, S. (1969). *A boy named Sue*. New York: N.Y. Evil Eye Music Inc.

Slote, M. (1983). *Goods and virtues*. Oxford: Oxford University Press.

Chapter 5
Enhancing the Capacity for Autonomy: What Parents Owe Their Children to Make Their Lives Go Well

Monika Betzler

5.1 The Parental Duty to Enhance the Autonomy of Their Children

According to common-sense morality, parents have duties toward their children *qua* parents that others, who are not parents, do not have. Enhancing their children's wellbeing, and thus, making their lives go well, is unquestionably among those parental duties. This does not preclude that other agents, such as the state, institutions, relatives, or even mere bystanders, have, in part at least, duties toward children too. But if there is such a duty to enhance the wellbeing of children, parents seem to have it more so, and in more particular ways, than any other agent. First, the duty asks parents for more in that it requires them to cater to their children's physical,[1] psychological,[2] and material needs almost all of the time and with an all-encompassing responsibility. Second, parents are required to meet children's needs with special attention. They are asked to love and care for their children in a way that is expressive of a close nurturing relationship.[3] Parents who do not fulfill this duty with regard to their children's needs are thought to be morally in the wrong, independently of whether or not we think that children have rights.[4]

---

[1] Such as their health and safety.

[2] Such as their sense of being cared for and loved in a nurturing environment.

[3] In what follows, I am concerned with parenthood as a social relationship (rather than a biological or legal one).

[4] I leave it open as to whether children have rights that correspond to these duties. See Archard (2003: Chap. 2).

M. Betzler (✉)
Department of Philosophy, University of Bern, Unitobler, 2. Stock,
Büro 210 Länggassstrasse 49a, Bern CH-3012, Switzerland
e-mail: monika.betzler@philo.unibe.ch

To better capture the content of the parental duty to enhance the wellbeing of children, we need a fuller understanding of what that duty involves. Here I will concentrate on one part of that duty, namely the duty to enhance the autonomy of one's children. The aim of this paper is to spell out *why* the autonomy of children falls within the scope of the parental duty to enhance their children's wellbeing, and *what kind of* autonomy parents are required to enhance. Furthermore, I will show *how* the autonomy of children can be enhanced.

There are two reasons why encouraging the development of children's autonomy is within the scope of parental duty. On one hand, leading an autonomous life just is constitutive of making a life go well. Let me call this the argument from wellbeing. On the other hand, parents are typically in a privileged position to enhance the autonomy of their children. Let me call this the argument from position. The arguments are jointly necessary for generating a parental duty.

As to the argument from wellbeing, there are many theories of wellbeing on offer, and I cannot defend any particular conception here. Suffice it to say that the duty to enhance the autonomy of[5] one's children is typically connected to the enhancement of their wellbeing, because, I suspect, we think that a good life is one led by someone who *regards* it as good, and thereby leads it according to his or her own conception of the good. Provided that this is correct, the duty to enhance one's children's autonomy is not independent of the duty to enhance their wellbeing.[6]

As for the argument from position, parents typically have a unique role as primary educators, and are best placed to help their children learn to lead a life of their own. But it is not just that they are causally privileged due to their proximity to their children. They are also normatively privileged in that they, as childrearers of a particular child, bear the responsibility of gradually helping her to learn to govern herself on her own.[7]

There are two broad explanations why exactly children need help in their development. Children are not only imperfect as rational deliberators and in understanding reasons.[8] Moreover, they lack knowledge about themselves and the world around them and are usually not able to evaluate the consequences of their actions, especially long-term consequences. This is connected to the fact that children do not have sufficient understanding of themselves as agents who persist over time.[9]

Apart from their deliberative and epistemic deficits, children do not have a stable volitional or evaluative outlook. They do not yet know what they 'really' value, but are more-or-less driven by their most urgent desires. In addition, they

---

[5] See Hurka (1987: 361–82; cf). Sumner (1996: Chap. 7, especially 156ff).

[6] But it leaves open the possibility that a non-autonomous life might not be worse overall than an autonomous one. This is the case because autonomy is but one constituent of a good life.

[7] This does not entail that the parental duty to enhance autonomy is weightier than other parental duties. I will not address the issue of how various parental duties can come into conflict, or how they might be balanced.

[8] See Schapiro (2003: 578), who thinks that children are unfit to govern themselves because they lack reason.

[9] Especially Noggle (2002: 101–10).

cannot assess what is of value, and are insufficiently able to critically reflect and question their motives.[10] Rather, children waver a lot between options and what they find important.

Claiming that children are not developed in their deliberative, epistemic, and evaluative capacities raises two worries that need to be addressed. First, one might wonder why children need help. Why not simply wait and see how they mature by themselves? Second, does this view of parental duties not also carry the danger that childhood is erroneously seen as a state of deprivation and thus underestimates its genuine value?

In response to the first worry, it is important to note that not helping children would of course endanger small children with regard to their health and safety, because they are unable to care for themselves. Trying and erring by themselves would also lead them into too many impasses, and would prevent them from cultivating the capacities necessary for autonomy. However, one could still claim that while this might hold true for young children, it does not hold for adolescents, who are better placed to learn from mistakes. Also, there are many adults who fail to attain autonomy, sometimes even more so than 16-year olds. So what would ground the duty to help teenagers to become autonomous, but not adults who lack autonomy? These questions not only highlight how difficult it is to draw a clear boundary between childhood and adulthood, but also reveal that childhood itself is a vague concept.[11] The concept refers to human beings with capacities that are developed to varying degrees. While babies are only motivated by their immediate desires, and barely (if at all) utilize their deliberative-epistemic and evaluative capacities, 16-year-olds have usually developed such capacities to some extent. Hence, the autonomy of a child develops with age, and is lower in small children than it is in teenage children.

Given that the concept of childhood is vague, the parental duty to enhance the autonomy of children co-varies with the development of any particular child.[12] This reflects the fact that there is no precise cut-off point that marks the transition from childhood to adulthood.[13]

Furthermore, in claiming that certain capacities are not fully developed in children does not suggest, as the second worry has it, that there is nothing intrinsically good about childhood. Since there are other intrinsic goods of childhood—such as imaginative play and being carefree—childhood is not merely a negative stage of

---

[10] See, e.g. Schapiro (1999: 730–1).

[11] It is only made precise for legal reasons by stipulating the age of majority. But this does not make it precise in other normative respects.

[12] It is a further question whether parents who lack autonomy themselves would be able to enhance the autonomy of their children. I am unable to sufficiently address that question here.

[13] I am unable to tackle the question why not-so-autonomous adults should not be interfered with at all, whereas the opposite seems to hold true for adolescents. Franklin-Hall (2013: 243), defends the view that different temporal positions in the life cycle can justify that minors and adults are held to different standards.

life that has to be overcome.[14] I am simply highlighting that children fall short of certain capacities that are necessary for autonomy, and hence need guidance in developing them. Also, once they have acquired the capacity of autonomy, children need support and encouragement to exercise and refine that capacity.

Let me briefly mention two related issues that I will sidestep in this paper. First, in focusing on the autonomy of children I will not tackle the problem of how much autonomy parents themselves should enjoy. I simply take it for granted here that parents should *not* have the freedom to *not* enhance the autonomy of their children. They only have *some* autonomy with regard to *how* exactly to fulfill their duty.

Second, in claiming that there exists a parental duty to enhance children's autonomy, I do not want to commit myself to any substantive normative theory. Suffice it to say that I believe that the parental duty in question might, in principle, be captured in consequentialist as well as in non-consequentialist terms.

With these qualifications in place, this paper proceeds as follows. First I will elaborate on the concept of autonomy that I think is appropriate here. Second, I will show that two problems loom if we regard children as not-yet-autonomous but think it appropriate to help them achieve autonomy by way of interference. To overcome these problems, I will concentrate in the third section on the question of what conditions of autonomy parents, in principle, can foster. In drawing from my work on the normative importance of personal projects I hope to make plain in the fourth section that helping children to come to value personal projects enhances their capacity for autonomy. I will close by discussing various objections against my view, in the fifth section.

5.2 What Autonomy?

According to a broad concept of autonomy, a person is autonomous if and only if she fulfills two conditions. These two conditions correspond the aforementioned epistemic-deliberative and evaluative capacities. Let me call the first the *control condition*, and the second the *condition of authenticity*.[15] As for the condition of authenticity, for a person to be autonomous she must have a 'self'. That is, she must have an evaluative perspective that is expressive of her deep commitments, which are 'her own'. The intuition behind this condition is the following: Only that which is expressive of a person's 'true' self and that is thus her own—many refer in this regard to attitudes with which she identifies or that are expressive of what she really cares about or values[16]—is informative as to how she can understand herself. Otherwise, she would lead a life that is not her own; she would be a mere bystander with regard to what she does.

---

[14] See A. Gheaus in this volume (2014). Cf. Brighouse and Swift (2014: Chap. 4).

[15] See, Betzler (2009); Christman (2009: Chap. 8). Cf. Dworkin (2010b: Chap. 12). Cf. Oshana (1998: 81f); Oshana (2003: 99ff).

[16] This does not require any self-reflective capacities.

As for the control condition, a person's attitudes can only be her own, and thus manifest her self-conception, if she is able to guide herself over time in light of these. That is, her attitudes, which are expressive of her self-conception, must remain stable, but also flexible in light of changing circumstances. She therefore needs deliberative capacities to achieve coherence among her attitudes, to think about the adequate means to realize ends she values, and to assess the implications of her valued ends. Moreover, she needs epistemic capacities to perceive (new) reasons and to reflect and re-assess her evaluative perspective in light of them. She must be able to differentiate between her immediate desires and her stable attitudes, and thus manifest what she really values. This entails that she might have to control the former with the latter. If she failed to do this, she would come to lead an instable and incoherent life.

Both the condition of authenticity and the control condition define the concept of autonomy, but different theories of autonomy spell them out differently. In addition, current theories of autonomy diverge with regard to whether further conditions must hold for a person to count as autonomous. Among those further conditions are sufficient self-esteem,[17] sufficient options to choose from,[18] and being engaged in supportive relationships.[19] My aim in this paper is not to defend a particular theory of autonomy. Rather, I presuppose a widely-shared, broad core concept of autonomy that underlies rival conceptions. Accordingly, for a person to be autonomous, she must have attitudes that manifest her own evaluative outlook. What's more, she must have the capacity to guide herself in light of these attitudes over time. In short, a person must fulfill the condition of authenticity and the control condition to be considered autonomous. Admittedly, this is a rough and ready view of what the concept of autonomy entails, but I take it to be uncontroversial enough to serve as a starting point in my investigation into how children's autonomy can be enhanced. But if we suppose that parents have the duty to enhance the autonomy of their children, and provided that the aforementioned concept of autonomy is adequate, we seem to be confronted with two connected problems.[20]

The first problem is about the compatibility of autonomy and paternalism. According to one received view, paternalism is interference with another person's liberty or autonomy against her will or consent, so as to protect her from harm or to promote her own good.[21] Parents precisely interfere with the choices and actions of their children in various ways all the time. For example, they determine what to do without asking their children for consent. They do things against the explicit will of their children. And they decide what is of value, persuade their children to have certain evaluative attitudes, and make important decisions for children's lives. Parents limit the options of their children, they do not share information, and they sanction children's behavior in multiple ways.

---

[17] Cf., e.g., Benson (1994: 650–68).
[18] Cf. Oshana (1998: 81–102).
[19] Cf. Mackenzie and Stoljar (Eds.), (2000).
[20] Cuypers and Haji (2007: 82), refer in this connection to the 'problem of authenticity'.
[21] See Dworkin (2010a).

If parents are thought to act paternalistically in these ways—and many of us will regard a great variety of these interferences as legitimate—they treat their children as non-autonomous beings. What remains elusive is how this could enhance their children's autonomy. To solve this problem we need to know what kind of interference is not autonomy-undermining, and thus, what the precise content of the parental duty in question is. One way to solve this problem might be by further differentiating whose autonomy is to be enhanced. If children as children are already regarded as having autonomy, which parents might therefore risk disrespecting, they should not be interfered with. But if only children as adults are thought to have autonomy, parents may well interfere with their not-yet-autonomous children as children. But on closer inspection, this way of differentiating the bearer of autonomy brings up a further problem: If autonomy is to be enhanced in children as children, how could this enhance the autonomy of children as future adults? And if children—as future adults—are thought to be the ones whose autonomy should be enhanced, does this not bear the risk of undermining their autonomy as children, thus preventing them from ever becoming autonomous adults?

Both problems thus manifest the puzzle of how parents can enhance the autonomy of their children by way of interference without undermining it. What needs to be shown is what kind of parental interference could help to develop autonomy. Once we make good the insight that neither childhood nor autonomy is static, that autonomy applies both *locally*—to single decisions and actions—as well as *globally*, that is, to 'a life', and we acknowledge that there is a difference between '*state-like*' autonomy and '*capacity-like*' autonomy, we will be in a better position to provide a solution.

To begin with, even though children are not yet in a state of autonomy, they have the capacity for autonomy. That is, they have an innate ability to learn how to guide themselves by gradually developing various mental competencies. The parental duty to enhance the autonomy of their children is both positive and negative and is directed towards the capacity for autonomy. Parents must support and encourage their children to develop their capacity for autonomy and they must not interfere with its development. But not interfering with the development of that capacity does not entail that parents must not interfere with any non-autonomous state their children might be in. Infants and very small children have not actualized their capacity for autonomy,[22] and more often than not are in a non-autonomous state. As such, parental interference is called for to protect them from harm. But the interference is constrained by conditions that guarantee the development of the capacity for autonomy. Parental interference would undermine children's autonomy if parents either did not ensure the causally necessary conditions for them to develop autonomy, or if they did not provide them the room to learn to fulfill both the authenticity and control condition.

---

[22] Even though it might hold locally from an early age. For example, even small children are able to autonomously decide which clothes to wear, but they are not yet able to decide (at least not fully) what school to go to.

As for the causally necessary conditions, parents can hinder or obstruct the acquisition of autonomy if they undermine their child's self-esteem by humiliating her verbally or by inappropriately punishing her. The same holds true if they do not provide various options and thus guarantee their child an open future,[23] or if they do not ensure a social environment with intimate relationships that allows the child to experience trust and to feel loved and cared for. Moreover, children would be rendered incapable of fulfilling the condition of authenticity if parents failed to live up to their own value commitments, and more importantly, if they hinder children in developing such value commitments by themselves—either by disrespecting their children's inclinations or by generally sanctioning value commitments that run counter to their own. In addition, parents can hinder their children in fulfilling the condition of control by failing to enhance their children's deliberative capacities and by impeding the child's perception of relevant reasons. This is the case, for example, if they do not listen to their child's attempts at reasoning, do not provide feedback on the appropriateness of their emotional perceptions, do not encourage them to practice deliberation on their own, and continue to decide on their children's behalf in matters that their children could, depending on their age, decide for themselves.

Parental interference is autonomy-undermining only if parents obstruct their children's capacity for autonomy that evolves gradually and in relation to age. Enhancing that capacity involves encouraging one's children to exercise their own evaluative perspective and rational capacities. To be sure, these are not strictly necessary or jointly sufficient conditions for autonomy to evolve. One might even point to methods of enhancing the autonomy of children by oppression, abuse, or degradation. Children who stand up against such illegitimately interfering parents, and who as a result develop a strong sense of autonomy by enhancing their self-reliance, might be cases in point. In response to this, however, I think it is plausible to assume that such children have experienced the above-mentioned kinds of support from other people, even if not from their own parents, and this has allowed their autonomy to develop. Hence, the conditions I mentioned are more than just causal, they are constitutive to the extent that they are a necessary condition for autonomy to develop. But they are not strictly necessary, in the sense that there is a set of various means to achieve that end. To the extent that the development of autonomy requires close nurturing relationships, however, and provided parents have a special obligation as childrearers to provide the conditions for that, parents have a duty to respect their children's capacity for autonomy. This requires interference where this capacity is not yet enabled, and it requires encouragement, support, and assistance in helping to make it work. If we appreciate the fact that children have the capacity for autonomy, but are often not in a *state* of autonomy, parents can respect their capacity for autonomy by interfering with their local non-autonomous states and with a view to enhancing that capacity further. This solves the first problem, and helps us envisage a solution to the second. Given that there is a parental duty to enhance and not interfere with children's capacity for autonomy, the duty is directed

---

[23] Cf. Feinberg (1980: 148–51).

towards that capacity at the appropriate developmental stage of the child. It is not directed at some fictitious autonomous state of the child as a future adult. To the extent that parents raise their children *only* with the purpose of turning them into autonomous adults, they might risk raising them in ways that undermine their capacity for autonomy.[24]

But this leaves the exact content of positive and negative duties with regard to the development of children's autonomy still rather open. In what follows, I will elaborate on one fundamental part of that duty: How can parents help their children to fulfill the condition of authenticity, thus assisting them in developing a personal sense of value that is expressive of who they are?

5.3 From Caring to Valuing

How can parents enhance their children's ability to exercise autonomy by fostering their acquisition of a more stable evaluative outlook? Since children cannot simply create an evaluative outlook out of nowhere, and since they do not know what to value themselves, it has been claimed that there is 'nothing intrinsically immoral or illiberal about giving the parent at least prima-facie permission to instill her own value system and the world-view on which it rests as an initial "default" position'.[25] This would not undermine the child's autonomy, because he does not yet have an authentic self.[26]

I agree that children cannot develop their own evaluative outlook in a vacuum, and that parents do have an important role both in guiding them to conceptions of the good as well as serving as role models for the appreciation of values. But just 'instilling' values in one's children is not the right way to respect their capacity for autonomy. If this capacity is to be taken seriously, we need to look for ways how children can develop an evaluative outlook *by themselves*.

I will therefore lay the ground for a more precise formulation of the condition of authenticity. I will then offer a proposal of how children can come to fulfill that condition. According to my view, an evaluative attitude can be deemed 'one's own' and thus manifest the value commitments that account for one's normative identity, if there is a relevant connection between a person's evaluative responses and the things or states of affairs of value she responds to. Her response proves successful, and thus in a relevant sense 'her own', if this is reflected in a complex and coherent connection of attitudes. This coherent connection accounts for stability and future guidance, as well as the person's vulnerability to what she herself evaluatively

---

[24] I therefore agree with S. Olsaretti's and P. Bou-Habib's criticisms in this volume (2014) of what they call the autonomy as end-state or achievement view.

[25] Noogle (2002: 113). He adds, however, that parents must not try to force the child to keep them forever. He remains rather unclear how parents can help their children to acquire their own values.

[26] See Noggle (2005: 101), where he refers to the apparent 'paradox of self-creation'.

responds to. It thus manifests her own perspective, and thus her authentic self. Somewhat more precisely, this connection accounts for a person coming *to value* a thing, a person, or a state of affairs that reflects her evaluative response—a response that is, in the relevant, autonomy-enhancing sense, 'her own'. Valuing X is a complex and coherent set of attitudes that involves:

(i) The belief that X is valuable
(ii) The susceptibility to various context-dependent emotions concerning X
(iii) The disposition to experience these emotions as appropriate
(iv) The disposition to consider certain X-related considerations as reasons for action in deliberative contexts[27]

The belief that X is valuable presupposes sufficient knowledge about what is valuable. Susceptibility to various context-dependent emotions concerning X expresses the commitment of the agent to what she takes to be of value. In addition to an evaluative judgment that some X is valuable, the person who values X is vulnerable to how X fares. For example, she may feel anxious if that which she values is doomed to failure. She may be liable to joy if she feels supported in what she values. That a person has become vulnerable in this sense, and therefore sensitive to the fate of what she values, is connected to the fact that she has come to develop a normative identity with a particular evaluative perspective. To the extent that she is conscious of that perspective and believes that what she values *is* in fact valuable, she experiences her emotions, and hence, her vulnerability, as appropriate. This is what the third condition expresses. Someone who understands himself as a person who values music, for example, has probably had many musical experiences in the past. That person also understands herself as someone who values these experiences. This explains why she considers them in relevant deliberative contexts and views them as reasons for action. That is, she views the fact that she values music as a reason to listen to music more frequently, and to renounce expensive clothes so as to have the financial means to take piano lessons.

If this is right, a person who values has an evaluative perspective of her own. She identifies with certain evaluative properties by being emotionally susceptible to them, and guides herself in light of them. Furthermore, not only is she emotionally susceptible, but she understands this susceptibility as an expression of her conception of the good, and hence as someone who guides herself in light of her own reasons and over time. Valuing thus expresses a person's 'own' response.

But even if we agree that valuing so understood accounts for the condition of authenticity, it remains elusive how children (especially small children) could fulfill it. After all, and contrary to the definition of valuing above, children have neither truth-conducive beliefs about what is of value, nor do they entertain a reflective stance with regard to their emotions, and they certainly do not test them for appropriateness

---

[27] Scheffler (2010: 29). There has been very little work done on valuing, and I draw heavily from Scheffler's proposal which he, however, makes independently from its normative importance for autonomy.

conditions. Neither do they engage in future deliberations about how to act in light of their acquired evaluative stance.

On closer inspection, however, children prove able to master a proto-version of valuing, and this seems to be precisely what parents need to attend to so as to encourage the development of an evaluative perspective that children can call their own. What makes it a proto-version is that it presupposes neither evaluative beliefs, nor knowledge, self-reference to one's own future, or a conception of one's own identity. This proto-version, which lacks reflexivity as well as justification or truth conditions, shares the following property with the aforementioned complex of attitudes dubbed 'valuing'. It is diachronic and stable instead of momentary and volatile (as in the case of mere desires). This is accounted for by the fact that it consists of recurring emotional connections that are directed at constant things or states of affairs. Due to this diachronic stability and representational character of these emotional connections (which are about some content), this proto-version expresses what the person in question finds important. This attitude, which I call a proto-version of valuing, can be individuated as 'caring'.[28]

Studies in developmental psychology haven shown, for example, that children as young as 2 years old are capable of caring. They try to comfort their mothers or to engage in a task, such as tying their shoelaces over and over again. Such attempts frequently fail. But by engaging in these attempts, children experience the joy of being the initiator of a change in the world—however well-targeted that change turns out to be. Children who are successful show enthusiasm, especially if their actions are responded to positively. And they show frustration, anger, and throw tantrums if prevented from engaging in such actions. Caring differs from mere desiring in that it involves a complex set of emotional attitudes that are indirectly connected, via their focus on the same object or the same state of affairs. They exhibit some kind of constancy in that they are frequently exhibited and reactivated. They are not blind impulses, but already presuppose a basic (albeit not higher-order or reflexive) sense of self, by way of these connections to the same object, its changing circumstances, and over time—with regard to oneself.

This is why caring already manifests, to some extent at least, evaluative attitudes that can be regarded as a child's own. In being directed to the same object or the same state of affairs over time in relation to its relevant context, a child not only develops her self-understanding, but her emotional attitudes also become intelligible as an expression of what she cares about. A small child, however, is able to care without being conscious of the fact that she cares and without possessing any concept of the good or valuable. Hence, caring manifests the second feature of the complex attitude of valuing that I introduced above.

The question that therefore needs to be answered is how children develop the attitude of valuing on the basis of their capacity for caring. Caring is a basic building block for the evaluative perspective of children. Children, however, frequently err in

---

[28] Jaworska (2007: 529–68), draws attention to the normative significance of 'caring'. She thinks that agents bear moral status due to their ability to care (which includes small children as well as Alzheimer's patients). I draw from her work to shed light on caring as a proto-version of valuing.

what they care about and how they care about it. They can care about things, persons, or states of affairs that do not merit a caring reaction.[29] In addition, they are unable to regard their caring as a normative source of their actions or to deliberately control themselves in light of it. Caring, however, is the basis of valuing because through it children guide their receptivity to the value of an object or state of affairs, in relation to their perspective, and in a more stable fashion. They thereby experience themselves as being susceptible and vulnerable to that object or state of affairs. To react to things or states of affairs that are indeed valuable, and to guide themselves in light of these (and against inclinations to the contrary), children need to acquire a better understanding of what is in fact valuable, how beliefs about what is valuable are justified, and what renders emotional responses appropriate. In short, they need to acquire conditions of rationality that apply to their caring. Only then are they in a position to fulfill the condition of authenticity that is central to autonomy. Only then are they able to understand their caring as justified, to orient themselves deliberately in light of it, and to develop a more reflective conception of themselves.

But this process does not happen automatically. I will therefore defend a view that takes seriously the claim that children need to learn how and what to value. This is only possible, I claim, because they have an innate ability to care. And it is their parents' duty to help them from early childhood to enhance their faculty for caring. This involves taking an interest in what children care about, encourage them in pursuing what they care about, empathizing[30] with them if what they care about gives rise to frustration, giving them critical feedback if what they care about is imprudent, immoral, or otherwise of disvalue, and helping them understand when their emotions are appropriate and their caring directed to something valuable.[31] Such supportive attitudes will help children come to acquire a better understanding of when their emotions are appropriate, and what justifies their emotional responses. They will thereby develop well-founded beliefs about value, and good judgments about the appropriateness of their emotional reactions in connection with their caring, so that they eventually enact their own ability to value.

But notice that children will develop the ability to value by themselves without having values instilled in them. What parents can help with is only building on their caring and presenting their children with various options that might be conducive to the development of caring—and eventually valuing—attitudes. They can also provide further rationale for their children's caring. But if they simply instill values in them, they will not enhance their children's capacity for valuing and thus for fulfilling the condition of authenticity. In the next section, and provided that I am on the right track, I will show how personal projects provide specific opportunities for children to acquire the ability to value.

---

[29] This does not rule out that adults can err in their carings too.

[30] Slote (2010: Chap. 9), defends the view that empathic concern is what respects the autonomy of children even while interfering with their will.

[31] This presupposes at least an intersubjectivist understanding of value which I cannot defend at any length here.

5.4 Personal Projects and Autonomy

If valuing is a complex web of attitudes that manifests a child's evolving perspective which gradually solidifies, children need opportunities to enact their valuing over time and in recurring ways. This will eventually enhance their coming to understand themselves as having such an evaluative perspective and help them acquire a normative identity.

The claim I wish to defend is that personal projects can provide such opportunities.[32] Provided parents have the duty to enhance the autonomy of their children, they have a positive duty to help their children pursue personal projects. Let me call this the Enhancing Autonomy Claim (EAC).

> (EAC) The parental duty to enhance the autonomy of their children entails the duty to enable them to pursue and come to value personal projects.

The (EAC) is based on the assumption that if parents provide their children with opportunities to pursue personal projects, they provide opportunities for their children to develop valuing attitudes. Since valuing attitudes manifest a person's own evaluative perspective, and personal projects help to enact them over time and solidify them in light of values, children who come to value personal projects finally come to fulfill the authenticity condition of autonomy. The (EAC) not only renders paternalism and autonomy compatible, it is also targeted at enhancing the autonomy of children as children. On one hand, it manifests parental interference to the extent that they shape their children's choices about projects, predetermine the entry and exit conditions of their pursuit, and monitor how their children's projects are pursued over time. On the other hand, this interference does not undermine their children's autonomy because its aim is to have children develop their own evaluative perspective from which they can guide themselves.

Children can thus actualize their capacity to value, which is based on their capacity of caring. They can learn that certain things are, or become, important to them, without being coerced. The pursuit of projects helps them to acquire justificatory conditions for their carings, to gradually understand themselves in light of what is important to them, and to have their valuing play a role in deliberative contexts.

To substantiate this claim, a better understanding of personal projects is required. I have shown in other work that careers, hobbies, other leisure activities, causes, ambitions, and so on are personal projects. Superficial differences notwithstanding, they can be characterized by the following three elements: Projects are complex goals that:

(i) Are norm-governed
(ii) Give rise to and are constituted by both interconnected recurring action types and forward- and backward-looking emotions with regard to the project, how it fares in changing circumstances, and how it affects the person pursuing it
(iii) Express an identity-constituting commitment

---

[32] In what follows I draw from Betzler (2013: 101–26).

A personal project, such as a hobby playing soccer, for example, is governed by norms that more or less determinately prescribe the constitutive aim of that project. Whoever engages in soccer thus needs to know what kinds of action-types are conducive to that aim, and needs to execute a relevant set of such action-types. For instance, a child pursuing soccer as a hobby will go to weekly practice, study soccer magazines, take interest in the games of soccer clubs, watch these games, and play in tournaments.

Once this project is pursued and these action-types are carried out, the child in question can come to emotionally respond to the various evaluative features of these action-types, and become emotionally vulnerable to how the project fares. Some of these emotions are directed to evaluative properties of the hobby in question, such as the satisfaction one enjoys when scoring a goal, when making a good pass, or simply when playing with others. Other emotions are directed to how the hobby fares in changing circumstances, thus affecting the person pursuing it in various ways. For example, a boy becomes sad if he falls ill and cannot make it to the weekly practice. He experiences frustration when his team loses, and he is excited at the prospect of the next tournament. These emotions jointly show that the hobby has gained importance for the child in question.

The more the child pursues a project and the more he emotionally responds to it, the more he learns to understand himself and to identify himself as a soccer player. He will come to judge his hobby as valuable as it gains importance for him. Moreover, he will deepen his understanding as to why he regards his project as valuable, and be able to refer to value-dependent reasons that explain it. This process is expressed, in part at least, by reflexive emotions, such as pride, self-trust, and self-esteem.

If this analysis—which would require a paper of its own, and is therefore, admittedly, short—is persuasive, and provided personal projects so understood can help children acquire and solidify the attitude of valuing, we now need to turn to the question of what the content of the parental duty consists in more precisely, so as to provide children with opportunities to pursue personal projects. Typically, parents are more familiar with the talents, dispositions, and preferences of their children than of other people. Based on their privileged access to this kind of knowledge about their children, parents can pre-select suitable projects and provide their children with the opportunity to try them out. In addition, they can foster and encourage the pursuit of projects that children come across by themselves, take an interest in them, and express their own valuation of their children's attempts to engage in them. They can also show children how to value by pursuing their own projects. Parents can exchange ideas with their children about the various evaluative properties of particular projects at hand, and pass on their knowledge and their experiences with a particular project. These are important and helpful ways for a child to learn to value projects.

Of course, not all projects are equally suitable for children. But there are a whole range of project-types, such as hobbies and leisure activities, or causes, ambitions, political activities, and many handy, sporty, and art activities—as well as friendships[33]—that provide cases in point and which children can come to value

---

[33] Mullin (2007: 542ff) argues that love of other people is a source of autonomy for children.

over time. I am not claiming, however, that projects are logically or strictly necessary for valuing, and hence for autonomy. And I do not need to claim that they are the only way to enhance valuing. But I think projects are particularly suitable for facilitating the development of a capacity to value.[34] The (EAC) passes muster if coming to value personal projects satisfies the authenticity condition. Personal projects fulfill that function in four different ways:

First, projects typically allow for the experience of multiple valuable properties, such as aesthetic, social, nature-related, technical, intellectual, or kinesthetic properties. They thus help children to connect up properties that are, in principle, valuable in multiple ways.

Second, given that projects are norm-governed and socially predetermined scripts for action they provide an intersubjective warrant for beliefs about their valuable properties and help children experience the emotions directed to them as appropriate.

Third, in providing opportunities for positive experiences as well as frustrations, projects can be seen as opportunities to learn to cope with adversities and overcome obstacles. Personal projects are thus conducive to developing certain virtues, capabilities and social competences. For instance, children can develop strength of will and persistence through pursuing a project under changing circumstances. In addition, they can improve their abilities by continuously or recurringly engaging in a project. They can see this improvement as the result of their own efforts and thus learn to value the properties borne by a project increasingly over time. This, in turn, results in the acquisition of knowledge about what is of value in various projects. Children thus develop self-knowledge with regard to who they are and what they can value, which further reinforces their self-understanding and self-esteem.

Fourth, in providing a source of reasons for action that children respond to over a longer period of time, personal projects are conducive to helping children acquire an evaluative outlook by which they can come to understand and control themselves.

I hope to have sufficiently shown that personal projects are very suitable sources of valuing. This is what makes them important building blocks for the realization of the condition of authenticity that is at the core of any conception of autonomy. If parents give their children the opportunity to pursue personal projects, encourage them in doing so, and show interest in them, they help them to develop valuings of their own that are directed at the valuable properties of that project. This is how children can appropriate values, even if they have not yet developed their rational capacities to the fullest.[35] The problem of autonomy is solved to the extent that it is children themselves who come to value projects, even if some of those projects are

---

[34] A. Mullin (forthcoming) draws attention to the importance of stable goals for autonomy. Projects as I understand them are a special kind of stable goal that gives rise to valuing.

[35] I take this to be a more substantive way of spelling out Callan's view, according to which becoming autonomous is 'as much learning autonomously to adhere to a conception of the good as it is learning autonomously to revise it'. Cf. Callan (2002: 137).

predetermined by their parents. Parents do not undermine their children's autonomy as long as it is up to their children to prove that they value these projects. That is, parents must neither coerce a child to pursue a particular project if a child is not able to value it, nor disallow projects they value if no strong reasons speak against them. Parental duty consists in creating opportunities for their children to try out projects and to encourage them in their pursuit so that they can develop their own valuing capacities. This is what the (EAC) entails.

5.5 Objections and Replies

So far, I have established my claim that the opportunity to pursue and eventually come to value personal projects is constitutive of encouraging the autonomy of children. I will further defend this claim by forestalling various objections.

5.5.1 Overdemandigness

One might object that my claim demands too much of children. Young children in particular do not, or at least rarely, possess the endurance nor the capacities and competence to engage in personal projects. More often than not, they start with an activity and soon leave it for other activities. They are thus much more exploratory in nature than personal projects would allow for. Demanding that they pursue projects is not only overdemanding, it also obviates their volitional and rational capacities as children.

I submit that (especially small) children do not fully pursue personal projects. Instead, small children, but also older children, pursue what I would like to call 'proto-projects'. Proto-projects are connected activities that, in principle, could amount to a full-blown personal project. But to the extent that a child might not come to value them, and not sufficiently engage in these activities, they simply remain *projects in the making*. That is, children try themselves out with different activities, they change from one proto-project to the next, and try to find out what their project could be. Trying out various proto-projects helps children in their development to acquire more stable valuing attitudes of their own. They have the opportunity to develop perseverance and bravery, to bear more setbacks, acquire more skills, and learn more about themselves—until they are finally able to commit themselves more strongly to a particular project. To be sure, this is also dependent on other facilitating factors, such as their character, the personality of their coaches and teachers, the social esteem of their projects among peers, or the role models that they can learn from. But independent of these factors there is a constitutive relation between personal projects and the condition of authenticity underlying our understanding of autonomy. For a child to become more and more autonomous, to be able to value on her own and acquire an identity-constituting basis to guide herself in light of what she values, she needs many opportunities to try out projects and thus engage in proto-projects. Projects in the making—such as a week-long swimming course, or a summer camp with disabled children—provide such opportunities. Typically, adolescents start to commit themselves more fully to personal projects. But to the extent that a child is given the opportunity to try out proto-projects, she is not put under any overdemanding pressure. Rather, she is introduced to pursuing projects and acquainted with the idea.

One might think, however, that my response is in danger of overstretching the concept of personal projects and blurring the distinction between projects and activities that do not fall under that category. To the extent that proto-projects become, if continued, either full-blown projects (like swimming as a hobby) or constitutive parts of projects (like mud-building as part of engaging in a creative building project), however, and are defined by the above-mentioned characteristics, they are different from other activities. But I submit that many activities can become building blocks of a larger project. If they are engaged in with a possible project in view, proto-projects so understood are basic forms of engagement that are conducive to helping children develop valuing attitudes.

My view, however, may be beset with a further problem. There are children, after all, who are very reluctant to pursue and value projects. Children diagnosed with ADHS might be a case in point. Are they thus doomed to remain non-autonomous? There are two answers to this problem. First, there is variation as to how many projects children should engage with, how strongly they should be committed to such projects, and how often they engage with and value both personal projects and proto-projects. There is nothing in my account that rules out somewhat more volatile projects. Second, if a child never manages to value a project (or proto-project), it follows indeed that she is hard-put to build an evaluative basis from which to guide herself autonomously.

5.5.2 Wrong Ways to Pursue Personal Projects

Even if I concede that children develop only gradually, so as to pursue and value personal projects over time, we are still confronted with a further worry that this might still undermine their autonomy. One reason for this worry is that overly ambitious parents—let me call them *Über*parents—might coax their children to pursue too many projects or to engage in one project too frequently. Problems commonly known as 'overscheduling' and treating one's children as 'future stars' are cases in point.

I agree that there is this danger that parents might not enhance their children's pursuit of personal projects in appropriate ways. It is therefore important to amend my initial claim. As it turns out, providing children with the opportunity to pursue personal projects is not an unqualified condition for enhancing the autonomy of children. What matters in addition is *how* the pursuit of a particular project or proto-project is enhanced. Not only do children need time for free and unstructured play, they also need room to try out proto-projects on their own. Creative play and the pursuit of personal projects are not mutually exclusive. Instead, they can meaningfully complement each other if neither kind of activity crowds out the other.

There is a further worry looming, however, according to which parents coerce their children into particular projects—either because they represent values that they themselves deem important or, and not independently, because they are socially acclaimed projects. And indeed, it is usual for parents to preselect projects for their children, and their social function may play a role in this selection. But what undermines their children's autonomy is not necessarily that parents predetermine projects (at least not, when their children are younger). Rather, their autonomy is undermined if parents, first, do not take their children's dispositions, talents, and interests into serious consideration (and to the extent there are no strong reasons against certain projects[36]). Second, autonomy is doomed if children are forced to continue to pursue a particular project even if they prove unable to value it or if this prevents them from engaging in imaginative play and other important activities. Third, paternalistic interference is illegitimate if parents choose projects simply to raise their own social prestige. Not only does this treat their children as a mere means, it also makes it very difficult for children to learn to value a particular project non-instrumentally. They will not receive the right kind of encouragement and support if they have to pursue a project for project-independent reasons, such as the prestige of their parents, and fear blame if they do not foster that prestige sufficiently. But it is important to note that, despite these malfunctionings and despite the fact that parents might act paternalistically in predetermining the projects of their children, this paternalism does not matter to the extent that children are, in principle, allowed to come to value a particular project.

5.5.3 Personal Projects Are Not a Necessary Means to Enhance Autonomy

An objector could also raise doubts about personal projects being either not generally accessible means or not the right means to enhance the autonomy of children. As for the first kind of criticism, one might think that personal projects are representative of a particular, but not universally shared way of life. It is a way of life that puts too much emphasis on goal-directedness, achievement and success as it is manifest in Western industrialized cultures. Personal projects could also be thought of as endeavours that only the upper stratum of society can afford, and often at the expense of others. In this vein, the parental duty to foster their children in pursuing personal projects could be viewed as inherently unfair. After all, only children of wealthy parents—that is, those who can afford expensive extracurricular activities—could thus become autonomous. Any remotely plausible moral theory cannot comprise duties that exclude a large group (namely, children of poorer parents and children in poor societies). My claim is not that children need to pursue and value particular *bourgeois* or consumer-oriented projects that only wealthy parents in highly-diversified societies

---

[36] This would be the case if these were immoral or risky projects.

can afford. I am only claiming that they should be helped in pursuing some kinds of project, whatever those projects may be. This neither entails expensive training nor highly specialized programmes. Even endeavours that seem to have nothing to do with goal-directedness and success, such as gardening, playing soccer, or building and re-building a tree house, can serve as projects—because they are sources for indirectly connected action-types and forward- as well as backward-looking emotions, with regard to which a child can, in principle, come to value. What my claim does presuppose is that children have sufficient spare time to pursue projects (among other things, such as imaginative play), and do not have to engage in child labour. It seems uncontroversial to think that children must not work. And to the extent that economic resources in fact further enhance whether children pursue personal projects, as they might more easily provide various opportunities, we just have a further argument for social equality from autonomy.

As for the second criticism—i.e. that personal projects are not the right means to enhance a child's autonomy—an objector might also point to the fact that many projects are immoral, imprudent, or otherwise bad to begin with. To claim that valuing any kind of personal project is autonomy-enhancing is therefore self-justificatory. Just because a child has come to value a particular project does not entail that she has a reason to continue with that project and thus becomes gradually more autonomous. Many adolescents pursue famously strange kinds of projects, and sometimes they make a point in keeping up projects where the value is not easily perceivable.

In addition, not only 'strange' projects, such as engaging in counterculture, but also personal projects, such as mistreating animals, could give rise to indirectly connected action-types and the relevant emotions that allow a child to value these endeavours. It is far less persuasive, though, to maintain that these kinds of projects form a basis from which to guide one's life. In response to this, I admit that there are sometimes very strong reasons—namely moral reasons, considerations from prudence, or other value-based reasons—that speak against such projects. My claim is both more modest and more ambitious than it might seem. What I want to defend is more ambitious in that I take any kind of project that gives rise to interconnected action types and emotions, and that accounts for coming to value these, as an important source of autonomy. It is more modest in that this does not suggest that valuing a particular project, albeit providing a platform for autonomy, can never be overruled by other and stronger reasons.

5.6 Conclusion

There are other objections that might be raised against the (EAC), and there are further qualifications that may be called for,[37] but I hope to have made some headway in maintaining that the parental duty to enhance the autonomy of their children

---

[37] This includes the defense of an intersubjectivist theory of value. It is only on the assumption of such a theory that we can preclude cases of fundamentalist indoctrination or cases of projects the value of which is more than questionable.

consists, in part at least, in providing the opportunity for them to come to value personal projects. It is through children coming to value a project on their own, and through being responsive to that project over time, that they pass the test for having acquired an evaluative basis that fulfills the authenticity condition of autonomy.

Defendants of different conceptions of autonomy might point out that pursuing and valuing a particular project is not sufficient for autonomy. I agree with this caveat. There are other relevant factors that are necessary for autonomy, such as freedom from manipulation, coercion, critical reflection, or the ability to imagine alternatives. My claim is only that personal projects provide *one* important basis for acquiring capacities that account for the authenticity condition of autonomy. One might also think that this is not all there is to helping children learn to lead a good life. Again, I agree. But my aim is not to defend a conception of wellbeing. I simply want to show what, in part at least, a parental duty to make a child's life go well can consist in. To enable children to come to value personal projects by themselves allows them not only to fulfill one condition of autonomy, but also one of the constituents of wellbeing.

As a result, much work still needs to be done to elaborate on what else parents are required to do to make their children's lives go well and ensure their wellbeing. But I hope to have shown that allowing them to value personal projects is part of their duty.[38]

References

Archard, D. (2003). *Children, family and the state*. Aldershot: Ashgate.
Betzler, M. (2009). Macht uns eine Veränderung unserer selbst autonom? Überlegungen zur Rechtfertigung von *Neuro-Enhancement* der Emotionen. *Philosophia Naturalis, 46*, 167–212.
Betzler, M. (2011). Erziehung zur Autonomie als Elternpflicht. *Deutsche Zeitschrift für Philosophie, 59*, 936–953.
Betzler, M. (2013). The normative significance of personal projects. In M. Kühler & N. Jelinek (Eds.), *Autonomy and the self*. New York: Springer.
Benson, P. (1994). Free agency and self-worth. *The Journal of Philosophy, 91*, 650–668.
Brighouse, H., & Swift, A. (2014). *Family values*. Princeton: Princeton University Press.
Callan, E. (2002). Autonomy, child-rearing, and good lives. In D. Archard & C. Macleod (Eds.), *The moral and political status of children* (pp. 118–141). Oxford: Oxford University Press.
Christman, J. (2009). *The politics of persons: Individual autonomy and socio-historical selves*. Cambridge: Cambridge University Press.
Cuypers, S. E., & Haji, I. (2007). Authentic education and moral responsibility. *Journal of Applied Philosophy, 24*, 78–94.
Dworkin, G. (2010a). Paternalism. In E. Zalta (Ed.), *The Stanford encyclopedia for philosophy*. http://plato.stanford.edu/archives/sum2010/entries/paternalism/. Accessed 25 June 2013.
Dworkin, R. (2010b). *Justice for Hedgehogs*. Cambridge, MA: Harvard Belknap Press.

---

[38] This paper draws from ideas that I developed in Betzler (2011), but it contains substantial elaboration. For valuable written comments on this version I am indebted to A. Bagattini, C. Budnik, A. Gheaus, A. Mullin, and N. Osborne. I am also grateful to A. Bagattini and C. Macleod for inviting me to revisit my ideas on enhancing children's autonomy.

Feinberg, J. (1980). The child's right to an open future. In W. Aiken & H. LaFollette (Eds.), *Whose child? Children's rights, parental authority and state power* (pp. 124–153). Totowa: Rowman & Littlefield.

Franklin-Hall, A. (2013). On becoming an adult: Autonomy and the moral relevance of life's stages. *The Philosophical Quarterly, 63*, 223–247.

Gheaus, A. (2014). The intrinsic goods of childhood and the just society. In A. Bagattini & C. Macleod (Eds.), *The nature of children's well-being: Theory and practice*. Berlin/New York: Springer.

Hurka, T. (1987). Why value autonomy? *Social Theory and Practice, 13*, 361–382.

Jaworska, A. (2007). Caring and internality. *Philosophy and Phenomenological Research, 74*, 529–568.

Mackenzie, C., & Stoljar, N. (Eds.). (2000). *Relational autonomy: Feminist perspectives on autonomy, agency, and the social self*. New York: Oxford University Press.

Mullin, A. (2007). Children, autonomy and care. *Journal of Social Philosophy, 8*, 536–553.

Mullin, A. (forthcoming). Children, paternalism and the development of autonomy. *Ethical Theory and Moral Practice*.

Noggle, R. (2002). Special agents: Children's autonomy and parental authority. In D. Archard & C. Macleod (Eds.), *The moral and political status of children* (pp. 97–117). Oxford: Oxford University Press.

Noggle, R. (2005). Autonomy and the paradox of self-creation: Infinite regresses, finite selves, and the limits of authenticity. In J. S. Taylor (Ed.), *Personal autonomy: New essays on personal autonomy and its role in contemporary moral philosophy* (pp. 87–108). Cambridge: Cambridge University Press.

Olsaretti, S., & P. Bou-Habib. (2014). Autonomy and children's wellbeing. In A. Bagattini & C. Macleod (Eds.), *The nature of children's well-being: Theory and practice*. Berlin/New York: Springer.

Oshana, M. (1998). Personal autonomy and society. *Journal of Social Philosophy, 29*, 81–102.

Oshana, M. (2003). How much should we value autonomy? *Social Philosophy & Policy*, 99–126.

Scheffler, S. (2010). Valuing. In *Equality and tradition* (pp. 15–40). Oxford: Oxford University Press.

Schapiro, T. (1999). What is a child? *Ethics, 109*, 715–738.

Schapiro, T. (2003). Childhood and personhood. *Arizona Law Review, 45*, 575–594.

Slote, M. (2010). *Moral sentimentalism*. Oxford: Oxford University Press.

Sumner, W. L. (1996). *Welfare, happiness, and ethics*. Oxford: Clarendon.

Chapter 6
Utilitarianism, Welfare, Children

Anthony Skelton

6.1 Introduction

Utilitarianism is the view according to which the only basic requirement of morality is to maximize net aggregate welfare. This position has implications for the ethics of creating and rearing children. Most discussions of these implications focus either on the ethics of procreation and in particular on how many and whom it is right to create,[1] or on whether utilitarianism permits the kind of partiality that child rearing requires.[2] Despite its importance to creating and raising children, there are, by contrast, few sustained discussions of the implications of utilitarian views of welfare for the matter of what makes a child's life go well. This paper attempts to remedy this deficiency. It has four sections. Section 6.2 discusses the purpose of a theory of welfare and its adequacy conditions. Section 6.3 evaluates what prominent utilitarian theories of welfare imply about what makes a child's life go well. Section 6.4 provides a sketch of a view about what is prudentially valuable for children. Section 6.5 sums things up.

---

[1] See, for example, Singer (2011) and Parfit (1984).
[2] See, for example, Sidgwick (1907: Book IV, ch. iii, § 3.), Broad (1971), and Brink (2001).

A. Skelton (✉)
Department of Philosophy, University of Western Ontario,
London, ON N6A 5B8, Canada
e-mail: anthonyjskelton@gmail.com

6.2 Preliminaries

Utilitarians are welfarists.[3] They believe that welfare is the only thing that one ought morally to promote for its own sake, and that therefore it is the exclusive concern of moral and political thinking. But in what does welfare consist? What makes a life go well for the individual living it? The purpose of a theory of welfare is to answer these questions. A theory of welfare provides us with an account of the nature of welfare. It tells us what characteristic(s) something must possess in order to make someone fundamentally better or worse off. It details what is non-instrumentally good or bad for an individual. More specifically, it measures prudential value: how well or poorly a life or part of a life is going from the point of view of the entity living it.[4]

The acceptability of a theory of welfare depends on its normative adequacy, or how appropriate it is for the purposes of moral and political reasoning, and on its descriptive adequacy, or how well it captures and explains our considered attitudes about welfare and related concepts.[5] The focus here will be on descriptive adequacy.

According to Wayne Sumner, there are four criteria of descriptive adequacy. First, a theory of welfare must be true to our core beliefs about the concept of welfare and our use of these in practical reasoning and in common-sense psychological explanations. Second, a theory must be general in two senses: it must explicate the range of welfare judgements that we routinely make, positive, negative, and so on, and it must cover the core subjects to whom these judgements are regularly applied, including non-human animals, children, and adults. Third, it must be formal: it must not provide merely a list of welfare's ingredients. It must tell us why certain things make us better off. It must give an account of what relation health, for example, must bear to us to be non-instrumentally good for us. Finally, a theory of welfare must be neutral: it "must not have built into it any bias in favour of some particular goods or some preferred way of life."[6]

Sumner is right that if a theory of welfare, whether for children or for adults or whatever, fails to plausibly capture and explain our most cherished pre-analytic convictions about welfare, this is a sign that something is awry. A theory of welfare must aim at fidelity to our core convictions. In addition, a theory of welfare must be general in the first sense: it must capture all of the "categories of judgement [about welfare] – positive and negative, of fixed levels and of changes in level."[7]

But an account of welfare need not be general in the second sense. It need not apply to all core subjects of welfare assessments. It might, for example, be perfectly adequate for children, but be inadequate for animals and for adults or vice versa. This

---

[3] Brink (1989: 217) and Sumner (1996: 186).
[4] Sumner (1996: 20); see also Griffin (1986: 31).
[5] Sumner (1996: 10–18); see also Haybron (2008: 43–58).
[6] Sumner (1996: 17–18).
[7] Sumner (1996: 13).

does not entail that it is false or deficient. It means only that the domain to which it applies is circumscribed. Yet it may still be true for those to whom it applies: it will depend on how well it fits with our considered convictions. This sense of generality is no constraint on a theory of welfare – *au contraire*. It has, it seems, led us to overlook the possibility that we fare well differently at different stages in life.

A theory of welfare need not, *pace* Sumner, aim at being formal. First, it is by no means obvious that our search for such a theory should, as Sumner puts it, be guided by the "regulatory hypothesis" that "however plural welfare may be at the level of its sources…it is unitary at the level of its nature."[8] The nature of welfare is not obviously the same for all core welfare subjects. Sumner himself denies that it is: he suggests that infants, small children and adults do not fare well in the same way.[9] It might be that a theory must be formal within distinct categories of welfare subjects. However, even this requirement seems too strong. It begs the question against positions making no attempt to deliver formal theories of welfare distinguishing between welfare's nature and its ingredients. That such views lack formality does not alone detract from their plausibility.

Finally, the neutrality requirement is inapposite when applied to thinking about young children's welfare. A theory that makes welfare dependent in part on the possession of particular goods in the case of non-human animals and young children is *prima facie* attractive. *A fortiori*, a theory of welfare needs to explain the fact that it is appropriate for parents to prefer for their children some forms of life over others on the grounds that this is what is prudentially good for them. A view of welfare must make room for the idea that paternalism is apposite in the case of some welfare subjects. Perhaps all Sumner's neutrality requirement amounts to is the claim that a theory of welfare should not presuppose a "concrete form of life", e.g., a life devoted to repose rather than to developing one's talents, to rigorous planning rather than to spontaneity. If Sumner means only to leave room for this variety of variability, there is no quarrel with him. Most reasonable views respect this weak form of neutrality.

A theory of welfare for children should, then, aim at fidelity to our intuitions about faring well as a child and at capturing and explaining the central categories of welfare judgement regarding children. It need not aim at being formal or at being neutral except in some weak sense. In what follows, the aim is to ascertain how well particular theories of welfare satisfy the criterion of fidelity.

It is important to note here a difficulty associated with working out a theory of welfare for children. There is a great degree of variability amongst the individuals called children. The average 16-year-old shares very little in common with the average 2-year-old, despite the fact that both are routinely called children. It is not possible therefore to work out a theory of welfare that fits all children. Doing so would ignore the fact that children develop quite significantly over time. A better way to proceed is to make a rough division between young children (e.g., toddlers) and older children (e.g., adolescents), and to work out different views for each. This paper focuses on young children.

---

[8] Sumner (1996: 17).
[9] Sumner (1996: 145, 146, & 178–179).

6.3 Utilitarian Theories of Welfare

Utilitarians have defended a range of views about welfare, including hedonism, life satisfactionism, objective-list views, and desire satisfactionism.[10]

Hedonism is the view that welfare consists in happiness, which consists in surplus pleasure. On this view, pleasure is non-instrumentally good for an individual, and pain is non-instrumentally bad for an individual. Pain is bad because of its painfulness, and pleasure is good because of its pleasurableness. The more surplus pleasure one has the better one's life is going. The more surplus pain one has the worse one's life is going.[11]

Martha Nussbaum notes that hedonism makes good sense of the "receptive and childlike parts of the personality."[12] The hedonists and especially Bentham understood "how powerful pain and pleasure are for children, and for the child in us."[13] Hedonism has a lot going for it as regards young children. It predicts many of our common-sense attitudes about their welfare, e.g., that alleviating their pain, letting them gain excitement from the prospect of a visit from the Easter Bunny, and the pursuit of their typical forms of disporting, is non-instrumentally good for them. It does seem that a child's life goes well to the extent that she finds her life pleasurable on balance.

One worry about the hedonist view is that it fails to capture the range of experiences that matter to a young child's happiness, and therefore to her welfare. Sumner argues, for instance, that states of mind other than pleasure and enjoyment matter to how happy we are, including everything from "bare contentment to deep fulfilment."[14] This is a persuasive criticism. A child is surely happy when she is merely contented with how things are going but not experiencing pleasure or enjoyment. A child is surely unhappy even though he is neither in pain nor suffering but is instead merely feeling glum or experiencing ennui.

To capture these judgements, Sumner advocates a more expansive notion of happiness that he thinks fits young children, namely, affective happiness: "what we commonly call a sense of well-being: finding your life enriching or rewarding, or feeling satisfied or fulfilled by it."[15] This involves judging that your life feels satisfying or rewarding or enriching to you. Together with the view that welfare consists in happiness, we get the position that welfare for young children consists in surplus satisfaction. What is non-instrumentally good for a young child is finding her life satisfying. What is non-instrumentally bad for a young child is finding her life dissatisfying. A child is faring well when her life is on balance satisfying to her.

---

[10] These are at any rate among the most prominent.

[11] On one interpretation, this is the classical utilitarian view; see Bentham (1996: chs. i & iv), Mill (1998: chs. ii & iv) and Sidgwick (1907: Book III, ch. xiv).

[12] Nussbaum (2004: 68).

[13] Nussbaum (2004: 68).

[14] Sumner (1996: 149).

[15] Sumner (1996: 146; also 147).

Like hedonism, this view predicts many of our attitudes about young children's welfare. However, it is more attractive than hedonism, for two reasons. The first, as noted, is that it is broader. It captures the full range of mental states relevant to happiness and welfare. The second is that it leaves room for the child's perspective to play a role in her welfare. We do ask children how various states of affairs would make them feel; and we take their judgement to be relevant to their welfare. Retaining the notion of satisfaction leaves some role in a child's welfare for a child's perspective and her judgement about how things are going affectively for her.

Sumner's view faces two challenges. One is that affective happiness as he characterises it contains several sophisticated concepts, including those of reward, enrichment, and fulfilment. It is not clear that young children have the capacity to judge that parts of their lives are fulfilling or rewarding. Such judgements may well be beyond the capacity of young children, for it is not clear that they possess these concepts.

In reply, Sumner can argue that he needs only a minimal notion of satisfaction, requiring no more than that a child have the capacity for some kind of judgement about the affective conditions of the parts of her life. Such responses might be gained from and confirmed using, among other things, verbal and behavioural evidence. It is not unrealistic to think that even a very young child can make a reasonably authoritative assessment of her affective condition.[16]

A second worry is more powerful. On Sumner's view, how well a young child's life is going depends exclusively on her experience of it. This follows from equating welfare with surplus affective happiness or with feeling happy on balance.[17] The more surplus satisfaction a child has the more welfare she has. But this leaves the view of welfare for young children vulnerable to a version of the experience machine objection. Robert Nozick asks us to imagine that scientists have invented a machine designed to replicate experiences associated with living a vast range of lives that one might desire to lead.[18] By plugging in, a child would experience the most robust and sophisticated satisfaction associated with rich friendships, a supportive, safe, and stimulating living environment, and loving parents. This life would of course not be real. But the child would not know this. Suppose the machine could provide more happiness on balance than life in reality. Would it be best for a child to plug in? If Sumner is right, then it seems the answer to this question is affirmative.

Many believe that the answer is not affirmative. One reason for not plugging a child in is that it would involve parents or guardians in violating a duty they have to care for their children. At least initially it seems wrong for guardians to give the care of their children over to a machine and the scientists running it.[19] Each parent has a responsibility to raise his or her child.

---

[16] This may not be true of infants, in which case their welfare may consist (at least in part) in some affective state not requiring judgment.
[17] Sumner (1996: 147, 149, & 156).
[18] Nozick (1974: 42–45).
[19] Except perhaps in extreme situations.

This does not refute Sumner's position, for parents might have this reason while it is still true that life inside the machine is better for the child.

There is another reason for not entering a child into an experience machine. It is not just that giving one's child over to a machine involves violating a duty to look after her. There is strong reason to want one's child to fare well. Were there nothing more to welfare than surplus satisfaction, one would feel that there was strong reason for a parent to want a child to plug in. One would feel significant tension between one's duty to look after one's child and one's duty to advance their welfare when confronted with Nozick's experience machine. That there is no such tension except in rare cases suggests that one reason we think it a bad idea for a child to live inside the machine is that there is more to faring well for a child than surplus happiness. The machine is unable to provide in addition to happiness, actual valuable relationships, actual play (physical and other kinds) and so on, things that any loving parent would want for his or her child for the child's own sake.

This argument has not convinced everyone.[20] Those who are unconvinced are keen to defend hedonism. The replies can be modified to defend Sumner's view.[21] There are two lines of defence. The first is to argue that the view can, despite appearances, capture and explain our intuitions.[22] The second is to cast sceptical doubt on our intuitive response to Nozick's thought experiment.[23]

The first line of defence involves noting that there is a strong connection between happiness and, for example, the pursuit of friendships, intellectual activity and play. Young children would be much less happy were they to eschew these things, and we take a dim view of the claim that these things are good for young children in the absence of happiness. The best explanation of this is that these things are good for children because they are instrumental to producing happiness. The defence goes on to note that pursuing these goods as though they are themselves non-instrumentally good is a way to solve the paradox of happiness. Children do better in terms of happiness if they pursue it indirectly rather than directly, by means of pursuing things other than happiness.[24]

In reply, one can argue that the happiness theory has trouble predicting our intuitions in some cases. Suppose your child has two options for what to do this afternoon. Both options involve equal amounts of happiness. In option one, the surplus happiness is taken in active engagement with your child's friends. In option two, the happiness is taken in passively watching TV. The happiness theory says we should be indifferent between these two options. We are not indifferent, however: the former is

---

[20] It should be noted that the experience machine objection does not show that Sumner's view fails as a theory of illfare. Illusory unhappiness seems to contribute just as much to faring poorly as real unhappiness.

[21] Sumner cannot avail himself of these arguments but this need not concern us here.

[22] For this line of defense, see Sidgwick (1907: 401–406), Crisp (2006a: 117–125) and Crisp (2006b).

[23] For this line of defense, see Hewitt (2010); see also Silverstein (2000) and Brandt (1989).

[24] For these thoughts, see, for example, Sidgwick (1907: 401–406), Crisp (2006a: 119–120), and Crisp (2006b: 637–638).

thought to be better for the child. Suppose further that there is no reason to think that one option is more likely than the other to make a greater contribution to your child's happiness over the long run. We still think that the former is better for the child. We do not have to await the outcome of a felicity calculus to yield this judgement. This suggests that there is more to faring well than surplus happiness.

The second line of defence is to argue that we should not trust intuitions suggesting that things other than happiness matter to welfare. The idea is that in rejecting hedonism we rely on what we want for young children and on intuitions about what is prudentially valuable for them beyond happiness.[25] For the argument to succeed we must be able to trust that such appeals reveal what is in fact prudentially valuable for young children. This, the argument continues, we cannot do, for our desires and our intuitions are shaped by factors (e.g., personal and cultural habits) that undermine their claim to reveal the truth about prudential value.

The best reply to this line of defence is to argue that appeals to what seem intuitively prudentially valuable and to what we desire are operative in arguments for the happiness theory. The traditional arguments for hedonism refer either to desire (Mill) or intuition (Sidgwick).[26] It is not clear what else one could appeal to in order to justify the happiness theory. If such appeals are *verboten*, then we end up with scepticism about prudential value in general.

It might be possible to respond by arguing that we are more directly aware of the prudential value of happiness than we are of the prudential value of other things. Sharon Hewitt, for example, argues that in experiencing happiness "we seem to be, in a very direct way, experiencing *goodness*." This is because goodness is a "phenomenal property of pleasure."[27]

The worry with this reply is that it does not tell us why we should trust what seems to be the case in this experience. Why not think that the appeal here to what seems to be the case is impugned by the same considerations that impugn our intuition that there are things other than happiness that matter to welfare? It may appear to us that happiness is good when we experience it, though this appearance or seeming is the result, as in other cases, of "pre-existing personal and cultural habits" and of a "preference for the familiar, as well as for what those around us are doing and/or approving."[28] Indeed, we might be fashioned to think this way about happiness because of the evolutionary advantages of doing so. We might think that happiness is non-instrumentally good for us because of its importance to the preservation of life and to reproductive fitness. We are in other words fashioned to think that happiness is prudentially good for us merely because of its instrumental importance. It is simply not clear how this seeming is any more reliable than what seems true in cases

---

[25] For Nozick's appeal to desire, see Nozick (1974: 43 & 45); for his appeal to intuition, see Nozick (1989: 106–107).

[26] Mill (1998: ch. iv) and Sidgwick (1907: 400–401).

[27] Hewitt (2010: 333n7; italics in original). Hewitt defends hedonism but the account of pleasure that she accepts makes her view essentially equivalent to Sumner's happiness view. See Hewitt (2010: 333n8).

[28] Hewitt (2010: 345).

where we have judgments that run contrary to the happiness theory. If the happiness theorist is to fend off this worry, they will rely on tools no less effective in defending the claim that things other than happiness matter to welfare.

There is no trouble free way around the experience machine objection. We should reject the claim that welfare for young children consists in happiness alone. However, we should concede that happiness is a necessary condition of faring well as a child. There are indeed good reasons for doing this. First, doing so captures the intuition that a child's perspective is at least partly relevant to her welfare at a time. Second, it provides us with a clear criterion for determining when something makes a difference to a child's welfare. Third, it explains why hedonistic and happiness theories have appeared compelling when thinking about young children's welfare. Fourth, it explains why books written for consumption by young children consistently focus on their happiness together with other things, e.g., friendships and play.[29]

Happiness is not the only thing that matters to welfare for young children. What more is required? In his discussion of the experience machine objection, Sumner notes that a view according to which only mental states matter to welfare is "too interior and solipsistic to provide a descriptively adequate account of the nature of welfare."[30] He thinks that this is true of hedonism. He does not notice that this is true of his own view of welfare for young children. He provides an account of welfare for adults that he thinks avoids this worry, which involves appeal to information and autonomy.[31] He rightly notes that appeal to these will not work in the case of young children.

How might one avoid this solipsism in the case of young children? One strategy is to impose a value requirement on welfare. A child's life goes well when her satisfaction or happiness is taken in something that is worthy of satisfaction, such as valuable relationships, intellectual activity, and play.[32]

Sumner is sceptical of such views.[33] His first worry is that it is difficult to determine which values matter to faring well. Whose views do we rely on? This worry is not insurmountable. He has encouraged us to take account of the most cherished of our common-sense attitudes about faring well. This puts us in danger of endorsing erroneous or biased views of welfare. The view we arrive at on the basis of this method may well turn out to be parochial. To avoid this, Sumner would presumably insist on relying on a broad set of views and sober reflection and on exposing one's views to analysis by relevant experts. There is no reason why an exponent of a value requirement on welfare for children could not avail themselves of the same tools in articulating their position.

---

[29] See, for example, Jeram (1999) and Clarke (2002).

[30] Sumner (1996: 98; also 110).

[31] Sumner (1996: 171–183).

[32] These things are described as "worthy of satisfaction" to avoid claiming that they are by themselves good for a child. The phrases "worthy of satisfaction" and "worthy of happiness" are to be treated as synonymous.

[33] Sumner (1996: 163–164).

A second worry that Sumner raises is that "a value requirement…seems objectionably dogmatic in imposing a standard discount rate on people's self-assessed" welfare.[34] He thinks that it is up to the individual to determine how well he or she was faring in the past, something an individual does when her values change over time. His view is that there is no right answer as to how an individual was faring previously: it is up to her to decide now. Things are different with happiness: there is a right answer to how happy one was. When thinking about some prior point in your life, he says: "You do not, and should not, reassess your level of happiness during that earlier stage of your life."[35]

There are three problems with Sumner's claim. First, his view equates children's welfare with their happiness, thereby imposing a "standard discount rate" on it. Second, his discussion is conducted in terms of changes in values and in terms of judgements and capacities that are well beyond young children. Third, it is certainly not obvious that one's adult self is in a position, normatively speaking, to determine one's welfare as a child on the basis of one's adult values. It might be that how well a child fares is fixed by the facts in the same way that everyone's happiness is.

Sumner is wrong to think that happiness is all that matters to children's welfare. One generates a more attractive view by endorsing a value requirement on children's welfare. On this view, a young child's welfare consists in taking satisfaction in activities that are worthy of satisfaction, that is, activities in which it is good for her to take satisfaction. Sumner has given us no reason to reject such a view. Providing it with a defence in part involves saying something about the sort of activities that are worthy of satisfaction for young children. A good place to begin such a defence is a discussion of the objective-list theory of welfare.

The general idea behind the objective-list view is that what is good for an individual does not (necessarily) depend on what satisfies her or her desires. What is non-instrumentally good for an individual is the possession of objectively valuable goods; what is non-instrumentally bad for an individual is the possession of objectively disvaluable evils and/or the lack of possession of objective goods. One's life is going well when one has on balance more objective goods than objective evils.

The most prominent utilitarian exponents of this view are David Brink and Richard Arneson.[36] Brink has the most developed version. He describes it as "objectivism about welfare."[37] According to Brink, what is non-instrumentally good for an individual "neither consists in nor depends importantly on…psychological states," e.g., desires.[38] There are in particular three primary components of welfare: development, pursuit and realization of an agent's admissible projects, certain personal and social relationships.[39] These are good for an individual in part because they involve the exercise of certain desirable traits and capacities. Pursing and realizing

---

[34] Sumner (1996: 165).
[35] Sumner (1996: 165; also 157).
[36] See also Hooker (2000: 43).
[37] Brink (1989: 231).
[38] Brink (1989: 221 & 231).
[39] Brink (1989: 221).

worthwhile projects involves practical reason: "the capacity to evaluate courses of action and decide what to do."[40] Forming, pursuing, and maintaining personal and social relationships involves our capacity for sociability and in particular our capacities "for sympathy, benevolence, love, and friendship."[41] These relationships express such capacities because they involve "mutual concern and respect" and "treating others as people whose welfare matters."[42]

Brink's view does not help us determine the nature of children's welfare. The problem with the view is that it relies on and emphasizes capacities and traits that young children typically do not possess in any reasonable and stable degree. This is especially true of Brink's understanding of practical reasoning. Children even at an advanced age seem incapable of engaging in the sort of practical reasoning that Brink describes, which involves, among other things, deep reflection, life plans and long-term projects.[43] The same is true of the other goods, for children do not realise and pursue the kind of personal and social relations that assume pride of place in his view. Young children do not for example engage in relationships that involve developing shared intentions, long-term planning, agreement, and bargaining (especially over how to solve conflicts between the principles governing mutual interaction), among other things. These are the relationships on which Brink focuses; they involve "agents" and "persons".[44]

Brink's objective-list view does not fit children. In addition, it is missing something that all agree matters to children's welfare, i.e., happiness. Arneson's list is more promising. He notes that love, accomplishment, friendship, pleasure and desire satisfaction would be on any plausible objective list.[45] Some of these fit children (pleasure and friendship); whether others do depends on how they are interpreted. In his discussion of love, for example, Arneson focuses exclusively on romantic love.[46] This is not the sort of love that appears to be worthy of satisfaction for young children. His discussion is at any rate conducted entirely with adults in mind.[47]

However, that advocates of the objective-list theory of welfare fail to develop views that fit children does not entail that their position is false. Arneson notes that some versions of the objective-list view accept that "there are different types of persons and a distinct list for each type."[48] He might be open to the idea that there is a distinct list for children, in which case all he needs to do is draw up a list of goods

---

[40] Brink (1989: 232).

[41] Brink (1989: 233).

[42] Brink (1989: 233; also 234).

[43] "The formation and pursuit of projects should be reflective; an agent's decisions should reflect a concern for her entire self. This requires that she attempt to integrate projects into a coherent life plan, one that realizes the capacities of the kind of being that normative reflection on human nature tells her she is." Brink (1989: 232).

[44] Brink (1989: 231 & 234).

[45] Arneson (1999: 119, 136, 140, & 141).

[46] Arneson (1999: 140).

[47] This is true of Hooker's view, which has a "central" role for "autonomy". See Hooker (2000: 43).

[48] Arneson (1999: 118). We can assume that "persons" here refers to "individuals".

that is specifically geared toward children. This requires no more than that he modify the list of the goods that he thinks form the nature of welfare.

What would such a list look like? An answer to this question will be provided in the next section. The view of young children's welfare that appears defensible to me includes a list of activities that are worthy of happiness. As some of the foregoing suggests, the possession of such things is part of the nature of children's welfare. It will suffice to maintain that the things most worthy of happiness for children are intellectual activities, loving and valuable relationships, and play, involving enjoyable mental and physical activity engaged in for its own sake.

The main difficulty with the objective list view is that it holds that one can fare well at a time without experiencing any happiness. This element of the view is dubious in the case of children. There are good reasons to think that happiness is necessary for faring well as a child. Hedonism and the satisfaction view appear to be too solipsistic and interior to be adequate views of children's welfare; they leave no room for things other than experiences to play a role in a child's welfare. The objective-list view has the opposite problem. It leaves too little room for the individual child. In particular, it leaves too little room for the seemingly important role that a child's own affective responses play in a child's welfare at a time. Of course, proponents of the objective-list view can and do include happiness and pleasure on their lists, but this seems insufficient to support the compelling idea that it is only when a child is happy that a child is faring well.

There is, however, a formidable challenge to the idea that happiness is necessary for well-being. Arneson claims that an experience requirement on welfare is refuted by the following case. Suppose that an individual desires strongly to write and publish a good novel and that this state of affairs obtains, but that it involves no "experience of any sort on the part of the desiring agent."[49] Arneson says that it is plausible to say that one is better off as a result of having this desire satisfied.

This is not persuasive. Suppose the state of affairs obtains while the person is an irreversible comma. Does the satisfaction of this desire really make the individual better off? It seems very hard to believe that it does.

This might be a strange example. Here is another, better one. Suppose that your child works hard to gain proficiency in ice hockey and that she takes great satisfaction in doing so. She acquires the skills of skating, puck control, stick handling, efficient passing, and so on. She gains these skills to such a degree that she is able to play hockey at a very high level thereby satisfying a desire of hers to do so. Suppose, however, that once she achieves her goal of earning a spot on the top team and is able to play with the best players, she experiences no happiness. The happiness she felt before is gone: she is left, as Arneson puts it, with no affective "experience of any sort."[50] It is highly plausible to think that up until she played with the top team she was faring well. It is less attractive to claim that she is now faring well. There is some reason to regard her current situation as less desirable. A reasonable explanation is that she is no longer faring well.

---

[49] Arneson (1999: 123).
[50] Arneson (1999: 123).

One might insist that what we really think is that the child is faring less well than she was. But there seems little basis for this claim: she is left absolutely affectively flat by the experience. The victory, we might say, is hollow. Suppose she wants to abandon playing, and I encourage her not to do so. When I do so I cannot really credibly claim to be doing so in order to promote her welfare if I know that she will gain no happiness. If I really thought she'd gain welfare in doing so I would try to find ways to get her to see that she will enjoy it either now or shortly with some effort. I might point to the fact that the other kids are enjoying it (if they are) or I might tell her to take a break and reconsider. If I really think that no happiness will be had, I might still, using a different tone, encourage her to continue. But in this case I might say that there is an important moral consideration to continue – you ought to finish what you started, your teammates are counting on you – or that it is important to pursue non-welfarist values, e.g., achievement.

At any rate, it is not obvious what is problematic in saying a young child cannot fare well in the absence of happiness. One can argue that some value other than welfare is being promoted when happiness is absent. However, saying that one can fare well in the absence of happiness is problematic. It involves ignoring a child's perspective about what matters to her. It ignores what resonates with her. It involves ignoring what all agree is salient to a young child's welfare.

I have been suggesting thus far that the most enticing view of welfare for young children is a hybrid view, combining elements of both the happiness view and the objective-list view. Before outlining it, it is important to note that the view stands in stark contrast to what is by far the most popular view of welfare amongst the utilitarians. This is the desire theory of welfare. On the desire view, the satisfaction of a desire makes one non-instrumentally better off; the frustration of a desire makes one non-instrumentally worse off. One's life is going well when one has on balance more of one's desires (adjusted for strength) satisfied than frustrated.

There is some dispute over which desires matter to welfare. Some believe that welfare consists in the satisfaction of one's actual desires.[51] In *Intelligent Virtue*, Julia Annas appears to suggest that this view fits young children.[52] The problem with the actual preference view, however, is that there may be too few actual desires to capture the range of things that matter to young children's welfare. Nozick suggests that one reason we might not think that one fares well inside the pleasure machine is that it fails to fulfil the range of one's desires. He is thinking in particular of the desire to be a certain person, the desire to do certain things and the desire to have contact with reality.[53] The problem is that children may not have these wants. They may not have in particular any clear desire for contact with reality or the desire to do certain things. If they failed to have these desires, we would not think that they would be better off plugging in. The problem is not that the set of desires that a child has is in some way corrupted or inauthentic. The problem is that the set of desires is not robust enough to capture all of what matters to a

---

[51] For a defense of this view, see Heathwood (2005).
[52] Annas (2011: 134).
[53] Nozick (1974: 43 & 45).

young child's welfare. This might be due to the fact that the set of desires is not mature or developed enough. That we think this is presumably why we encourage children to develop desires for certain things.

Some of the worries about the actual desire satisfaction view might be deflected by adopting the view that welfare for children consists in the satisfaction of the desires one would have were one fully rational, i.e., informed and free of logical errors. R. B. Brandt's version of the view is that a desire is rational when it survives cognitive psychotherapy; otherwise, it is irrational. A desire survives cognitive psychotherapy when one possesses it after one has at the right time repeatedly and vividly exposed one's desire to all of the available empirical facts that are relevant to its formation.[54]

The purpose of relying on cognitive psychotherapy is to discover what one truly wants or what is truly good for one. It has its greatest attraction in cases where one is making a decision about what to do with one's life.[55] The idea seems to be that one has an evaluative profile, and that all one needs to do to find out what it truly dictates is to undergo cognitive psychotherapy. The problem is that in the case of a child we have no reason to think that the outcome of this process – in the event that it is (a) possible and (b) consistent with treating a child properly – is one we have reason to think will reveal a robust evaluative profile. The problem with this position is that it assumes that the individual in question has a reasonably developed value-system. The aim is to find out what of the things you value is really good for you from your perspective. The function of cognitive psychotherapy, according to Brandt, is to help the agent in question "find his [her] ideal value-system."[56] But do young children have reasonably developed or "ideal" value-systems? The answer seems to be negative. This is because a child's value system is still under development. Even were some value system to emerge it would lack the characteristic that such a system of values possesses in the case of adults, namely, a presumption of authority.[57]

Peter Railton's version of the desire theory might be more suitable. He maintains that what is good for one is what one's fully informed self would want one to want in one's actual situation. This is referred to as the ideal advisor view, for the advisor is an ideal version of you. She is more informed and therefore more authoritative. She tells you what is good for you, rather than what is good *sans phrase*. The idea is that

---

[54] Brandt (1979: 110–129).

[55] See, for example, Brandt's discussion of the professor deciding where to work. Brandt (1979: 125–126).

[56] Brandt (1979: 114).

[57] Brandt may be willing to grant that this view does not fit young children. In an article, he suggests that some individuals might not be "sufficiently mature to engage in the reflective evaluation characteristic of 'cognitive psychotherapy'." Brandt (1989: 40). In Brandt (1979), he argues that happiness consists in net or surplus enjoyment, and that "obviously in the case of children, animals, and mental defectives we want to make them happy and avoid distress." He is clear that he thinks that this is all we want for them. His position seems to be that this is a closed question in the case of children, though not in the case of adults. Brandt (1979: 146, 147, & 252). It's not clear how he squares these claims with his account of the concept of welfare.

one's good is determined not by what one's fully informed self wants for herself in her position. The satisfaction of such wants might not be good for one in one's actual situation. Instead, as Railton puts it, "an individual's good consists in what he would want himself to want, or to pursue, were he to contemplate his present situation from a standpoint fully and vividly informed about himself and his circumstances, and entirely free of cognitive error or lapses of instrumental rationality."[58]

This is not a plausible view about what is good for young children. How do we inform a child so that she is in a better to position to judge what is good for her in her actual situation? The trouble is that informing a child to the right and proper degree seems to involve turning her into an adult, for, it seems, being vividly informed in this way is inconsistent with what it is to have the perspective of a child, which is the relevant standard for determining a child's welfare. This suggests that there is something incoherent about thinking of a child's good as consisting in what a more fully informed version of a child would recommend to herself in her actual circumstances. Even if this worry were avoidable, it is still meaningful to ask whether the ideal advisor's desires would be a normatively adequate standard for a child. Why think that we should trust that this informed version of a child is the right standard for the child? After all, what the ideal advisor might want is for a child to do things that are good for the future adult the child will become rather than the child herself. Indeed, since there is no requirement that the advisor care about the individual in question there is a real possibility that the advisor may (arbitrarily) discount the child's good relative to the future adult's good.

We might add here that the worry that arises for Brandt also arises for Railton. The problem is that Railton's view seems to presuppose that there is some set of authentic desires or some set of desires that truly reflect one's autonomous self that the process of informing and freeing from error terminates in. But there is no such set of desires in the case of children and there is no presumption that this set of desires, even if it did exist, would be worthy of respect. To put the point another way, the desire view aims to preserve the individual's authority to determine what is good for her. But there is no such authority to be preserved in the case of a child, suggesting that this view is applicable only to adults, where the presumption of authority makes sense. We should therefore reject the desire theory as an adequate account of children's welfare.

6.4 Welfare as Satisfaction in What Is Worthy of Satisfaction

It was suggested above that a child's welfare consists in being happy in what is worthy of happiness. A child is better off when she is both happy and her happiness is taken in something that is worthy of it. This is a hybrid theory of welfare. Some utilitarians defend this sort of position, though none has applied it to children.[59]

---

[58] Railton (1986a: 16); see also Railton (1986b).
[59] See, for example, Parfit (1984: 500–501) and Kagan (2009). For a similar view that is explicitly applied to children, see Kraut (2007: 131–204). Kraut is not a utilitarian. For a critical evaluation of Kraut's view, see Skelton (2014).

Something has already been said about the nature of the happiness that is integral to this position. It is plausible to follow Sumner in holding that happiness consists in something like satisfaction.[60] But what things are worthy of a child's happiness? It was suggested in the previous section that it is possible to draw up a list of activities worthy of happiness for children. A promising list includes intellectual activity, loving and valuable relationships, and play. It is important to say more about these activities.

One can do so by dwelling on Thomas Scanlon's view of welfare. He argues that welfare consists in success in one's worthwhile projects, valuable personal relationships, and desirable consciousness.[61]

The last of these fits the case of children. It is captured in the claim that happiness is a necessary condition of welfare.

The second of Scanlon's goods also fits children. However, the relationships or friendships that matter to how well a child's life is going are different from the ones on which Scanlon focuses. The sorts of friendships and relationships that are worthy of satisfaction for children are not the same as those that Scanlon thinks are good for adults, because the latter seem to presuppose attitudes (reciprocity) and abilities (mutual and shared cooperation over time) that are beyond young children.[62] Scanlon also claims that the prudential value of valuable relationships *depends* in part on the fact that they constitute the achievement of a worthwhile goal. A happy and loving monogamous marriage is prudentially valuable both because it is a valuable relationship and because it is the concrete realization of the goal that two people share of living together happily. In the case of children, it is not possible to make this kind of dependency claim. This is due to the fact that success in one's worthwhile goals has to do with the desirability of one's "choices and reactions" and with "how well…[one's] ends are selected and how successfully they are pursued."[63] There are no such standards that govern young children for they cannot make the sort of sober choices and take the actions that seem to matter to the pursuit of worthwhile goals. They cannot be held responsible as adults can for making certain choices or for pursuing certain ends.

The relationships that are worthy of satisfaction for children are, first, loving, engaging relationships with adults with whom the child is closely bonded, socially speaking (e.g., a parent or grandparent). These should take on a particular shape. They need not be based on reciprocity or on robust attitudes of equal concern and respect. They should involve the child being loved by a caregiver or parent where this involves a life-shaping desire on the part of the caregiver to nurture and guide the child by means of reasonable moral and other principles. It should involve a deep desire to engage and support and love the child for her own sake and to provide the child with the environment in which to express him or herself honestly

---

[60] For a different view of happiness, see Haybron (2008: 105–151).
[61] Scanlon (1998:120–123); see also Scanlon (2011).
[62] For what appears to be Scanlon's view of friendship, see Scanlon (1998: 88–90).
[63] Scanlon (1998: 125).

and in which the child can develop the skills for success in adulthood. It should, however, not necessarily include complete candidness on the part of the adult. Finally, the child should recognize the adult as someone to whom she or he should defer and as someone who he or she can trust and from whom he or she can seek assistance or care.

Another, second set of relationships is worthy of satisfaction for children, namely, valuable friendships with other children, including siblings (if any). It is hard to characterize these in any detail. They can take on myriad forms. Generally, they are worthy of happiness when they involve at least some form of cooperation, effective communication and the use of skills to create situations that are to the mutual benefit of the children in question. These seem to be worthy of satisfaction even if they last only for a short period and even if they are pursued largely at the discretion of a child's parent(s).

In addition to desirable consciousness and valuable relationships, Scanlon argues that success in one's worthwhile aims or goals makes one better off. As suggested above, this seems not to fit young children. However, it is possible to argue that there is something in the vicinity of this item that does fit children, namely, the development of the sorts of capacities and the activities that are integral to and that enhance success in one's rational aims in the future. One such good is that of intellectual activity, the use and development of one's intellect or intellectual powers. This should not simply be equated with the acquisition of knowledge, which may be entirely passive, or simply with what is required for success in one's goals in adulthood. What matters is something like intellectual striving and growth. This encompasses a broad range of things, including curiosity, learning, artistic activity and creation, understanding, appreciation, reasoning, and so on. It is important that we do not think that intellectual activity is worthy of satisfaction only because it is relevant to/connected with success in one's rational aims in the future. It can be good for a child to happily develop his aesthetic appreciation and abilities even when this has little or no impact on his abilities in later life.

A final item is that of play. This is missing from Scanlon's list. It seems integral to faring well as a child. What is of particular importance is the sort of play that is unstructured and spontaneous, and which might involve playing with friends, animals, or one's parents, or playing a game. The basic idea is that what is worthy of satisfaction for a child is to be free from what Moritz Schlick describes as purposes. This is, in his view, the essence of play: "free, purposeless action, that is, action which in fact carries its purpose within in itself."[64] This is a pursuit that is distinct from that which connects with success in one's future goals or aims. There is also another form of play that is worthy of happiness. This is the sort of thing that John Stuart Mill says he lacked in his childhood: "the accomplishments which schoolboys in all countries chiefly cultivate." Mill is referring primarily to physical activities involving "feats of skill or physical strength" and "ordinary bodily exercises."[65] The free use of one's physical abilities for no purpose or goal by, for example, playing

---

[64] Schlick (1979: 114).

[65] Mill (1981: 39).

in a park, swimming on one's back, swinging on a swing, or riding a bike, is an activity that is worthy of satisfaction for a child.

My view, then, is that when these activities are objects of satisfaction or when a child finds herself happily engaged in one of these activities, this is prudentially good for her. When a child has a surplus of satisfaction or happiness in an activity that is worthy of happiness her life is going well for her.

This account has virtues that are worth highlighting briefly. First, it is attractive on its face and avoids some of the errors of the views discussed above. Second, it seems to possess the kind of weight or importance that a normatively adequate view of welfare should possess. The account makes it clear why children's welfare is worth promoting. Third, it is a view of welfare that involves the engagement of the full range of a child's capacities, active and passive, intellectual and physical. Fourth, it is not obviously in tension with views of welfare that seem to be plausible in the case of adults.

This view does, however, face some objections, three of which will be addressed here. The first is that it fails to capture the fact that sometimes happiness appears by itself to enhance a young child's welfare. Surely, when a child enjoys a sweet drink or laughs at a mindless joke, the happiness she receives from this makes her to some extent better off. It is certainly better for a child to plug into an experience machine in cases where all other options lack happiness or produce only suffering. It is hard to deny that there are cases in which happiness in the absence of things worthy of happiness is sufficient for welfare. But the sort of welfare that this happiness forms is going to be of a low form, compared to the welfare represented by the hybrid view defended above. It is low welfare or low fare. Thinking of it this way explains the intuition that being in a machine and eating sweets are not as good for a child as are situations in which the same quantity of happiness gained from these is taken in things worthy of happiness. The view of welfare defended here is full welfare or full fare.

The second objection targets the account of full welfare. Roger Crisp argues that it is mysterious that the activities worthy of happiness do not count towards welfare in the absence of happiness but that they do count when they are found with happiness.[66] This does not, however, strike me as especially mysterious. Some of the mystery is dispelled by noting that the hybrid view captures many of our intuitions about what it means to fare well (fully) as a young child, and by noting that it involves the unity of things that we think are in some way independently desirable.

The third objection claims that the view defended here cannot capture important intuitions about the following kinds of situations. Suppose a child believes that her classmates love her when in fact they do not. They routinely mock her when she is not present. She derives a lot of (surplus) happiness from her mistaken belief. One might think that since the account of welfare defended here denies that the possession of things worthy of happiness in the absence of happiness make one better off, the account cannot accommodate the judgement that this child's life is going less well than it would be were she not being mocked.

---

[66] Crisp (2006a: 123) and Crisp (2006b: 640).

The account given here does capture this judgement. It claims that while the happiness makes a positive contribution to welfare, the fact that it is not taken in something that is worthy of happiness means that it counts for much less welfare value than it would were it to be taken in something that is worthy of happiness (e.g., loving friends).

It is important to end by emphasizing that the view developed here is an account of welfare for young children who are not properly autonomous. It may not, then, be suitable for older children who have developed at least some capacity for agency and autonomy. A theory of welfare for older children who possess more robust forms of agency should include some space for that in the core elements of the position. This is not to suggest that the view defended here leaves no room for choice and for exercises of proto-agency. Because a child fares well when she takes happiness in intellectual activity, which involves choice and the articulation of some limited aims, and in play, which often involves at least primitive thoughts about the desirability of various pursuits and the need to make choices, faring well as a young child seems to involve the acquisition of just those skills that are necessary for the execution of agency and autonomous decision making in the future.

6.5 Conclusion

This paper discussed a number of theories of welfare to which utilitarians have been attracted. Some imply a view about what it is to fare well as a child, including hedonism, Sumner's happiness view, and the actual desire satisfaction view. I have argued that these views are not descriptively adequate. Some views fail to imply anything about children's welfare, including fully informed desire views. Some views fit children but only with modification. This is true of objective-list views. But, it was argued, even with modification these views are not acceptable. A hybrid view of welfare for young children according to which welfare consists in happiness in activities worthy of happiness appears most defensible. In some cases, however, happiness is sufficient for welfare, though this welfare is inferior to the welfare that results when a young child takes happiness in activities worthy of happiness.[67]

References

Annas, J. (2011). *Intelligent virtue*. Oxford: Oxford University Press.
Arneson, R. (1999). Human flourishing and desire satisfaction. *Social Philosophy and Policy, 16*(1), 113–143.

---

[67] Thanks to Anne Skelton, Roger Crisp, Wayne Sumner, Ariella Binik, Anca Gheaus, Lori Kantymir, the editors of this volume, audiences at the Ethox Centre, Oxford University and at the Centre of Medical Law and Ethics, King's College London, and (especially) Carolyn McLeod for helpful comments on previous drafts of this chapter.

Bentham, J. (1996[1789]). In J. H. Burns & H. L. A. Hart (Eds.), *Introduction to the principles of morals and legislation*. Oxford: Oxford University Press.
Brandt, R. B. (1979). *A theory of the good and the right*. Oxford: Oxford University Press.
Brandt, R. B. (1989). Fairness to happiness. *Social Theory and Practice, 15*(1), 33–58.
Brink, D. (1989). *Moral realism and the foundations of ethics*. Cambridge: Cambridge University Press.
Brink, D. (2001). Impartiality and associative duties. *Utilitas, 13*(2), 152–172.
Broad, C. D. (1971). Self and others. In D. Cheney (Ed.), *Broad's critical essays in moral philosophy* (pp. 262–282). New York: Humanities Press.
Clarke, G. (2002). *Max and the rainbow rain hat*. London: Andersen Press.
Crisp, R. (2006a). *Reasons and the good*. Oxford: Oxford University Press.
Crisp, R. (2006b). Hedonism reconsidered. *Philosophy and Phenomenological Research, 73*(3), 619–645.
Griffin, J. (1986). *Well-being: Its meaning, measurement, and moral importance*. Oxford: Oxford University Press.
Haybron, D. (2008). *The pursuit of unhappiness: The elusive psychology of well-being*. Oxford: Oxford University Press.
Heathwood, C. (2005). The problem of defective desires. *Australasian Journal of Philosophy, 83*(4), 487–504.
Hewitt, S. (2010). What do our intuitions about the experience machine really tell us about hedonism? *Philosophical Studies, 151*(3), 331–349.
Hooker, B. (2000). *Ideal code, real world*. Oxford: Oxford University Press.
Jeram, A. (1999). *Bunny my honey*. London: Walker Books.
Kagan, S. (2009). Well-being as enjoying the good. *Philosophical Perspectives, 23*(1), 253–272.
Kraut, R. (2007). *What is good and why: The ethics of well-being*. Cambridge, MA: Harvard University Press.
Mill, J. S. (1998[1863]). In R. Crisp (Ed.), *Utilitarianism*. Oxford: Oxford University Press.
Mill, J. S. (1981[1873]). Autobiography. In J. Robson (Ed.), *Collected works of John Stuart Mill* (Vol. I, pp. 1–290). Toronto: University of Toronto Press.
Nozick, R. (1974). *Anarchy, state, and utopia*. New York: Basic Books.
Nozick, R. (1989). *The examined life*. New York: Touchstone.
Nussbaum, M. C. (2004). Mill between Aristotle and Bentham. *Daedalus, 133*(2), 60–68.
Parfit, D. (1984). *Reasons and persons*. Oxford: Oxford University Press.
Railton, P. (1986a). Facts and values. *Philosophical Topics, 14*(2), 5–31.
Railton, P. (1986b). Moral realism. *Philosophical Review, 95*(2), 163–207.
Scanlon, T. M. (1998). *What we owe to each other*. Cambridge, MA: Harvard University Press.
Scanlon, T. M. (2011). *Ideas of the good in moral and political philosophy*. Routledge lecture in philosophy, Cambridge University. http://www.dspace.cam.ac.uk/handle/1810/240489. Accessed 22 July 2014.
Schlick, M. (1979). On the meaning of life. In H. L. Mulder & B. F. B. Van De Velde-Schlick (Eds.), *Moritz Schlick: Philosophical papers volume II (1925–1936)* (pp. 112–129). Dordrecht: Reidel.
Sidgwick, H. (1907). *The methods of ethics* (7th ed.). London: Macmillan.
Silverstein, M. (2000). In defense of happiness: A response to the experience machine. *Social Theory and Practice, 26*(2), 279–300.
Singer, P. (2011). *Practical ethics* (3rd ed.). Cambridge: Cambridge University Press.
Skelton, A. (2014). Two conceptions of children's welfare. Unpublished manuscript.
Sumner, L. W. (1996). *Welfare, happiness, and ethics*. Oxford: Oxford University Press.

Part II
Children's Well-Being and Authority

Chapter 7
Paternalism in Education and the Future

Dieter Birnbacher

7.1 Introduction: Forms of Paternalism

Paternalism is a recurrent theme in applied ethics because of the enduring tensions that make themselves felt between the principles of autonomy and beneficence in areas of societal concern such as public health, consumer protection and education. In all these areas the question arises to what extent policies should be allowed to go in arrogating to themselves the right to act against the manifest will of persons in the best interest of these persons. Recently, discussions of paternalism have received new impulses especially from an influential and widely acclaimed version of paternalism called "libertarian paternalism" by its authors and claiming to further the good of persons without interfering with their liberty of choice by orienting their choices by "nudges" rather than by social pressure or force (Thaler and Sunstein 2008). At the same time, the debate on the extent to which paternalism can be ethically justified (starting in the 1970s) has produced a number of important theoretical results, among them fruitful distinctions between various forms of paternalistic interventions, each one with a different moral profile. One such distinction is that between *direct* and *indirect* paternalism (cf. Kleinig 1983: 11). *Direct* paternalism is the practice (and the doctrine justifying it) of directly making a person do what is in his or her best interest against the person's will. *Indirect* paternalism consists in the prevention of potentially harmful influences on the person by coercing others not to do something that might harm the person, without exerting pressure or coercion on the person himself. Examples are the legal ban on drug trafficking or the legal protection for children and young persons concerning films and other media. Ethically, these forms of paternalisms are not on a par. Differently from the direct form of

D. Birnbacher (✉)
Department of Philosophy, University of Düsseldorf,
Gebäude 23.31, Ebene U1, Raum 64, Universitätsstr. 1, 40225 Düsseldorf, Germany
e-mail: Dieter.Birnbacher@uni-duesseldorf.de

paternalism the indirect form can be justified not only (in Beauchamp and Childress's parlance, cf. Beauchamp and Childress 2013) by the principle of beneficence but also by the principle of non-maleficence because the provider of opportunities of self-harming is at least partly causally responsible for the harm.

Another and ethically more far-reaching distinction is that between a *broad* and a *narrow* concept of paternalism (cf. Schickhardt 2012: 191 ff.). The *broad* interpretation of paternalism corresponds to the "classical" definition of paternalism by Gerald Dworkin:

> By paternalism I shall understand roughly the interference with a person's liberty of action justified by reasons referring exclusively to the welfare, good, happiness, needs, interests or values of the person concerned. (Dworkin 1972: 65)

This definition leaves open whether the "liberty of action" restricted by a paternalistic intervention is the liberty of a person fully autonomous in its choices ("strong" or "hard" paternalism) or not ("weak" or "soft" paternalism, cf. Feinberg 1979: 450; 1986: 12). It applies to fully autonomous persons in the same way as to persons with no or diminished autonomy, including children, the mentally ill and other mentally decapacitated persons. The *narrow* interpretation of paternalism restricts the concept to interventions, for the sake of their own interests, in the liberty of fully autonomous persons. The motivation of those who thus restrict the concept (e. g. Tom Beauchamp and the present author in a former publication, cf. Beauchamp 1977; Birnbacher 2010) is clear: They wish to concentrate ethical attention on those controversial cases in which there is a particularly sharp conflict between, on the one hand, the principle of autonomy understood as a right to self-determination, and the principle of beneficence understood as acting in a person's best interest.

Though there is a good point in distinguishing the broad and the narrow concept, making the distinction does not imply that the broad concept generates genuine moral problems no less than the narrow one. It is true, there must be particularly good reasons (such as the presence of fatal ignorance, as in Mill's famous example of the man entering a bridge that is going to collapse) to exert force (or its weaker analogue, deception, by misinformation or otherwise) to prevent a person from seriously harming him- or herself. But even in such extreme cases, paternalistic interventions constitute a breach of an important right. That does not mean, however, that there are not also moral problems with cases of paternalism in the broad sense that are not, at the same time, cases of paternalism in the narrow sense, i. e. cases in which full autonomy is absent. Though there is, in these cases, not the same kind of conflict between the right to self-determination and the principle of beneficence as in cases of paternalism in the narrow sense, there is still a conflict. Even if the preferences and choices of a person are not fully voluntary or not fully autonomous, paternalistic interventions involve a conflict of values, viz. between the undisputed value of acting in a person's best interest, and the value of the person's negative freedom, the freedom to act on his or her own preferences. Thwarting the will of a person by acting against his or her preferences is always axiologically worse than acting in conformity with his or her preferences. Freedom to act according to one's will is a value even in the absence (situational or enduring) of the capacity to act freely. Autonomy as a *right* is not the exclusive privilege of whosoever possesses autonomy as a *capacity*. Therefore, paternalistic interventions in not fully autonomous persons stand in need of justification no less than paternalistic interventions in fully autonomous persons. Even in the absence of autonomy, paternalistic interventions are normally felt as frustrating, or worse, as an exercise of control and coercion. E. g. fixating demented patients in their beds overnight in order to prevent them from harming themselves by uncontrolled strolling in the ward is clearly morally problematic as a form of evident compulsion quite independently of the degree of autonomy that can be attributed to the respective patients. The same holds for fixating the hands of small children to prevent thumb-sucking and consequent dislocation of teeth. Interestingly, even courts now increasingly recognize the right to negative freedom on the part of non-autonomous patients, e. g. by denying liability of hospitals and nursery homes for the costs of treatment in case of accidents due to non-fixating (cf. Damm 2010: 459).

It should be noticed that the particular disvalue of frustrating whatever one wants is *additional* to the other disvalues the respective act or state may imply. It is one thing to voluntarily suffer some deeply unpleasant state or to engage in a deeply unpleasant activity. It is quite another thing to suffer the state or to engage in the activity involuntarily. After all, one of the most fundamental and far-reaching findings in the psychology of risk acceptance is that voluntary risks are tolerated to a far higher degree than involuntary risks, irrespective of what the risks consist in in terms of potential harm and probability. Even if one must assume that voluntary risks are judged to be less of a threat than involuntary risks (otherwise they would not have been taken), the facts suggest that the quality of being involuntary is an independent factor making involuntary risks appear much less acceptable than their voluntary counterparts.

Of course, to exhibit this special kind of disvalue, a paternalistic intervention must in some way, directly or indirectly, enter the consciousness of the person frustrated by the intervention, and it must be experienced as frustrating. Though it does not need to be recognized specifically as a *paternalistic* intervention it must be seen as some form of restriction of freedom. It does not suffice for a paternalistic intervention merely to limit the options open to a person to count as a disvalue in this sense. A limiting of options for paternalistic reasons is not necessarily experienced as frustrating. On the contrary, it may go completely unnoticed. The same holds for acting for a young child's best interest without the child's explicit consent. So far as the will of the child is not yet fully autonomous, this can be an act of paternalism only if it contradicts the child's explicit or implicit will or wishes. It cannot count as an act of paternalism if the parents or others can reasonably assume that the child would not object to the action if asked. It would clearly be an inflation of the concept of paternalism to apply it to the plethora of decisions made and actions done in the life of a family involving a child without the child's explicit approval (cf. Giesinger 2007: 138).

7.2 What Is Problematic About Paternalism in Education?

There is a wide consensus in liberal circles that paternalism is primarily a problem with adults and not with children. Paternalism with adults, if at all legitimate, always stands in need of justification, whereas paternalism with children does not, or at least to a much lesser extent. With adults there is only a very limited number of conditions and situations in which acting against a person's explicit or implicit will seems to be justified, e. g. in cases of mental illness, in cases of mental crisis with a high risk of short-sighted acting-out (like attempts at suicide or self-mutilation), in cases of extreme affect like love-pain and existential loss, and in situations of fatal ignorance or misinformation. In contrast, the very idea of upbringing and education seems to bound up with paternalism. Since the inherent purpose of both is, among others, to form a character that is not yet fully formed, the child's will, expressing this not yet fully formed character, cannot claim the authority and sovereignty of the will of the adult. Forming a character will in general not be possible without some degree of resistance on the part of the child's "immature" character. The chisel of the sculptor can be expected to meet with resistance from the unformed stone out of which a statue is going to be formed, and it is only natural that this resistance has to be overcome to successfully achieve the sculptor's task.

On the other hand, it follows from our introductory considerations that paternalism constitutes a moral problem with children no less than with adults. Children are subjects of wants and wishes in the same way as adults, and among these are many wants and wishes that are liable to be frustrated by educative action. That is not to say that education is inherently paternalistic or that educational aims can be attained only by paternalistic means. A child may love to go to school so that pressure or coercion to attend lessons are completely uncalled for. But though not strictly necessary, paternalism is a *typical* phenomenon of education, and especially in the education of young children. On the other hand, education is more than paternalism. The values it pursues are not exclusively prudential. Education also deploys the values of the community to which the child belongs. To some extent at least, education forces a certain community's values on the child irrespective of whether this conformity is in the child's own best interest. But it seems that at least a great part of education can be explained (and justified) by best interest considerations. To the extent that a child resists what others conceive to be in its best interest, conflicts between self-determination and paternalism seem unavoidable.

There is a wide consensus that paternalistic interventions in education are legitimate if not morally required. There are a great number of national and international documents in which the right of parents and the state (in so far it acts *in loco parentis*) to paternalistic interventions in children is affirmed. Even the UN Convention on the Rights of the Child of 1989 is quite generous in legitimizing paternalistic interventions. In article 12, it says:

> States Parties shall assure to the child who is capable of forming his or her own views the right to express those views freely in all matters affecting the child, the views of the child being given due weight in accordance with the age and maturity of the child.

This is far from giving children a right to actively participate in decisions concerning them. The only right it grants to children is to freely express their opinions about what they think is good for them. It leaves it to the discretion of parents and administrations to define the "due weight" of these opinions in relevant decisions and procedures. As the case may be, this weight may be naught so that children have to content themselves with protesting against what they are made to do or to suffer. The same conclusion follows from article 5 of the Convention where the accent lies again not on the rights of children but on the rights of parents to "direct and guide" the child, and not only of parents but even of the "extended family or community":

> States Parties shall respect the responsibilities, rights and duties of parents or, where applicable, the members of the extended family or community as provided for by local custom, legal guardians or other persons legally responsible for the child, to provide, in a manner consistent with the evolving capacities of the child, appropriate direction and guidance in the exercise by the child of the rights recognized in the present Convention.

That means that even the right to express opinions about what is in his or her interest is not absolute. Even this right is restricted by what others think is in conformity with established social standards. By leaving the interpretation of the rights accorded to children to "local custom", the Convention does not only give plenty of leeway to the *exercise* of paternalism in education but also to the determination of the *content* and *purpose* of paternalistic intervention, i. e. to what is held to be in the child's best interest. One wonders what remains of the children's rights granted by the Convention if adults and their cultures are given the right to interpret these rights as freely as this article allows. In this respect, I am unable to agree with the opinion expressed by Brighouse (shared by the majority of commentators) that the Convention "is an almost entirely positive document" (Brighouse 2003: 694).

It may seem that the legitimacy of paternalism in education is so universally recognized that the question arises whether there is a moral problem at all. Unless "paternalism" is taken as an inherently depreciatory expression (which seems inappropriate given the close connection between education and paternalism) there seems to be no point in questioning paternalism in education. This impression, however, cannot stand up to closer scrutiny. Even in education, paternalism necessarily involves a conflict of interests and values that has to solved in one way or other.

My purpose in the following is to explore how far paternalism should be allowed in the context of education and by what other considerations it is limited. My further purpose is to formulate a number of rules ("tendency rules") that may be of help in deciding this question.

7.3 Best Interest: The Time Dimension

An ethical assessment of how far educative paternalism is legitimate depends on many factors. One, and a crucial one, is the time-frame of the benefits paternalistic interventions are expected to realize for the child. In fact, temporal scope is the most important dimension by which paternalism in the upbringing and education of children differs from other varieties of paternalism, and especially from paternalistic interventions in the elderly. The main aims of paternalistic interventions in children – protection from harmful external influences and development of autonomous self-control – are expected to have an impact on a person throughout his or her lifetime. This consideration stands, however, in a certain contrast to what is commonly thought about justified paternalism. In general, short-term benefits carry much more weight as justifiers of paternalistic interventions than long-term ones. Think of everyday examples like holding back a child from eating attractive kinds of food expected to have detrimental health effects. It seems much more obvious that parents are justified in preventing their child to eat poisoned or rotten foodstuff with a high risk of producing immediate stomach pain or vomiting. It is much less clear that parents are justified to prevent their child to eat sweets known to produce obesity, bad teeth and, in the long run, diabetes. In both cases a balance is struck between the frustration of the child's present wishes and the benefits expected from this frustration. These benefits, however, are situated at different points of the time-axis. In the first case, the benefits are expected to come about in the near or immediate further, in the last case, in a farther away and, in consequence, more uncertain future.

It is mainly this balancing of present bads with long-term goods, of "immediate" with "future interests" (Brighouse 2003: 699) that makes paternalism a problem. Mill's example of the man entering a bridge that is about to collapse is highly tendentious and, ultimately, misleading. It appeals to the common intuition that paternalistic coercion for the sake of the prevention of an immediate bad is fully legitimate. The controversial question, however, concerns paternalistic interventions for some temporally more remote (and purely probabilistic) good, such as the prevention of harms caused by car collisions in the case of compulsory seat-belts.

The ethical problem about paternalism in the long-term case is, therefore, threefold: (1) Is a balancing of the costs of present frustration with the benefits expected to accrue from it later in principle legitimate? (2) If yes, what are the stakes that have to be taken into account in balancing? (3) Is the asymmetry customarily assumed to exist between immediate and temporally distant benefits legitimate? These are controversial and, indeed, wide-ranging issues transcending the narrow sphere of upbringing and education. But they have to be answered if we want to have not only a common sense practice of educational paternalism but also a more or less well-founded theory of it.

There is a strong presumption that the first question has to be answered in the positive. So much, at least, follows from the consideration that the extremes on both sides are inacceptable: that only the future or only the present counts morally. The view that only the future counts morally and that there is no limit to which present interests of the child can be sacrificed for the sake of future benefits was common in German petty bourgeois circles after the Second World War. It left deep traces in the generation (my own generation) that was subject to it and no doubt was one of the factors in the unexpected rise of Germany's economy after the breakdown of 1945. Upbringing and education were conceived as essentially future-oriented. Everything was done to secure a better future for the children born after an era of moral and non-moral disaster. The period of childhood was only rarely seen in the Rousseau-like perspective, as a period of life having a value in its own right. It was rather seen as a purely preparatory stage in which the competences were to be developed that were expected to flourish and come to fruition later in life. Enjoyment and spontaneity were generously sacrificed to prudential considerations. The only or at least primary moral consideration guiding upbringing and education was care for the well-being of the future person. Moral or other transpersonal values played practically no role, except to the extent that their observance was expected to further the child's future prospects. For example, church going was held to be important, but neither for the sake of the formation of the child's character nor for reasons of religious observance but for the sake of securing a higher degree of acceptance of the future adult in society at large. As might have been expected, many of these well-intentioned educational "investments" proved, from the future person's perspective, a waste of effort. But this is not true of all of them. Some of them proved to be highly welcome in later years. What was remarkable, however, was how little attention was given to the moral costs of paternalism that were taken into account. These costs were considerable even in the early period of childhood in which there cannot yet be question of autonomy. After all, each single paternalistic act constitutes a violation of the child's interests, and if protracted and intransparent, a violation of the child's self-respect. On the assumption that a child can be attributed four distinct kinds of vulnerability: interest vulnerability, moral vulnerability, autonomy vulnerability, and education vulnerability (Giesinger 2007: 23 ff.), continued frustration of the child's interests for paternalistic reasons is problematic not only in the dimension of interest vulnerability but also in the dimension of moral vulnerability. By being frustrated the child gets used to the thought that its interests count for nothing. It not only feels devalued but will easily take over this devaluation from parents and care-givers in the form of self-devaluation and feelings of shame. The message conveyed by paternalistic coercion is consciously or unconsciously taken over by the child and made one of the building-blocks of its self-image. Moreover, continued paternalism can be a massive obstacle to the development of autonomy and self-determination including the freedom to learn form one's own mistakes (cf. Buchanan and Brock 1989: 231). Self-determination does not fall from heaven, but must be practiced in the same way as other capacities, and practicing self-determination in early years is hardly thinkable without risks. Exaggerated and one-sided efforts to further the long-term well-being of the child at the cost of short-term satisfactions can thus have the paradox effect of generating heavy burdens for the child's future self.

In contrast, the view on the other side of the spectrum, the view that only the present (or more adequately: the present and the immediate future) counts and that paternalistic interventions are never morally justified, seems likewise inacceptable. Among the philosophers of education, it was Schleiermacher who gave the first elaborate defense of this extremist position (cf. Giesinger 2007: 130 ff.). In his lectures on pedagogics of 1826 he explicitly raises the question how far we are morally allowed to sacrifice the bad of one life-moment to the good of another, and especially how far we are morally permitted to make a child do what it does not want to do (or suffer what it does not want to suffer) in order to secure some later good for the child. This good, Schleiermacher assumes, can consist either in one of the general aims of education, e. g. the development of basic cognitive, social and emotional competences, or in the development of the child's specific talents. He further assumes that the paternalistic intervention in the child is a purely negative magnitude for the child, i. e. that its value consists only in its expected consequences (Schleiermacher 2000: 51). Interestingly, of the four arguments Schleiermacher offers against the legitimacy of sacrificing "one moment" for later moments, only one is definitely outdated. The others have been taken up and elaborated, in one way or other, by later authors.

Schleiermacher's outdated argument is that the purpose of paternalistic interventions in education will often be missed due to the high risk that the child dies at an early age. Apart from being, fortunately, outdated, this is a curious and highly tendentious argument. Though, in Schleiermacher's time, children died more frequently than today, they often died at an age at which the kind of paternalistic measures in question played only a minor role in bringing them up. The life expectation of a 4- or 5-year old child was much higher than that of a newborn, so that is was far from evident, even in those times, that paternalistic measures were not worth the while. No doubt, Schleiermacher would have had a better argument if he had referred to another factor involved in any sacrifice of the present for the future, the uncertainty whether these sacrifices will have any effect on the future well-being of the child. What is uncertain, is first, whether the paternalistic measure will have any significant effect on the later life of the child, and, second, that the harms they are designed to prevent do not occur or the goods they are designed to produce will not be needed. The only exception are all-purpose goods like good health, physical fitness, and basic cognitive and social competences.

Schleiermacher's second argument is of limited plausibility because of its question-begging dogmatism. Schleiermacher simply asserts that "the ethical task consists in supporting each singe life-moment as such", which is taken to imply that any sacrifice of one life-moment for a later one is morally ruled out (Schleiermacher 2000: 52). By insisting on this axiom, Schleiermacher, again, polarizes and unnecessarily closes the door to mediating positions. One such position would be one that allows for paternalistic interventions that sacrifice not the "life-moment" as a whole but only part of it, or, in other words, that do not frustrate the child's will drastically but moderately, in a way that balances the frustration of the child's present wishes with the probable contribution of the paternalistic act to the child's later well-being. In contrast to Schleiermacher's assumption that paternalistic measures leave no room for positive side-effects and are experienced by the child as purely negative, frustration of present wishes is no yes-or-no affair but admits of grades. Everyday educational practices are full of such gradations and compromises, and their rationale is no other than an implicit intertemporal balancing. Such practices must have been well known to Schleiermacher, a father of four children, himself.

The third argument has the same ring of dogmatism, or even sophistry, and is of interest mainly as an anticipation of similar arguments that have been propounded by philosophers of education in the wake of Derek Parfit's "deconstruction" of personal identity (cf. Parfit 1971, 1984: ch. 15, Hügli 1983). Schleiermacher argues that the individual who is harmed by paternalistic interventions is "not identical in the strict sense" with the individual benefited by it. Because of the ultimate non-identity of the earlier and the later person paternalism is at bottom heteronomy, the subjection of one person to the purposes of another. Correspondingly, the more rigorous rules for *inter*personal balancing of harms and benefits apply instead of the more generous ones for *intra*personal balancing. Given that paternalistic measures have a purely negative value as far as the present moment is concerned, imposing such measures on a child implies something analogous to an act of instrumentalizing the present person to the future person, which, according to Kantian ethics, is unethical. Indeed, Schleiermacher suggests that paternalistic measures are not only morally wrong but absolutely and irretrievably wrong in treating the present life-moment of the child "only as a means" to its future well-being, thus violating its dignity or, as Schleiermacher implies, not treating it "as a human being" at all (Schleiermacher 2000: 56). Paternalism, it is implied, comes to no less than the negation of the human quality of the child.

These are strong words, but we should not be overly impressed by them. Their conceptual basis is too weak to carry Schleiermacher's emphasis.

First, even if we accept the view that the person of the child subjected to paternalistic measures is not "strictly" identical with the later person expected to benefit from it, and that imposing the bad of paternalism would constitute a case of using the child-at-present "only as a means" for the child-later, this would constitute a violation of human dignity only in drastic cases, such as the infringement of basic rights to bodily integrity, freedom and psychic integrity. Not every case of "instrumentalizing" a person for the sake of another person's well-being constitutes a violation of human dignity or excludes negotiation with the good of others, especially not in persons with severely reduced autonomy. Think, again, of the widespread practice of fixating demented patients in nursery-homes. This is done, in part, not for paternalistic reasons but for the reason of preventing hurtful attacks on other patients. Though this act makes the respective patient a "mere means" and is surely morally problematic, it seem far from constituting a violation of human dignity, at least in a sense that makes such violations non-negotiable with any other good or value.

Second, nothing in Schleiermacher's argument suggests that it applies only to paternalistic interventions aiming at the more distant future (as Parfit's analogous objections suggest, cf. Parfit 1984: 347). Instead, it seems to apply even to the near and immediate future. If we follow him, the objection of treating someone as a "mere means" would even apply to the act of holding back a person from an imminently dangerous irrationality (like a panic suicide), which seems absurd.

Third, and most importantly, the premise of non-identity on which Schleiermacher's argument rests seems to be confused. Identity of persons is perfectly compatible with a change, even a thoroughgoing change in mental properties or selves. Even the "perfect identity" that Thomas Reid in the 18th century opposed to Hume's reductionist view of personal identity (cf. Reid 1975: 111) is compatible with a change of character traits and preferences and even with what in dramatic cases may be called a change of "selves". Paternalism is defined in terms of persons, not of character stages or selves. It presupposes identity of persons, not identity of selves. Its very point is that a person as a unit persisting through time (however analyzed) might profit from a paternalistic act that involves the exercise of coercion on a former self for the sake of the well-being of later selves. A view that confuses persons and selves clouds the issue by substantializing selves. Moreover, by assuming that later selves differ qualitatively from former selves (or, in Parfit's terms, that later selves lack psychological continuity with former selves) it generates additional confusion. The moral problem of paternalism is not that paternalistic interventions put the burden of coercion on self A for the sake of a qualitatively different self B but that they put the burden of coercion on a person for the sake of later temporal stages of the same person. Paternalism is a problem even if self A does not change but remains identical through time not only numerically but also qualitatively.

7.4 Legitimate Paternalism

Schleiermacher's criticism of paternalism in education leaves only one way open to a future orientation in education, namely making what is, in the view of others, in the child's best interest (over the whole of its future life) coincide with its own present will, so that the satisfaction of the expected future interest is at the same time a "satisfaction of the present" (Schleiermacher 2000: 55). The wording here is, I think, significant, since it makes clear that nothing much depends on whether what is done or not done to the child has the child's explicit consent. This is relevant to the recent debate on paternalism in so far as it is sometimes postulated or implied – possibly under the inspiration of the concept "informed consent" in medical ethics – that any act that is burdensome to a person but in its long-term best interest should be classified as paternalistic if it is not explicitly consented to. The consequence is an undesirable inflation of the concept of paternalism. It is definitely not sufficient for an act to be classified as paternalistic that the act is done to a person without his or her explicit consent. In the majority of cases in which someone is burdened without explicit consent paternalism is absent since it is clear from the situation that the act corresponds to the will of the person. For example, most medical acts (except those carried out for research purposes) are carried out without the patient's explicit consent. This does not make them paternalistic as far as they are in conformity with the patient's wishes. They would be paternalistic only if the patient is coercively made to suffer them (as, e. g. psychiatric patients by being fixated or drugged against their will) or is denied something he wants by someone who is in principle able to provide it to him (as, e. g. a drug addict during withdrawal treatment).

In other words, *presumed* consent is a sufficient condition for the absence of paternalism in the same way as is *prior* consent, as, e. g., in Ulysses contracts (Elster 1979) or advance directives. In consequence, both conditions are without the problems of moral justification specific to paternalism. Much more problematic are the two principles by which paternalistic acts are standardly justified in practice: the *Principle of Hypothetical Rational Consent* and the *Principle of Subsequent Consent*

(VanDeVeer 1986: 70 ff.). Both principles are a rather unreliable basis for paternalistic interventions, especially in the sphere of education.

The *Principle of Hypothetical Rational Consent* legitimizes paternalistic acts to the extent that they would be consented to by the person under the hypothesis that he or she judges with full rationality. What is problematic about this principle is that it is highly normative and presupposes a standard of rationality of which it is doubtful whether it is shared by the future adult. Moreover, it is unclear whether a standard of rationality is able to adjudicate between different educational strategies as far as it is an open question what rationality amounts to in this context. Given that religion is irreducibly "irrational", is religious education per se illegitimate by this criterion? Atheists might want to follow Rousseau in arguing that choice of a religious creed should be left to the adolescent and not be prejudged at a stage of immaturity. On the other side, religionists might argue that religious forms of education are not only legitimate on this criterion but even to be recommended, given the anthropological facts about the chances of firmly established religiosity to provide basic feelings of security and belongingness for a lifetime. According to many philosophers, including Schopenhauer, the one cannot be had without the other. To a certain extent, religion must be "irrational" if it is to have these desirable effects, at least for the common run of people.

While the *Principle of Hypothetical Rational Consent* suffers from semantic underdetermination, the other popular justifying principle, the *Principle of Subsequent Consent* suffers from the risk of circularity. What paternalistic interventions a child can be expected to retrospectively consent to depends at least partly on what kind of education is has been subjected to. Consider, again, the example of religious education. Given a sustained religious education, there is a good chance that the child will be religious enough as an adult to approve having been subjected to religious education against its will. Analogously, a person for whom a certain mastery of a musical instrument is a central component of his or her satisfaction with life my well approve of having been driven to lessons at an age at which alternative pastimes were more attractive, but would not otherwise do so. There is thus a high chance that the criterion of subsequent consent is self-fulfilling. Even more important, however, is the uncertainty about whether the child will later approve of what was forced upon it. Parents may be partial in projecting their own values, convictions and ideals onto the child who later on feels resentment against parents or caregivers for having been pressured on a route that he or she would not think of taking as an adult.

How might a more appropriate criterion for paternalist intervention look like?

I propose to answer this question on two different levels: on a theoretical or *ideal* level on which we take the liberty to abstract from a number of factors we have to confront under real-life conditions; and on a *practical* level at which we have to content ourselves with rules of thumb that provide an approximation to what is morally required and which do not in every case amount to clear and unambiguous recipes. I do not believe that rules can be formulated that, as, e. g. Buchanan and Brock expect their "guiding principles" to do, give "substantive direction" how decisions should be made (Buchanan and Brock 1989: 88). The rules that can be formulated are not suited to give definite answers in individual cases. They rather have the form of *tendency rules* (Birnbacher 2010: 19; Schickhardt 2012: 204) designed to serve as an inspiration and orientation for decision-making, leaving room, on a case-for-case basis, for good judgment.

The ideal principles of legitimate paternalism are, I think, two and straightforward:

1. Paternalistic interventions are justified if and only if the infliction of harm by frustrating the will of a child combined with the possible harm of the act independently of its involuntariness as well as their present and future consequences for the child are evidently less grave than the harm done by not preventing the later evil the paternalistic intervention is meant to prevent or by depriving it of the later good to which the intervention is meant to contribute. "Evil" and "good" are here understood to be defined in terms of the person's subjective interests. What has to balanced, on the ideal level, is, on the one hand, the gravity of the frustration and violation of the child's present interests, and the value of the opportunities thereby created for the interest satisfaction of the later person. Paternalistic intervention is justified whenever there is a clear disproportion between the extent to which the interests of the child are frustrated and the extent to which this frustrating is necessary to prevent harm or to create positive opportunities.
2. Future goods and bads should not be discounted for reasons of time preference. In contrast to a widespread tendency to hypothetical discounting in longitudinal comparisons (Ainslie 1975), future goods and bads should be treated in exactly the same way as present ones.

The trouble with this theoretical answer is that it offers concrete and practically useful advice only in extreme cases: first, if the later harm to be prevented by paternalistic intervention is beyond a certain threshold of gravity, or if the later good that is made possible by the intervention is of the kind of an all-purpose means like health, physical fitness, and basic intellectual and social competences, i. e. capacities from which the child is certain to profit later in life irrespective of the turn its personal preferences take; second, if the intervention is of negligible gravity, short of coercive measures like the use of force or deception, e. g. warning, admonishing, or confronting the child with the prospects of ex-post-facto regret.

These extremes leave plenty of room for intermediate cases where a decision is more difficult and more controversial. In these cases the applicability of the ideal principles is severely restricted by uncertainty, both about the *direction* the interests of the child will take in the future and about the *value* the future person will attribute to their satisfaction. This double uncertainty, however, will in some cases be greater than in others. Coercing a child into protective medical measures against a late-onset debilitating disease with grave symptoms in adulthood and old age seems the more justified the more certain it is that there is no alternative means to avert or at least to postpone the outbreak of symptoms. Coercing a child to develop a capacity for which to all appearances it is specifically talented (e. g. playing the violin) has a greater probability to result in opportunities that will be welcomed by the grown-up person then investing the same educational efforts (including coercive or deceptive measures) in an untalented child only for the satisfaction of its parents' ambitions. Even in this case, however, it is doubtful whether the probabilities are sufficient to justify paternalistic measures. After all, there remains a considerable risk that the grown-up child will have lost interest in making use of its particular talent or will have developed different values.

7.5 Tendency Rules

Tendency rules are understood here as rules of thumb that do not strictly determine decisions about the legitimacy of paternalistic interventions. They should serve as inspirations rather than recipes. Nevertheless they can, I believe, be useful in the practice of education and especially in situations in which a balance has to be struck between the child's prospective long-term welfare and its right to self-determination.

A first tendency rule that extends beyond the sphere of education concerns the preferability of *indirect* to *direct* paternalism. Indirect paternalism involves restrictions of freedom no less than direct paternalism. But though indirectly paternalistic acts may involve coercive measures (like the safety regulations for toys or the sanctions for drug trafficking) these measures do not affect the child directly and are therefore morally less problematic than direct coercion.

A second tendency rule is that the burden of proof for paternalistic measures of a *furthering* nature should be higher than for paternalistic measures of a *protective* nature. Interventions intended to further a child's cognitive and affective growth (like making an unwilling child learn to play an instrument) should, in general, give way to the child's right to self-determination, whereas measures intended to protect the child from indubitable harm (such as preventing it from engaging in pastimes with a considerable danger for life) should, in general, not, or to a lesser extent. As was said above, children are vulnerable both in the dimension of bodily integrity and in the dimension of self-respect, and there will often be situations in which it is impossible to do justice to both dimensions simultaneously. Moreover, each dimension can by itself lead to conflict because both extend into the future. A violation of self-respect now can be a necessary to secure self-respect later on (e. g. by pressuring an intimidated child into a public performance), and a momentary violation of bodily integrity can be necessary for life-long health gains (like inoculation against infectious agents). From this perspective, the opposition sometimes postulated between "protective" and "directive" forms of educational paternalism (cf. Benporath 2003: 136) should be rejected. What is "protective" in the long term may under certain conditions appear as "directive" (in the sense of being contrary to the child's self-determination), whereas protecting the child's situational self-determination would simply mean to act irresponsibly. This tendency rule is, in fact, nothing but a variation on the familiar principle that harm avoidance should have priority over furthering the good, with the corollary that the more harm or risk a paternalistic act is able to avoid the more probable it is that the act is justified. The other side of the coin is that paternalistic acts of a furthering kind, designed to increase the opportunities of the later child, cannot be justified but under very narrow conditions, e. g. when it is certain that the child will later profit from having been subjected to some unwanted regime. Since the future is in general more uncertain than the present there will be a certain presumption against paternalistic interventions even for future harm prevention, at least in the sense that the burden of proof lies with paternalism and not the other way round. There are a large number of procedures, especially concerning health and diet, to which the children of my generation were subjected without sufficient proof that they would do any good, let alone prevent harm.

An example for how this rule might work in practice is the illegitimacy of forcing religious education on a child under circumstances in which the parents are not themselves regular church-goers or under which it is improbable that a child will live, as an adult, in a religiously committed social environment. In both cases, it is not to be expected that the child will profit from a religious education. In the first case, the prospects are poor that religion forms part of its bonds to its family and enables the child to experience that kind of intimacy with its family that is a condition of later emotional security and autonomy. In the second case a religious education risks that the child will in later life experience conflict rather than harmony with a predominantly secular social environment. Since religious education is mostly intended to further the future person's good rather than avoiding harm, it is already on that account insufficient to legitimize paternalistic coercion or pressure. In this respect, I disagree sharply with the view of Brighouse and Swift that parents should have an (unconditional) right to make their child attend a church (Brighouse and Swift 2006: 102) or the view of the German constitution that allows the state to make religious education a regular part of the school curriculum from which the child can dispense itself only at a certain stage of maturity (14 years).

A third plausible tendency rule is that paternalistic measures like coercive measures or measures involving deception should be acceptable only if milder forms of intervention like encouragement or admonition are unavailable or if the protective aim of the measure does not suffer delay so that it cannot be realized by postponing it until the child is more likely to agree to it, wills it on its own accord, or will have attained a level of autonomy that allows it to decide for itself. Milder measures or postponing should be preferred even if these involve higher costs or opportunity costs. In any case, the severity of the coercion exercised on the child has to be balanced against the probable gains in long-term protection against harm. Thus, though an early operation to fix the sex of a child with ambiguous sex characteristics may involve less costs in terms of violation of bodily integrity, suffering and financial expenses, it seems preferable either to wait with the operation until the child has grown up to a stage in which it is autonomous enough to decide on its sex (or its hybrid status) by itself or to enable the child to make an autonomous decision by specifically qualifying it for such a decision. In less dramatic cases, waiting is often the strategy of choice because the child's interests may be unstable and dependent on changing situational factors. Irreversibility, on the other hand, is a strong reason in favor of paternalistic intervention, at least in the case of certain and severe harm. The less grave the harm is and the less certain it is, the less plausible is the justification from irreversibility. Preventing a child to have a tattoo is less urgent than preventing drug addiction, though both may be equally irreversible. Moreover, irreversibility is, again, gradable. Neither drug addiction nor tattoos are strictly irreversible, though reversible only at considerable costs.

A fourth tendency rule is that the moral gravity of paternalistic acts should be graded not only by the intensity of coercion involved but also by the degree of the child's growing autonomy. Though autonomy as a *capacity* is not necessary for possession of the *right* to autonomy or self-determination, paternalism becomes the more morally problematic the higher the level of autonomy the child has reached in its respective stage of development. This level must be judged on a strictly individual basis. For example, it is well known that the capacity to decide on medical interventions may be much more "mature" in children with chronic diseases requiring repeated burdensome medical treatment than in healthy children of the same age generally.

7.6 Conclusion

The conclusion to be drawn from what has been said is that a certain amount of paternalism in education seems in principle morally legitimate, and indeed required, but only under severe restrictions. These restrictions are not generally taken account of in practice. They can be given the form of tendency rules that give orientation for practical decisions on the part of parents and caregivers, leaving, however, plenty of room for discretion and good judgment.

References

Ainslie, G. (1975). Specious reward: A behavioral theory of impulsiveness and impulse control. *Psychological Bulletin, 82*, 463–496.
Beauchamp, T. L. (1977). Paternalism and biobehavioral control. *Monist, 60*, 62–80.
Beauchamp, T. L., & Childress, J. F. (2013). *Principles of biomedical ethics* (7th ed.). New York: Oxford University Press.
Benporath, S. R. (2003). Autonomy and vulnerability: On just relations between adults and children. *Journal of the Philosophy of Education, 37*, 127–145.
Birnbacher, D. (2010). Paternalismus im Strafrecht – ethisch vertretbar? In A. von Hirsch, U. Neumann, & K. Seelmann (Eds.), *Paternalismus im Strafrecht. Die Kriminalisierung selbstschädigenden Verhaltens* (pp. 11–26). Baden-Baden: Nomos.
Brighouse, H. (2003). How should children be heard? *Arizona Law Review, 45*, 691–711.
Brighouse, H., & Swift, A. (2006). Parents' rights and the value of the family. *Ethics, 117*, 80–108.
Buchanan, A. E., & Brock, D. W. (1989). *Deciding for others. The ethics of surrogate decision making*. Cambridge: Cambridge University Press.
Damm, R. (2010). Medizinrechtliche Grundprinzipien im Kontext von Pflege und Demenz – "Selbstbestimmung und Fürsorge". *Medizinrecht, 28*, 451–463.

Dworkin, G. (1972). Paternalism. *Monist, 56*, 64–84.
Elster, J. (1979). *Ulysses and the Sirens. Studies in rationality and irrationality.* Cambridge: Cambridge University Press, Editions de la Maison des Sciences de l'Homme.
Feinberg, J. (1979). Legal paternalism. In R. Wasserstrom (Ed.), *Today's moral problems* (2nd ed., pp. 434–451). New York: Macmillan.
Feinberg, J. (1986). *Harm to self.* New York: Oxford University Press.
Giesinger, J. (2007). *Autonomie und Verletzlichkeit. Der moralische Status von Kindern und die Rechtfertigung von Erziehung.* Bielefeld: Transcript.
Hügli, A. (1983). Lernzwang zum Wohle der Kinder? Aspekte des Zeitlichen im menschlichen Dasein. In *Vierteljahresschrift für Heilpädagogik und ihre Nachbargebiete* (Vol. 52, pp. 172–181).
Kleinig, J. (1983). *Paternalism.* Manchester: Manchester University Press.
Parfit, D. (1971). Personal identity. *Philosophical Review, 80*, 3–27.
Parfit, D. (1984). *Reasons and persons.* Oxford: Oxford University Press.
Reid, T. (1975). Of identity. From T. Reid, Essays on the intellectual powers of man (1785). In J. Perry (Ed.), *Personal identity* (pp. 108–118). Berkeley: University of California Press.
Schickhardt, C. (2012). *Kinderethik: Der moralische Status und die Rechte der Kinder.* Paderborn: Mentis.
Schleiermacher, F. (2000). Grundzüge der Erziehungskunst (Vorlesungen 1826). Texte zur Pädagogik. In M. Winkler & J. Brachmann (Eds.), *Kommentierte Studienausgabe* (Vol. 2). Frankfurt am Main: Suhrkamp.
Thaler, R. H., & Sunstein, C. R. (2008). *Nudge. Improving decisions about health, wealth and happiness.* New Haven: Yale University Press.
VanDeVeer, D. (1986). *Paternalistic intervention. The moral bounds of benevolence.* Princeton: Princeton University Press.

Chapter 8
Anti-perfectionist Childrearing

Matthew Clayton

An important problem that every parent faces concerns how she should exercise her authority over her children. In this paper, I address one aspect of that problem: how we should judge whether a parent's conduct as a parent is more or less successful. Since I hold a reasonably controversial view about how we should understand the morally appropriate relationship between parent and child—which I call *parental anti-perfectionism*—I begin by setting out that view by contrasting it with some alternative—perfectionist—conceptions of the morality of parenting. The anti-perfectionist view is that parents act illegitimately if they enrol their child into religious practices that are controversial within society. Thereafter, I sketch some aspects of an answer to the central question of what successful anti-perfectionist parenting is, and I respond to three objections that might be raised against it, namely, that the view is too vague or too insipid, and that it permits parents to neglect the well-being of their child.

8.1 Parental Perfectionism

There are moral limits to the extent to which parents and others are morally permitted to promote a child's well-being. Some of those limits are generated by the claims of third parties. As in other domains of morality, it is generally impermissible to use other people in certain ways to advance one's child's well-being. For example, although my child's well-being might be improved if I kidnapped an effective mathematics tutor or cricket coach and forced her to perfect my child's arithmetic

---

M. Clayton (✉)
Department of Politics and International Studies, Social Sciences Building,
The University of Warwick, Coventry CV4 7AL, UK
e-mail: m.g.clayton@warwick.ac.uk

or spin bowling, I am not morally permitted to do so. A second limit relates to parents whose concern for their child leads them to perform acts that set back the interests of others as a side effect. Suppose that taking my child for a walk in the woods to enhance her understanding of the natural world would foreseeably release hundreds of wasps that would inflict harm on other people near the wood. If the harm done to others were disproportionate, I would not be permitted to improve my child's well-being in that way. The interests and claims of third parties, then, limit the extent to which parents are permitted to advance the well-being of their child.

Are there limits to the extent to which parents are permitted to promote their child's well-being that are grounded in the interests and claims of the child herself rather than the interests or claims of third parties? I shall call those who claim that there are no such limits *parental perfectionists*. Their view can be stated in more or less demanding ways. The most demanding parental perfectionist view asserts that, bracketing moral questions concerning third parties, parents are *morally required* to act in a way that *maximises* their child's well-being. The demanding perfectionist view is too demanding, however, because it requires parents to make huge sacrifices with respect to their own well-being if that would generate merely minor improvements in their child's well-being. On any plausible view of morality, parents have interests as adults that are separable from those of their child, and their reason to pursue these interests is not always defeated by their reason to promote their child's well-being.

A more plausible, less demanding, conception of parental perfectionism asserts that, bracketing their duties to third parties, parents are *morally permitted* to act in ways that maximise their child's well-being. Some might object that this view needs some revision, because parents are not morally permitted completely to sacrifice their interests as non-parents for the sake of their child. This objection seems to have some force. For example, some think that we have self-regarding duties. If I have a duty to live a dignified life, then it seems impermissible for me to accept an offer of employment in which I am dominated or abused in a way that is inconsistent with my dignity even for the sake of enhancing my child's well-being.[1]

Accordingly, a plausible account of parental perfectionism will claim that, bracketing duties to third parties and provided they do not violate their self-regarding duties, parents are morally permitted to act in ways that maximise their child's well-being. However, this is an incomplete description, because perfectionists say that it is often the case that parents have a *duty* to promote their child's well-being. For that reason, they need to supply an account of when parents are morally required, and not merely permitted, to promote their child's well-being. Since I reject parental perfectionism, it is sufficient for my purposes to interpret perfectionism as a permissive view. However, those who embrace parental perfectionism need to offer a more complete account of the rights and duties of parents than has so far been provided.

Some embrace parental perfectionism because they assume that it permits parents to enrol their child into the practices and goals they (the parents) deem

---

[1] For a discussion of dignity and self-respect that suggests this view, see Dworkin (2011: pp. 202–209).

worthy of pursuit. That assumption is mistaken, because perfectionism is a *fact-* or *evidence-relative*, not a *belief*-relative, view. For example, if we suppose that a religious life is unworthy of pursuit, is it morally permissible for Christian parents to raise their child to be devout? If a Christian upbringing would diminish the child's well-being then the reason that motivates parental perfectionism—that, other things equal, parents ought to act to improve rather than diminish their child's well-being—suggests that it may well be morally impermissible to raise one's child in that way. Perfectionism is a set of claims about what we ought to do given the facts, or the evidence available to us. In the case above, it does not permit parents to raise their child as a Christian merely because they *believe* that a Christian life is good for her; to be permissible their belief must be correct or indicated by the available evidence.[2] Thus, parental perfectionism might condemn many practices that are commonly thought to be acceptable, such as parents pursuing their ethical goals with their child.[3]

It is not my aim to set out the most plausible version of parental perfectionism. If a version of parental perfectionism were adopted we would need to know more about well-being. In particular, we would need to understand well-being at different parts of the life cycle. As others have suggested, there might be certain goods that can be enjoyed only, or particularly, in childhood (Macleod 2010). On the other hand, childrearing involves imparting the beliefs and desires that will enhance the child's enjoyment of goods in her life as an adult. Furthermore, if there are different life-cycle-relative goods that cannot all be reconciled, then questions arise as to whether trade-offs can be made between them and, if so, which trade-offs should be made. These are questions that parental perfectionist must address. However, because I believe parental *anti*-perfectionism to be the right view, I shall not address those questions here.

8.2 Political Anti-perfectionism

A different kind of perfectionism that has received considerable attention in normative theory is *political* perfectionism. The question here is not whether *parents* are morally permitted or required to act in ways that maximise their child's well-being, but whether the *government* is morally permitted to interfere in society, by regulating the family or educational institutions, to promote the well-being of its citizens. Although political perfectionists accept that the government might have other reasons for action that sometimes compete with and, perhaps, override its reason to advance

---

[2] The distinction between the three different kinds of permissibility draws on Parfit (2011: pp. 150–151).
[3] Brighouse and Swift (2009) set out a conception of familial relationship goods, which might be thought to rescue the compatibility of perfectionism and parents sharing their values with their child. However, it is not obvious that the value of parents and children having common goals is wholly independent of the intrinsic value of the goals that they pursue together.

its citizens' well-being, they claim that there is no principled reason for it to disregard this consideration (Raz 1989: p. 1230). *Anti-perfectionists* reject this view. They claim that the government has principled reasons not to take a stand within certain debates, such as those about religion, and, accordingly, should not use its powers to maximise the well-being of its citizens. Consider the example of Christianity again. Suppose it were true, and the government knew, that living a Christian life is always worse for individuals than living some alternative life. In those circumstances, would it be morally permissible for the government to use its legal powers over educational institutions to promote suitable non-Christian lifestyles, if such promotion were shown to be successful in enhancing the well-being of its citizens? Anti-perfectionists claim that the government should refrain from promoting non-Christian lifestyles even if Christian belief and practice is worse for people and their well-being might be enhanced by the political promotion of non-Christian practices.

One prominent argument for anti-perfectionism proceeds from the ideal of *independence*, which asserts that each person should endorse the rules that govern how she lives her life. With respect to our personal goals, for example, independence requires that we decide for ourselves what ends we pursue during our lifetimes, rather than have our ends set by other people. Standardly, however, the fact that we live in political relationships poses a problem for independence, because we are born into a society with legal, social and political institutions that force us to do various things and exercise coercion over us. In short, we do not choose which political ends we serve. A central question of political philosophy, identified by Rousseau, is how to reconcile our independence with the fact that our relationship to the state is both non-voluntary and coercive. Rousseau's solution to this problem is that political authority and independence can be rendered compatible if legal and political institutions are regulated by principles that every citizen endorses. In that way, each can view herself as governed by ends she sets for herself (Rousseau ([1762] 1978, Book I, Ch. vi–viii).

Rousseau's solution is developed by Rawls who argues that we have duties of justice to arrange our social institutions so that they distribute social goods and bads fairly. Legitimate political institutions, he argues, will protect a range of familiar civil and political freedoms—democratic rights, and the rights of free expression, association, and conscience—as well as distribute social and economic goods so that everyone has the opportunity to be healthy and the wherewithal to pursue her goals. Rawls notes that if such institutions are maintained then a diversity of convictions about what he calls 'comprehensive' ends will inevitably develop. Comprehensive ends include, for example, religious goals, occupational aims, and conceptions of the kinds of family and sexuality that are worthy of pursuit. Individuals who think about these issues under conditions of freedom are, he claims, bound to disagree over which comprehensive ends are worthy of adoption and pursuit. Given that we have a weighty reason to arrange political institutions in a way that is compatible with the maintenance of independence, it appears that those institutions should not be motivated by or directed to serve any particular comprehensive end. Because citizens disagree about religion, for example, if the government adopted and promoted a particular view of religion, then those citizens who reject that view would no longer be constrained by rules they endorse. The upshot of this argument is political anti-perfectionism. It is not the government's role to promote the well-being of its citizens, because that would jeopardise the independence—Rawls calls it 'political autonomy'—of many of its citizens (Rawls 2006).

8.3 The Case for Parental Anti-perfectionism

What are the implications of political anti-perfectionism for what parents are permitted to do to or for their children? The most *popular view* articulated by those who subscribe to political anti-perfectionism is that, within certain constraints, it is legitimate for parents to raise their child according to a religious view even if that religious view is not widely shared within society. Provided that they educate her so that she has the wherewithal to live an independent life as an adult and they observe other constraints such as the duty not to inflict physical harm on her, parents may legitimately raise their child as they choose. Among the constraints placed on this permission are that parents must raise their child in a way that enables her to understand the various ends she might pursue and to deliberate rationally about which ends she ought to embrace, and they must impart to her the mental and physical wherewithal to pursue those ends rationally.[4]

On this view parents are permitted to maximise their child's well-being subject to the constraints discussed above involving duties to third parties and to parents' own self-regarding duties. They are also permitted to act in ways that fail to maximise their child's well-being. According to the popular view, anti-perfectionist political morality refuses to engage with the question of which comprehensive ends are worthy or pursuit and, thus, it gives parents rights over their child that permit them to act in ways that make their child's life go worse than it might with an alternative upbringing.[5]

I reject the popular view of the implications of political anti-perfectionism for parental conduct.[6] I claim that if anti-perfectionism applies to the relationship

---

[4] Many liberal educational theorists endorse what I call the popular view. Perhaps the most prominent statement of it is Feinberg (1992).

[5] For the observation that this view permits parents to encourage their child to adopt goals that diminish her well-being, see Fowler (2010). Perhaps it is consistent with the popular view for the state to prohibit parents acting with an inappropriate *attitude* towards their child. For example, suppose I am a devout Christian but regard my child as not entitled to an upbringing that introduces her to Christianity, because children are morally inferior to adults and, therefore, their well-being matters less. In that case, the state might legitimately claim that I have the wrong attitude towards my children that is revealed by the fact that I refuse to offer my child the opportunity to pursue what I take to be the right way to live. That attitude might be wrongful and, perhaps, an appropriate basis for creating a criminal wrong, even if refusing my child an introduction to Christianity does, in fact, improve her life (because, suppose, Christian lifestyles diminish people's well-being). For discussion of the right to an attitude, as applied to human rights, see Dworkin (2011: pp. 335–339).

[6] Here I summarize and clarify the argument of Clayton (2006, Chap. 4).

between state and citizen, then it should also govern the relationship between parent and child. Like citizens, children are also born into families that have significant effects on their life-chances and the values they adopt. Parents also force their children to do various things. If the ideal of independence requires us to arrange unchosen coercive political arrangements so that they can be affirmed by citizens whatever the particular comprehensive ends they endorse, then the activities of parents should be similarly constrained. For these reasons, parental anti-perfectionism appears to be a required extension of political anti-perfectionism.

An obvious objection to the parallel case argument described above is that there is a morally relevant difference between the relationship between adult citizens and the state, on the one hand, and that between children and parents, on the other. Because adults reflectively endorse their religious convictions, making them worship or live under laws that promote religion involves requiring them to act *against their reasoned convictions*. By contrast, parents who make their child worship do not thereby require her to act in ways she reflectively rejects. The child, at least when a young child, does not possess appropriately formed beliefs and desires that constitute the basis for principled moral constraints on how parents may treat her. True, she is entitled to certain kinds of treatment that serve her various interests. However, unlike a mature citizen whose reasoned convictions operate as principled constraints on how the state can legitimately act, the child lacks the properties that make her convictions morally relevant in that way. The exercise of parental power, the argument goes, need not, therefore, be regulated by ideals and principles that are acceptable to the child. On this view, parents are off the hook with respect to the anti-perfectionist restraint that characterises political morality: perfectionist parents do not wrong their child in the way the state wrongs a citizen when it enrols her into a particular comprehensive practice.

The response to this objection is that it is mistaken to claim that the child cannot reject her religious enrolment on the basis of morally relevant—reasoned—convictions. Granted, she cannot offer that kind of rejection as a young child. Nevertheless, she can object to her enrolment in the right way when she becomes an adult and evaluates her upbringing *ex post*. She is capable of giving or withholding *retrospective endorsement*.

When evaluating *ex ante* how they ought to raise their child—that is, before their child has developed the mental powers to give or withhold endorsement—parents must accept that if they enrolled their child into a religious practice their child might, and it is likely that the child will, retrospectively reject that enrolment. The explanation of this non-normative fact appeals to Rawls's observation of the 'burdens of judgement': disagreement about comprehensive matters is an inevitable consequence of people forming beliefs and desires under free institutions (Rawls 2006: pp. 54–58); furthermore, if political morality demands an education that provides individuals with the capacity to decide for themselves which comprehensive ends are worthy of adoption and pursuit, then we can add that which of the diverse comprehensive ends any particular person will adopt is unpredictable.

Accordingly, the revised argument for parental anti-perfectionism is as follows. Because (i) retrospective rejection is morally troubling and they have weighty reasons to raise their child in a way that avoids it, and (ii) they know that their child might retrospectively reject her religious enrolment as a child, and (iii) there are adequate alternative ways of raising their child that do not involve comprehensive enrolment, parents have a weighty *ex ante* reason not to enrol their child into a religious practice.

Several objections have been raised against parental anti-perfectionism. Some argue that I overstate the similarities between state-citizen and parent-child relationships, others that respect for independence is not incompatible with the comprehensive enrolment of children (Morgan 2009; Cameron 2012). I have responded to some of these objections elsewhere (Clayton 2009, 2012). In the remainder of this paper, I turn to certain concerns about anti-perfectionist childrearing that centre on considerations of the child's well-being. One worry about parental anti-perfectionism is that its implications for evaluating whether parents and other adults raise and educate children well or poorly are unclear. It is reasonable to expect parental anti-perfectionism to provide a positive account of how children should be raised given its claim that parents (and other adults) should not regard their role as encouraging the child to adopt comprehensive ends that will enhance her well-being. Secondly, it might be thought that the view allows for only an insipid upbringing, because it seems to rule out many different activities that make for a rich and stimulating upbringing and, thereby, fails to prepare the child for adulthood or simply makes her suffer a drab childhood.

And, finally, there is the fundamental objection that anti-perfectionism denies parents the moral resources to protect their child from falling into comprehensive activities that are harmful and from forming false beliefs that make her life go worse, either instrumentally or intrinsically. A prominent issue that might be thought to illustrate this powerful objection to parental anti-perfectionism is the teaching of biology. In some societies—the USA is a prominent example—the truth of evolution as an account of natural history is widely contested, and many embrace creationism or intelligent design as a superior explanation. Does it follow that parents and teachers who teach that intelligent design is demonstrably false violate the norm of anti-perfectionism? Should they instead teach natural history in a way that does not take a stand on the dispute between the evolutionary biologists and creationists? The objection I shall consider claims that, because they must be committed to the view that parents and teachers ought not to take a stand on which version of natural history is correct, anti-perfectionists are wedded to educational norms that set back the interests of children.

To respond to these three worries about vagueness, insipidness and negligence, I shall first set out the principal elements of a positive account of upbringing that is compatible with parental anti-perfectionism and, thereafter, try to show that such an upbringing is neither vague nor insipid. I shall finish with some remarks on whether the failure to promote the child's well-being is a decisive objection and the specific issue of whether parents can legitimately encourage their child to reason scientifically.

8.4 An Anti-perfectionist Conception of the Currency of Parental Concern

Parental anti-perfectionism asserts that it is not a legitimate aim for those responsible for raising a child to enrol her into particular comprehensive practices. In what follows I shall discuss the example of religious enrolment, but it is worth noting that parental anti-perfectionism is not hostile to religious enrolment alone. It holds that resolute atheists who encourage their young child to reject theism and religion also act illegitimately; the prohibition on enrolment also applies to other comprehensive ideals, such as controversial conceptions of sexuality and occupational choice, and views about which personal goals are worthy of pursuit. Thus, although I illustrate the view I articulate by reference to religion, this should not be taken to imply that religious enrolment is uniquely problematic.

According to parental anti-perfectionism, religious parents are not permitted to enrol their child into particular religious practices. The term 'enrolment' is shorthand for a number of activities. It covers the following: baptising one's child thereby making her a member of a church and undertaking religious commitments on her behalf; encouraging her to pray and perform as other believers do; and encouraging her to believe and affirm particular religious views. These activities constitute enrolment when the aim of parents is to raise their child as a Christian, Hindu, Muslim, Jew, and so on, by shaping her beliefs and desires such that the child is motivated to affirm the central doctrines of the religion and to participate in its practices. Moreover, as I argue elsewhere (Clayton 2006, 2012), enrolment is wrong even when parents also educate their child such that later in life she can autonomously decide to continue with or reject the religion into which she has been enrolled.[7]

The impermissibility of the religious enrolment of children implies that parental perfectionism is mistaken. Consequently, the morality of childrearing cannot simply be read as the answer to the strategic question 'what kinds of upbringing would make children's lives go well?' If we have reason to respect individuals' independence then, like states, parents should not understand their role as seeking the truth about well-being and encouraging their child to act in ways that enable her to maximise her well-being as a child or adult, or across her life.

If parental concern for their child should not be understood exclusively in terms of promoting her well-being, then how should it be understood? Plainly, parents can perform their role more or less successfully. Our question is: how should we understand the *currency* or *metric* by which we identify the successes or failures of parents if the child's well-being is not the appropriate currency?

---

[7] One objection to my focus on enrolment is that it rests on the controversial view that the permissibility of acts is not independent of the aims that motivate the agent. For a critique of that view, see Scanlon (2008). I lack the space to deal with this objection here. However, I simply note that, like its political counterpart, anti-perfectionist parenting is primarily an account of the reasons that ought to motivate individuals. The precise relationship between parental motivation and the permissibility of their actions, I leave to discuss on another occasion.

In what follows I attempt to offer a response to that question, albeit an incomplete one. I characterise an account of children's *advantage*, which consists of those items that are the proper object of parental concern. An account of advantage is commonly used by liberal political philosophers who want to specify a conception of interpersonal comparison for the purpose of guiding social and political institutions in a way that avoids controversial judgements about well-being. Those philosophers identify a metric that gives appropriate guidance with respect to whom to help and how to help those who are entitled to help. For example, a prominent account of advantage is Rawls's account of *primary social goods*. In his conception, individuals are identified as more or less advantaged by reference to their enjoyment of certain basic liberties, the educational and employment opportunities available to them, their level of wealth and income, and whether they live in social conditions conducive to their self-respect. Those who favour parental anti-perfectionism must articulate a similar account of parental concern.

The currency of parental concern also provides an account of what parents may do to or for their child. That account is constrained by the considerations that favour parental anti-perfectionism. Parents are not permitted to enrol their child into particular comprehensive practices. Part of the task, then, is to figure out the implications of the prohibition on comprehensive enrolment and to identify what parents are permitted or required to do for their child.

8.5 The Implications of the Ideal of Independence

Our questions are: (1) what are parents permitted or required to do for their child if they are not permitted to enrol her into a religion? And (2) on what bases are we to evaluate the success or failure of different kinds of parenting if well-being is not the appropriate metric? In response, I suggest that the foundational ideal of *independence for everyone* that motivates anti-perfectionism offers a significant, if incomplete, basis for answering these questions. Here, I summarise two different ways in which independence might be elaborated as a conception of children's advantage, that develop Rawls's account of our basic interests as 'free and equal' persons.

8.5.1 *The Capacity for a Conception of the Good*

In the first place, as I understand it independence requires adults to set their own goals in life rather than have them set by others. If they are to set their own goals individuals must have what Rawls calls 'a capacity for a conception of the good': the capacity to deliberate rationally about the various goals, projects and relationships that are available to them and the intellectual and physical wherewithal to pursue the ends that they come to endorse.

It is clear that we can use the capacity for a conception of the good as the foundation for judging whether parents and teachers are effective in raising a child. Plainly, for the purposes of developing a public guide to evaluate individuals in these roles we would need to disaggregate several different features of the capacity. For example, the capacity for rational thought needs further elucidation. Is the child rational only if her thought conforms to the requirements of expected utility theory, or are the requirements of rationality for the purposes of conferring independence less demanding? Second, the intellectual and physical capacities that constitute the capacity for a conception of the good might be characterised in more detail. Is it better from the point of view of independence if the child has an advanced understanding of mathematics or literature, for example, or better to the extent that she is physically stronger or faster?

I cannot give complete answers to these questions. However, it should be noted that the rational, intellectual and physical powers required for ethical independence are satiable. Independence requires that individuals have enough of these powers: just because Bertrand is a better philosopher, logician, linguist and mathematician than Barry does not mean that his life is more independent, because Barry might possess sufficient rationality and intellectual and physical capacity to satisfy the conditions for independence. The capacity for a conception of the good demands a certain threshold of capability with respect to rationality: individuals should understand that their goals are nested in structures in which certain goals serve others, and they should have the ability to avoid adopting mutually inconsistent goals and to choose effective means of realising their fundamental goals. The rationality required for this capacity need not, then, be the kind of rationality that is demanded by certain variants of decision theory in which individuals maximise their expected preference-satisfaction. The rationality required for independence is less demanding and consistent with individuals adopting different attitudes towards preference-satisfaction. They may be satisficers rather than maximisers, or be averse to certain kinds of risk, or regard their practical reasons as given by their duties to others regardless of their preferences, without jeopardising their independence. What matters is that their goals are chosen in a way that faithfully reflects their own ambitions.

Below the threshold, we might say that individuals might deliberate and act more or less rationally and, accordingly, be closer or further away from independence. One example of this concerns the development of children. In our infancy, when we lack well-developed deliberative and rational powers, independence is absent and others must control our lives and conduct so that we acquire these capacities. As we develop deliberative and rational powers, that control lessens until the point at which we have sufficient powers to develop and pursue our own goals according to the standards of independence (Locke [1690] 1988: II. 55). In addition, we might evaluate different kinds of parenting and education to assess whether they are well designed to assist the development of these powers such that individuals acquire them in a timely fashion: parenting arrangements that fail to facilitate their acquisition or that take longer to do so might be subject to criticism or reform (Hannan 2011).

Independence, I have argued, requires possession of the capacity for a conception of the good. But some have suggested that the capacity is itself a conception of the good and, therefore, if it is illegitimate to enrol children into religious conceptions then surely it is also illegitimate to shape the child's life so that she is able and willing rationally to choose and pursue the particular goals that strike her as worthwhile. The objection is that anti-perfectionist childrearing cannot without contradiction advocate the development of the child's capacity for a conception of the good.

This objection can be rebutted by observing that it overlooks the fact that anti-perfectionism operates with a distinction within ethics. It asserts that there is a set of ethical ideals—in this account, comprehensive ideals—with respect to which adults should take no stand in their capacity as carers or educators of children. But that does not mean that this set of ethical ideals includes *every* ideal. It is a coherent to hold that there is an ideal—independence in this conception—that should guide the choices of parents and, at the same time, hold that parents should not be guided by other ethical ideals, such as those involving religious claims. Indeed, the argument above is that the ideal of independence, which demands that the individual sets her own ends, explains and justifies the distinction that is drawn within ethics. Independence is possible only if we are able rationally to adopt and pursue our own goals. That explains the importance of the development and exercise of the capacity for a conception of the good. An upbringing that goes further and enrols the child into a particular conception of the good is not inconsistent with her acquisition of that capacity, but it is ruled out by a further requirement of independence: that others do not force her to serve ends she later reflectively rejects.[8]

8.5.2 A Sense of Justice and Morality

The second important educational implication of independence for everyone is the good of the development of a sense of justice and morality. The reason is straightforward: if everyone is to lead an independent life then we must constrain our behaviour towards others such that we do not jeopardise their independence. My independence is lost if others manipulate or coerce me to pursue ends they set for me; and it is lost if I lack the opportunity to pursue my own ends due to the intentional or unintentional conduct of others: if they steal the property I was counting on to lead my life, for example, or pass laws that criminalise the pursuit of my religious convictions.

The ideal of independence generates the need for a set of moral and legal arrangements that are familiar within liberal democratic societies. These arrangements are stably realizable only if individuals operate with appropriate convictions about what is owed to each other—a sense of justice that regulates how we choose our

---

[8] I am conscious that the position I expound here differs in many important respects from the way in which Rawls deploys the capacity for a conception of the good. For an examination of those differences and an argument for departing from Rawls, see Clayton (2006: pp. 24–27).

important legal, political and socioeconomic institutions, and a sense of morality that shapes how we interact with others where the law is silent.

Although the preconditions and requirements of independence have implications for the kind of justice and morality we ought to adopt it does not fully determine their content. For instance, independence restricts the extent to which we are morally permitted to act in ways that make another's pursuit of her goals more costly or difficult. However, it does not tell us whether we owe others *equal* or *sufficient* opportunity to pursue their goals or, if we adopt an egalitarian interpretation, how to judge whether equality obtains.

Interesting questions are raised by the fact that independence is compatible with different conceptions of distributive justice. Is it a violation of independence if parents and teachers aim to impart particular moral and political convictions to the children they raise? If it is a violation are we morally forbidden from imparting such convictions? Is it morally impermissible to raise one's child to be an egalitarian, supposing equality to be more plausible as a moral and political ideal compared to sufficientarian views, say?

Several different responses might be offered to these questions. The response I favour is that our reason to respect individuals' independence is conditional: setting one's own ends, and endorsement of the ideals that motivate the legal rules that constrain one, are normatively important provided one honours one's duties to others, at least reasonably well. On this conditional view we have no reason to refrain from imposing liberal democratic principles on fascists; similarly we have no reason not to shove Arthur into a pond to save a drowning child at small cost to Arthur—assume that shoving Arthur is the only way of saving the child's life—just in virtue of the fact that Arthur does not believe he has a moral duty to save the child. In these cases, we should say that our reason to respect an individual's independence is cancelled because she proposes to commit a serious injustice. Our claim to be governed by institutions that we endorse is conditional upon our views conforming to certain standards of morality. These claims can be extended to address questions of upbringing: parenting is less successful to the extent that it fails sufficiently to develop the child's understanding and motivation to comply with the demands of morality. The child herself has certain duties to others and successful parenting involves taking steps to ensure that she recognises and fulfils those duties. The independence case for anti-perfectionism, then, does not rule out enrolling children into justice-promoting practices or the cultivation of various moral dispositions.

There are further issues of detail to be resolved in this account. For example, a sense of justice might be given a more or less determinate specification. Consider Rawls's distinction between the properties of a reasonable conception and the details of a particular reasonable conception, such as his own conception of *justice as fairness*. In his view, reasonable conceptions of justice are constituted by their endorsement of basic liberal rights and their priority, and of the provision of the material wherewithal for citizens to make use of their freedoms; and he sets out some quite demanding institutional proposals that follow from these requirements, including basic health care for all and society underwriting employment for everyone (Rawls 2006: lvii–lx). However, although reasonableness with respect to political morality seems to rule out many views that are widely held in contemporary society—such as libertarian views, for example—it does not choose between, say, Justice as Fairness and Dworkin's resourcist account of justice. Our sense of justice might be legitimate—it might be permissible to act on it in public life—even if it is not entirely right. If we apply that observation to parenting, we might say that parents are morally required to cultivate a sense of reasonableness in their child, but they should not try to perfect their child's sense of justice.

8.6 Too Vague?

I hope I have outlined enough of its positive conception of upbringing to rebut the charge that anti-perfectionist childrearing is too vague to operate as an ideal of parental morality. The charge is founded on the worry that the impermissibility of religious enrolment is a wholly negative injunction telling parents what they may not do, and it offers little guidance on the question of what they ought to do for their child. Setting out the positive requirements of anti-perfectionism—the cultivation of a sense of justice and providing the wherewithal for the child reflectively to decide religious matters for herself—dispels that worry.

A more interesting elaboration of the vagueness worry is that anti-perfectionism is primarily a view about which kinds of reason can legitimately guide parental conduct. While I have argued that it is incompatible with religious enrolment, that is because enrolment is an activity in which parents aim to align their child with a particular faith. But if that is so, the worry is that legitimate aims can be expressed in action in several ways and anti-perfectionism cannot choose between those different ways of raising or educating children. For example, one set of parents, cognisant of their duty to avoid religious enrolment, might send their child to a secular school; another set might give their child an education in a religious school in the belief that such an education compensates for her exposure to the commodifying norms that saturate the background culture of society. Despite the profound differences in the way they raise their children, neither set of parents, it seems, violates the constraint against religious enrolment.

Observations such as these, however, raise open questions that call for further investigation, rather than confirm the worry that anti-perfectionist childrearing is hopelessly vague. I do not know whether parents who choose to send their child to a religious school on the grounds that it gives them a different perspective to the dominant culture do the right thing for their child. True, such parents need not count as enrolling their child into a particular viewpoint; their aim might simply be to expose their child to a wide range of comprehensive viewpoints from which to make an informed choice. But there are other requirements of the liberal anti-perfectionist view on the basis of which we might evaluate the success of their decisions, such is whether the education they choose serves the child in acquiring a sense of justice and the wherewithal to decide for herself which comprehensive ends to pursue.

Whether or not their parenting is fully adequate according to those requirements is a separate question. Of course, in the final analysis there may remain many different ways of satisfying the anti-perfectionist liberal conception of upbringing. To the extent that that is the case, the conception is permissive rather than vague.

8.7 Too Insipid?

Two versions of what I shall call the insipidness worry about anti-perfectionist childrearing might be distinguished. The first worry is that, because parents are not permitted to enrol their child into a particular religion, the child will not develop the right kind of understanding of the rich meaning of religious commitment that can be gained only from being immersed within a set of religious practices. Children will be left directionless, the argument goes, and not develop a sense of commitment to a project, which is a necessary feature of leading an independent life. In short, then, the objection is that enrolment is necessary preparation for an independent adulthood.[9]

The second version of the concern is not that anti-perfectionist childrearing serves our interests as adults less well than a regime that permits religious enrolment; rather, it fails to serve us as children. Childhood should not be theorised simply as preparation for adulthood; the child's enjoyment of certain goods makes her life go well *as a child* irrespective of whether those goods also prepare her well for life as a free and equal adult. However, because these goods—what Macleod (2010) calls the 'intrinsic goods of childhood'—are not universally valued and, indeed, might be rejected by one's child when she reaches adulthood, it appears impermissible to enable one's child to enjoy them.[10] If that is the case, then parental anti-perfectionism condemns too much, because it does not permit parents to offer their child a childhood in which she can experience and partake in the activities that are particularly valuable for children.

In response to the first worry, it is worth noting that although anti-perfectionist childrearing finds comprehensive enrolment and immersion problematic, it allows and, indeed, requires *political* enrolment and immersion. If Rawls's account of moral development is right, the acquisition of a sense of justice seems to require an upbringing in an intimate family and relevant associations that enable the child to cultivate an appropriate understanding of morality and justice, and to acquire the motivation to comply with their demands. That can be viewed as developing a sense of commitment to particular moral ideals, a sense of permissible and impermissible conduct, and fitting attitudes towards moral success or failure. To the extent that the objection is premised on the claim that parental anti-perfectionism leaves individuals incapable of understanding fully what it means seriously and responsibly

---

[9] See, for example, McLaughlin (1984); worries of this kind are also expressed by Callan (2002).

[10] Consider, for example, 1 *Corinthians* 13: 11, 'When I was a child, I spoke like a child, I thought like a child, and reasoned like a child; when I became a man, I gave up childish ways'.

to pursue goals, the moral and political demands of liberal citizenship give assurance that this kind of orientation to life will not be lost. Religious enrolment is, therefore, unnecessary to give individuals an understanding of what it means to adopt, reflect on, plan and execute a life plan, because that understanding is provided via the development of a sense of justice.

The second worry—the loss of childhood goods—appears more threatening. It is not merely that theorising children's advantage in terms of the development of a sense of justice and the wherewithal to lead an autonomous life is, as Macleod argues, incomplete in virtue of not offering a conception of what is good for children as children. The possibility of retrospective rejection seems to make it impermissible to encourage one's child to engage in imaginative, adventurous and carefree play or to provide opportunities for valuable aesthetic experience, athletic success, fun and amusement. If so, then the charge is that an anti-perfectionist upbringing is incapable of delivering the intrinsic goods of childhood: it restricts parents to providing a dreary or insipid upbringing on pain of retrospective rejection.

Because I lack the space fully to consider this objection, I shall simply offer some suggestions about how an anti-perfectionist might respond to it. In doing so, I shall assume that there are certain types of activity that are appealing to us as children but which we might find disagreeable as adults. Even so, it does not follow that parents must prevent their child from engaging in those activities. In virtue of its focus on the reasons that motivate parents, the non-enrolment requirement treats the intention/foresight distinction as morally relevant. Parents who allow their young child to engage in uninhibited dance knowing that she might later develop puritanical convictions that condemn dance as ungodly, do not thereby wrong their child. Even if her later rejection of the activities she pursues in childhood were foreseeable, that would not be sufficient to render her parents' conduct illegitimate. Anti-perfectionist childrearing objects to parenting that tries to shape the child's life in accordance with a particular religious doctrine, not indiscriminately to any upbringing that happens to involve the child engaging in activities that she may retrospectively reject.

Suppose, then, that the child is introduced to a range of different activities, including different kinds of sport, music, art, and literature. Part of the justification of that exposure appeals to the child's interest in developing the two moral powers reviewed above—a sense of justice and the wherewithal to lead an independent life. However, it is also the case that living within the particular background culture of a free society makes it inevitable that the child will experience a variety of those activities. Suppose, in addition, that her parents notice that their child is attracted to a certain activity and face the decision of whether to facilitate or encourage her pursuit of it. Of course, they will take various considerations into account, such as the nature and strength of the child's preferences, whether her pursuit of that particular activity needs to be balanced against other developmental considerations, risks to her psychological well-being (if the activity in question has a significant competitive element, for example), and so on. But in this story, there need be no violation of the non-enrolment constraint, because it is the child's preferences and her developmental needs that determine the shape of her childhood.

Anti-perfectionist childrearing is compatible with parenting that delivers the goods that some take to be distinctively good for children: a childhood involving adventure, play, and creativity. True, it does not justify such parenting on the grounds that it enhances the well-being of children. It is not obvious, however, how many of the intrinsic goods of childhood are lost in virtue of the impermissibility of enrolment. It appears that many of these goods—carefree, imaginative, and uninhibited play, for example—are goods that young children choose to pursue without any parental guidance. To the extent that that is the case, parents need only facilitate their pursuit and, perhaps, share their child's enthusiasms. The imposition of ends is not required. More needs to be said to flesh out the anti-perfectionist view of the child's advantage as a child, but I hope its central features are reasonably clear.

8.8 Too Negligent?

The final set of criticisms I shall consider develop those discussed above into a direct challenge to anti-perfectionist childrearing. The central objection is that it makes parental negligence a moral requirement. The proper role of parents is to act in ways that promote rather than neglect their children's long term flourishing. Because it sets out a principled objection to that conception of parenting, anti-perfectionist childrearing is mistaken.

For an illustration of the concern, consider the dispute about the teaching of Darwinian evolution as science. The public debate about that issue is whether the science curriculum in schools ought to give students the opportunity to learn about creationist and intelligent design theories as alternatives to Darwinian natural history. It appears to some that anti-perfectionist liberals who neither affirm nor deny the truth of particular religious conceptions of the world or universe must be committed to the view that public money should not be used to promote a sectarian irreligious conception of natural history. Critics insist that this case vividly reveals the counter-intuitive implications of this kind of liberal political morality. Not only are creationism and intelligent design demonstrably false, they claim, a schooling that presents them as a genuine alternatives to Darwinian accounts makes a mockery of science education and allows impressionable children to form the belief that scientific understanding can be gained from reading The Bible. Permitting those outcomes is, they insist, detrimental to individuals to the extent that holding veridical beliefs makes their lives go better, and worse for society in virtue of setting back the project of scientific progress, which enhances our collective ability to deal with many pressing problems.

Similar, perhaps stronger, objections of this kind might be raised against parental anti-perfectionism. The critic claims that parents have a weighty reason to attend to their child's interest in leading a flourishing life. Compliance with that reason supports imparting to their child an understanding of the methods and current state of scientific knowledge. Such an understanding is instrumentally beneficial for the child, for it enables her to form her beliefs and desires on the basis of reliable non-normative facts, and it is, for some, a constituent of living well. Since parents have a special and, arguably, very weighty reason to attend to their child's interests, it is surely a dereliction of their duty if they fail to take a stand on important issues such as the dispute between Darwinian and creationist conceptions of biological change. Parental anti-perfectionism does not merely permit parents to offer their child a non-scientific education, it requires parents not to take a stand on the debate between ID and Darwinian evolution as accounts of natural history. In other words, it requires parents not to promote their child's interests, or so the critic argues.

Parental anti-perfectionists might offer two responses to the charge that their view requires parents to neglect their child's interests. First, they might soften the objection by pointing out that while parents may not adopt and promote a controversial comprehensive doctrine, such as a particular religious or irreligious doctrine, they are permitted, perhaps morally required, to educate their child according to the requirements of public reason. In the context of the debate about natural history, for example, parents might have weighty reasons stemming from their duty to promote their child's sense of justice to provide an education in science that conforms to well-established standards of inquiry and knowledge. In that way, it might be that parents have reasons other than the promotion of her well-being to encourage their child to adopt certain true or justified beliefs.[11] To the extent that that is the case, the differences between anti-perfectionist and perfectionist accounts of childrearing are smaller than they might at first appear and the charge of negligence loses some of its force.

The softening response depends on the soundness of the claim that public reason requires an education that imparts an adequate understanding of biology and natural history, or at least one that denies the assertions of those who advance creationist or ID accounts. That response depends, in turn, on showing that one's responsibilities as a citizen are better fulfilled if one possesses a more accurate understanding of science. I lack the space to offer a complete justification of that claim. The prima facie case for it is that citizens are duty bound to attend to the interests of their fellow citizens with respect to health or energy, for example, and those interests are likely more effectively to be served through public institutions that are responsive to reliable science, just as individuals' interests in securing socioeconomic goods are better served if citizens' deliberative and electoral activity rests on good reasoning and evidence about society or the economy. Anti-perfectionists may take a stand on the soundness of claims that are relevant to our status or conduct as free and equal citizens.

The second response to the negligence claim is to bite some bullets. The softening response goes only so far, and it must be accepted that in some cases anti-perfectionist childrearing does indeed require parents to refrain from promoting their child's long term flourishing as much as they might. In that respect, parental anti-perfectionism is on a par with its political counterpart, which claims that it is impermissible for

---

[11] This is a familiar strategy within liberal thought. For an analogous argument for prohibiting trade on Sundays, see Mill ([1859] 2008: Ch. IV, par. 20).

citizens to use the legal powers of the state to advance the well-being of other citizens. Parents may hope that their child's life goes well, but respect for her independence limits the extent to which they can legitimately make that happen.[12]

References

Brighouse, H., & Swift, A. (2009). Legitimate parental partiality. *Philosophy and Public Affairs, 37*, 43–80.
Callan, E. (2002). Autonomy, child-rearing, and good lives. In D. Archard & C. Macleod (Eds.), *The morality and political status of children* (pp. 118–141). Oxford: Oxford University Press.
Cameron, C. (2012). Clayton on comprehensive enrolment. *Journal of Political Philosophy, 20*, 341–352.
Clayton, M. (2006). *Justice and legitimacy in upbringing*. Oxford: Oxford University Press.
Clayton, M. (2009). Reply to Morgan. *Studies in Philosophy and Education, 28*, 91–100.
Clayton, M. (2012). The case against the comprehensive enrolment of children. *Journal of Political Philosophy, 20*, 353–364.
Dworkin, R. (2011). *Justice for hedgehogs*. Cambridge, MA: Harvard University Press.
Feinberg, J. (1992). The child's right to an open future. In Feinberg (Ed.), *Freedom and fulfillment: Philosophical essays*. Princeton: Princeton University Press.
Fowler, T. (2010). The problems of liberal neutrality in upbringing. *Res Publica, 16*, 367–381.
Hannan, S. (2011). *Balancing parental authority and children's autonomy rights: A role-based solution*. Oxford: Oxford University D. Phil.
Locke, J. ([1690] 1988). In P. Laslett (Ed.), *Two treatises of government*. Cambridge: Cambridge University Press.
Macleod, C. (2010). Primary goods, capabilities, and children. In H. Brighouse & I. Robeyns (Eds.), *Measuring justice: Primary goods and capabilities* (pp. 174–192). Cambridge: Cambridge University Press.
McLaughlin, T. H. (1984). Parental rights and the religious upbringing of children. *Journal of Philosophy of Education, 18*, 75–82.
Mill, J.S. ([1859] 2008). In J. Gray (Ed.), *On liberty and other essays*. Oxford: Oxford University Press.
Morgan, J. (2009). Critical review of justice and legitimacy in upbringing. *Studies in Philosophy and Education, 28*, 79–89.
Parfit, D. (2011). *On what matters*. Oxford: Oxford University Press.
Rawls, J. (2006). *Political liberalism*, paperback edition. New York: Columbia University Press.
Raz, J. (1989). Facing up: A reply. *Southern California Law Review, 62*, 1153–1236.
Rousseau, J.-J. ([1762] 1978). In R. Masters (Ed.), *On the social contract*. New York: St. Martin's Press.
Scanlon, T. M. (2008). *Moral dimensions: Permissibility, meaning, blame*. Cambridge, MA: Harvard University Press.

---

[12] For their instructive written comments, I thank Alex Bagattini, Sarah Hannan, Colin Macleod, Tom Parr, and Andrew Williams. I am also grateful for valuable discussions with Paul Bou-Habib, Chiara Cordelli, Tim Fowler, Hugh Lazenby, R. J. Leland, Adam Swift, Debra Satz, Victor Tadros, and audiences in Oxford and Stanford.

Chapter 9
Respecting Children and Children's Dignity

Holger Baumann and Barbara Bleisch

9.1 Introduction

It is striking that the concept of human dignity is almost entirely absent from philosophical discussions about the ethics of childhood. This is all the more remarkable because human dignity plays a prominent role in debates about other vulnerable groups, such as demented, disabled or 'unborn' persons. Likewise, as a group, children are almost completely neglected in the ongoing discourse on the meaning and conceptualization of human dignity, while again, it is precisely vulnerable groups that are often taken into consideration by dignity theorists in order to test and sharpen their respective theories.

How can this be explained? Does it simply make no sense to speak of the 'dignity of the child'? Or is human dignity clearly applicable to children, but not in any particularly interesting way which would ask for an in-depth discussion regarding the dignity of the child? Or is the concept of human dignity simply not needed in discussions about how to treat and respect children – i.e. of no theoretical or practical use in debates concerning the ethics of childhood?

In this paper, we attempt to show that there is a meaningful way to speak of children's dignity, and that considering children as a group can also be illuminating for

---

H. Baumann (✉)
Centre for Ethics, University of Zürich, Zollikerstrasse 117, 8008 Zürich, Switzerland
e-mail: baumann@ethik.uzh.ch

B. Bleisch
Centre for Ethics, University of Zürich, Zollikerstrasse 115, 8008 Zürich, Switzerland
e-mail: bleisch@ethik.uzh.ch

dignity theorists who attempt to conceptualize what respect for (and violations of) human dignity amount to in general.[1] More importantly, we will argue that taking the concept of dignity into account in the ethics of childhood can enrich the debate, especially with regard to the question of what it means to *respect children*. In our view, these discussions remain incomplete if they are restricted to the concept of a child's well-being or her autonomy.

In order to develop our idea of filial dignity (on which we will build our idea of what it means to respect a child later in the paper), we will firstly elaborate on possible reasons why the debates on human dignity and the ethics of childhood have been conducted almost entirely separately (Sect. 9.2). In the main part of the paper, we will then – against this background – introduce our idea of filial dignity and illustrate it by looking at several cases of what we consider to be violations of children's dignity.[2] By drawing upon a proposal made by Norvin Richards,[3] we will maintain that respecting a child's dignity means above all respecting her *activity*, which is expressed by having and developing a *perspective of one's own*, and which is an essential prerequisite of developing an *identity* or *self*. In the course of our argumentation, we pay particular attention to distinguishing concerns about children's dignity from concerns about their well-being and their autonomy, and demonstrate how the notion of dignity helps to articulate certain concerns that cannot be captured adequately by these other notions (Sect. 9.3). In the last section, we will finally take a step back from the debate about the ethics of childhood and point to some possible conclusions for the debate about human dignity. We indicate how the understanding of human dignity that has evolved from our discussion of children's dignity could provide a fresh perspective on discussions about what it means to respect the dignity of demented or mentally impaired persons (Sect. 9.4).

9.2 Some General Concerns with Filial Dignity

There are several possible reasons why the notion of human dignity has been mostly neglected within debates about the ethics of childhood,[4] and why children as a group have been more or less ignored by dignity theorists so far. Our aim in scrutinizing some of these reasons is twofold: On the one hand, we would like to identify the (implicit) assumptions and views about dignity and/or about how children should be regarded and treated; on the other hand, we thereby want to map several challenges that must be met by anyone who wants to speak reasonably about filial dignity.

---

[1] It is often noted that the group of children is too diverse to constitute a homogenous group. In the following, we will be particularly concerned with children of the age around 2–12 years, for reasons that will hopefully become clear in the course of the paper.

[2] The negative-inductive approach to human dignity, which starts from looking at paradigmatic examples of violations of human dignity, is explicitly defended by Stoecker (2010).

[3] Richards (2011).

[4] One noteworthy exception is Giesinger (2012).

Let us begin, then, with an investigation of what we take to be the most important reasons why the notion of dignity is very seldom referred to within discussions about the ethics of childhood: *First*, we believe that this neglect is at least partly due to the *widespread general scepticism* about the very concept of human dignity. Many philosophers share the concern that human dignity is a notoriously vague notion that has no distinct content at all and is, therefore, particularly prone to ideological abuse. Several authors have argued that the whole 'dignity-talk' either obstructs rational discussions on what we owe to each other and what we are allowed to inflict upon others; or that the concept of dignity can be substituted without loss of content with clearer notions such as 'autonomy' or 'moral rights'.[5] The reference to the notion of dignity in the U.N. convention on the rights of the child,[6] (rare) references to it in the philosophical literature about children,[7] as well as (frequent) references to it by children funds and relief organisations for children, might even nourish this scepticism, because the concept of filial dignity is more often used as a rhetorical device or political key word than as a systematically elaborated concept. *Second*, and relatedly, we suppose that most philosophers working on the ethics of childhood might think that the concept of human dignity is just *unnecessary*. They can point to increasingly detailed and sophisticated debates about the well-being and the autonomy of children during the last decades, and question that there are, in fact, any practically relevant cases that cannot be addressed within the already established framework. In their view, the concept of human dignity simply adds nothing of theoretical and practical value to the existing debates.

Taken together, these doubts about the general concept of dignity or its relevance with regard to children provide an important challenge to anyone who wants to insert the notion of dignity into the ethics of childhood, and to thereby enrich its moral vocabulary: The notion of dignity has to be given distinct and specific content; it has to be clearly distinguished from other notions such as well-being or autonomy; and it has to be shown that there are relevant cases that cannot be adequately dealt with without invoking the notion of dignity.

Turning now to the question of why dignity theorists have mostly neglected children as a group, we believe that there are two very different explanations at hand. This can be brought into focus by drawing on some linguistic evidence: It seems that some find it rather natural to speak of children's dignity, while others think that it is artificial and only a manner of speech or a rhetorical device to emphasize the abomination treating children in certain ways. These diverging linguistic intuitions can be traced back to two different understandings of human dignity.[8] Against their

---

[5] Cf. Macklin (2003); Pinker (2008). A similar critique has been raised with regard to the 'rights-talk' which is sometimes used as a rhetorical means without elaborating on the proper normative foundations of moral rights.

[6] Cf. UN Convention on the Rights of Children (1989); for a commentary, which does not really clarify the meaning of dignity in the UN Convention, see Melton (1991).

[7] For an example see George (2009); Reed et al. (2003) attempt to give dignity a clear meaning, but their contribution illustrates rather how diversely the concept of dignity is used.

[8] Cf. Dworkin (1994).

background, two further reasons can be given why even dignity theorists – who believe that the notion can, in principle, be given a clear meaning and is indispensable in certain normative domains – have not paid much attention to children and filial dignity until now.

On the first understanding, the notion of human dignity designates the inherent value of human beings or the 'sanctity of human life'.[9] If one holds such an inherent value account of dignity, the reason why children have been neglected so far is rather obvious. Since every human being is said to have human dignity, and since there is no disagreement that children belong to the class of human beings, children as a group are just not *particularly interesting*. Proponents of such a 'human-centred' understanding of human dignity are above all interested in creatures at the border of human life, and in questions about life and death – e.g. when does human life (in a morally significant sense) begin and when does it end?

In recent discussions, this understanding of human dignity as inherent value has received much criticism: it is asked, e.g., in virtue of what are human beings attributed dignity? If this attribution is explained by reference to the human species only, one seems to commit either a naturalistic fallacy, or to fall back into a highly contested speciesism. Moreover, what follows from such a broad conception of human dignity is dubious. On the one hand, it seems to be rather difficult to cover paradigmatic cases of violations of dignity, such as torture or humiliation, because it is at least unclear how their inherent value is violated by such acts. On the other hand, every act of killing or letting die seems to constitute a violation of dignity, according to such accounts, and this is regarded as rather counterintuitive and normatively inadequate by many. Furthermore, the notion of human dignity seems to be redundant and unnecessary in such a theoretical framework, because it may be reduced to the view that human beings have inherent value or that human life is sacred; there is, thus, no need to add yet another concept.[10]

Drawing on these and related criticisms, a different understanding of human dignity has become predominant in recent debates that can be labelled as *'personhood accounts of human dignity'*. These accounts relate dignity to some kind of personhood or agency of human beings. Human beings are then said to have dignity because they are – to mention just the most prominent proposals – able to claim rights,[11] to provide justifications for their actions,[12] to govern their own lives autonomously,[13] or to have self-respect.[14] The dignity of a person is, accordingly, violated if she is treated as if she is not a legitimate maker of claims, not owed any justification for what is inflicted upon her, not allowed to exercise control over

---

[9] Cf. Kass (2002).

[10] Cf. Waldron (2012) who argues against accounts of dignity as inherent value.

[11] Cf. Feinberg (1970).

[12] Cf. Forst (2009).

[13] Cf. Griffin (1998) (dignity as autonomous agency) and Schaber (2010) (dignity as having normative authority).

[14] Cf. Margalit (1996); Stoecker (2003).

important domains of her life, or if her self-respect is violated by acts of humiliation or degradation.

In our view, defenders of personhood accounts fare much better with regard to the criticism applicable to defenders of 'inherent value-accounts'. Human dignity is linked to certain normatively relevant properties or abilities of human beings and is thus not arbitrarily ascribed; proponents of such accounts can provide rich explanations why, e.g., torture, humiliation or slavery are considered to be paradigmatic violations of dignity; and they are careful to give the notion of human dignity a specific and irreducible content. In other words, defenders of personhood accounts attempt to give a sound foundation and justification of dignity, and their approaches are specific enough to capture paradigmatic cases of violations of dignity.

Within personhood accounts, children are not neglected because they are uninteresting as a group. The reason why children are not paid much attention is rather that the concept of human dignity seems to be not (yet) applicable to them. Children are neither able to claim rights, nor to respect the claims of others reciprocally and exchange reasons for their actions; nor they are able to autonomously govern their lives. More generally, they are not aware of their own dignity, and of the dignity of others, and thus they cannot be violated in their dignity, so it is argued.

While personhood accounts can do justice to paradigmatic cases of violations of dignity, and at least attempt to give the notion of dignity a distinct and specific content, the exclusion of children reveals what many consider to be a specific weakness of such accounts: they tend to be exclusive in that they are only applicable to *adult* humans, whilst other human beings that do not yet (or no longer) fulfill the necessary personhood conditions are excluded from having dignity. In other words, personhood accounts are often criticised for failing to meet the adequacy condition that the concept of human dignity should be applicable to *all* human beings, including old and mentally impaired persons as well as children.

In light of the above considerations, the following general challenge can be formulated: anyone who wants to bring together the debates about the ethics of childhood and about human dignity has to show that the notion of human dignity can be meaningfully applied to children without resorting to an understanding of dignity that is too vague to be of any normative relevance or that falls back into a highly controversial naturalistic view of human dignity. Furthermore, it has to be shown that the notion of dignity that is formulated in the light of these challenges is of theoretical and practical value to the debates about the ethics of childhood.

9.3 Children's Dignity: Being Active and Relating to the World

As mentioned above, personhood accounts relate human dignity to certain capacities that are regarded as normatively relevant and that are distinctive to certain ways of existing. The concept of a 'person' is thus, in this context, always and from the very beginning a normative concept. These theories come in different varieties, and they have various advantages as compared to theories which interpret human dignity as inherent value (see above). But for whichever type of personhood account one is opting, certain human beings are excluded from having dignity. Children, as a case in point, do not have (or have not yet developed) the relevant normative capacities – dignity, thus, cannot be ascribed to them, and children cannot be violated in their dignity respectively.

In the following, we attempt to show that this line of argument is not convincing and that the notion of dignity can also be applied to children, without falling back into an account of dignity that is too broad or vague to be of any practical and theoretical relevance. In a nutshell, we will argue that the basic (and plausible) idea underlying personhood accounts can be reconstructed in a way that opens up the possibility of also applying the notion of dignity to children. In this regard, we maintain that the crucial principle of personhood is a certain concept of *activity*:[15] persons are persons, and have dignity, due to the fact that they are in a specific way active rather than passive. This characteristic trait of being active is accompanied by having and developing a *perspective of one's own*. To our view, it is precisely because human beings are active and have a perspective of their own that they are owed respect for their dignity – that we should not treat persons as mere things or as puppets. Being active and having a perspective are thus normatively relevant, because they prohibit us from treating beings with these capacities in ways that deny that they are *persons*.

This prohibition is, of course, anchored in the different varieties of personhood accounts mentioned above. However, none of these accounts explicitly declares 'activity' as the core idea of personhood; and all of them understand activity in a very narrow way that is informed by the specific ways in which *adults* are active, e.g. by being able to claim rights, by governing their lives autonomously, or having self-respect. Whilst we believe that there is something essentially right about personhood accounts of dignity, we want to argue that common accounts improperly focus on very specific and limited ways of being active and of having a perspective of one's own. By adopting a broader concept of activity, we will make room for the relevant alignments we emphasized above.

Let us, against this background, start by having a closer look at what we mean by 'activity' and 'perspectiveness' as core features of personhood: Being a person means, in our view, having a perspective on the world; experiencing oneself as *regarding* the world and not only as *being a mere part of it*. One feature of perspectiveness is, thus, capturing the 'first person-perspective': viewing the world from a standpoint and thereby relating to the world. The second feature of perspectiveness comprises *developing an identity* or a *self*: experiencing oneself as someone who has not only impressions, but also convictions, interpretations and carings. Perspectiveness in this sense enables human beings to come into action, to influence what is happening 'out there' and to shape the life of which they are part. We contend that this is exactly what makes 'persons': they are able and strive to experience

---

[15] As we have already mentioned, we draw upon a suggestion made by Norvin Richards, whose account we will explain and put into perspective below.

themselves as part of the world, but also as divided from the world – since they are capable of changing and impacting on their surroundings and relationships. Perspectiveness is, thus, the prerequisite of being active; of shaping and mapping one's life and not only of coping with what life brings to you. Respecting the dignity of persons and also of children means, in general terms, to treat them as active beings who already have, and actively strive for having a perspective of their own and who need to be supported in this endeavour.

In order to elaborate on this general idea of what it means to respect children's dignity, let us introduce a somewhat similar proposal that has been put forward by Norvin Richards.[16] In developing his account, Richards draws on the case of a 14-year-old boy suffering from a deadly failure of the respiratory system. His parents decide together with an expert panel to refrain from further treatment, and the discontinuation of treatment is considered to be in the 'best interest' of the affected boy. The boy, however, is neither involved in the decision making process, nor informed about his state of health. As Richards points out, this preclusion is usually justified in the following way: Firstly, the boy's parents fear that the information about the approaching death would stress the boy too heavily; and secondly, the boy is not able to understand the complex information sufficiently. His decision with regard to treatment would therefore not be competent.

Both arguments are, of course, worth considering and controversial. With regard to the first argument, which points to welfarist considerations and aims at establishing that the boy is harmed in addition to his already poor condition, it can be asked whether the boy is really harmed by receiving the information about his condition, and of what exactly this harm consists. It seems true that coping with dreadful news is a hard task for every individual – for children as well as for adult persons. But we nevertheless believe that, in general, persons have a right to be informed (about important matters regarding themselves), independently of whether the information is good or bad. Defenders of the welfarist argument must thus explain why the boy, in contrast to adult persons, should not have a right to be informed about his situation. As to the second argument, it could be questioned whether children really lack autonomy. Especially with regard to teenagers from the age of 15 years on, it seems rather narrow-minded to conceive of autonomy as being applicable to adults only, since teenagers do generally seem to be able to fulfill the conditions that are demanded of adult persons.

Richards does not engage with these discussions about the meaning and importance of well-being and autonomy, but rather assumes that withholding the information from the boy can be justified along these lines. However, he does believe that some wrong is done to the boy by withholding information, and at this point introduces his notion of dignity. According to Richard, the boy has a right to adequate and honest information because he is entitled to experience his situation adequately and to interpret what is happening to him. Only by perceiving and interpreting his situation on his own can the boy escape being a mere bystander to his own dying. And, according to Richards, this is what respect for dignity demands. He states:

---

[16] Cf. Richards (2011).

"Insofar as the source of human dignity is our ability to be *active* rather than passive, our interpretive way of experiencing is a source of that dignity."[17] He thus relates human dignity to being active, and he understands this activity as an *interpretative capacity and way of living*. Respecting the dignity of children means, on this view, to take seriously the fact that children are beings who are capable of experiencing and interpreting the world by themselves.

Richards' argumentation resembles the line of argument we want to put forward, and his emphasis on the capacities of *experiencing* and *interpreting* the world as relevant to a child's dignity is illuminating and helps to give content to our general idea of the importance of a person's being active and developing a perspective of her own. Partly due to his example, however, Richard's account seems to be incomplete in defining what it means to respect children's dignity: First, Richard provides no guidance in how to distinguish between cases in which it is permissible (and not a violation of dignity) to withhold information or to 'bypass' the interpretive capacities of a child, and those cases in which it is not. Second, withholding information is just one way to violate children's dignity, as we will illustrate by discussing further examples below. Third, Richards' account remains fragmentary insofar as he considers only the epistemic dimension of interpreting the world or of perspectiveness. But perspectiveness comprises an *epistemic* as well as an *evaluative dimension:* by the first, we mean that persons and even young children can (and strive to) get a grasp on the world, to understand it as a sound system and an understandable and secure interplay of actions and incidents. By the evaluative dimension, we bear in mind that even children from very early on begin to care about persons or things, they attempt to understand the rules that guide interpersonal relations, and aim to build up relationships on their own. With regard to both dimensions, having and developing a perspective of one's own is a prerequisite to being active; only from a perspective are we able to find epistemic and evaluative orientation. In order to flesh out this still vague idea, let us have a closer look at further examples.

What Richards objects to – i.e. that children's dignity is disrespected by neglecting their specific ways of being active – is not limited to the case of withholding information. One important case in point is the common practice of habitually lying to children. As a recent study with parents in the US and China has shown, a vast majority of parents lie to their children regularly to obtain behavioral compliance. The practice of lying most frequently takes the form of falsely threatening to leave a child alone in public if he or she refuses to follow the parent.[18] Parental lying is often due to considerable stress associated with the child's noncompliance. Other parents lie to their children when they feel the truth would be too difficult for them to understand, such as concerning the family budget. Still other parents appear to be focused on the immediate goals they hope to achieve. Lying is, thus, seen by many

---

[17] Cf. ibid.
[18] Cf. e.g. Heyman/Hsu/Fu/Lee (2012).

as an appropriate means to an end.[19] The study leaves open the question when, if ever, parental lying is justified, but indicates there is a need for further research.[20]

In our view, habitually lying to children amounts *(prima facie)* to undermining their activity and is thus a violation of their dignity. Lying means eroding a child's standpoint because she cannot have and develop a perspective of her own without understanding the world in an ordered manner – which is impossible if the world is presented to her in a way that is incomprehensible and unsteady, and that precludes experiencing and interpreting the world as it is. In this way, a child becomes a mere bystander who is passive with regard to her surroundings, left far behind in ignorance, in an unsecure world which is not understandable, but rather hostile in its erratic and enigmatic disorder. Since children are very dependent upon others to have and develop their own standpoint, they are particularly vulnerable in their ability to grasp the world.[21] For this reason, lying to them, and thereby treating them as if they were passive beings that do not have a perspective of their own, constitutes a violation of their dignity. Similar considerations apply to the case in which parents take an *overly protective* attitude towards their children, by shutting them off from having new experiences or by constantly correcting their interpretations of the world. Doing so amounts to treating children as if they were puppets instead of conscious beings that strive to understand the world on their own.

Of course, we do not want to argue that lying to children or protecting them from having certain experiences is always a violation of their dignity.[22] This refers back to the question we have raised with regard to Richards' account: How are we to distinguish cases in which it is permitted to withhold information (to lie to children or shut them off from making certain experiences) from cases in which this constitutes a violation of their dignity? As we have already mentioned, children are particularly vulnerable with regard to relating to the world actively and developing their own standpoint. This means that we should refrain from distorting their activity by making it impossible for them to get a grasp of the world. The important point to note, however, is that in certain cases lying to children or withholding information is precisely a means to secure this very activity. If parents know that their child is unable to cope with certain information or experiences, because it cannot (yet) process these and relate it to other experiences or information, exposing it to such

---

[19] Cf. ibid. p.7.

[20] Cf. ibid. p.8.

[21] Since adult persons normally have internalized this experience and security, it is not possible to lie to them as it is with regard to children. Grown-ups are able to align new information to a stable picture of beliefs; they are not daunted so easily. Children, by contrast, live in a threshold region between a growing picture of 'reality' and fantasy. Habitually lying to children thus incapacitates them and holds them back in this childlike threshold region.

[22] One might argue, for example, that it is certainly permitted to tell children the story of Santa Claus or the myth of Easter bunny. Whether upholding such traditions and rituals – which seem to be part of our culture and belong, at least for many, to infancy – is tantamount to lying is open to dispute. But even if this was the case, this type of lie is different from the examples above. Such 'cultural lies' are better described as 'social games' comparable to organising by surprise a birthday party for a friend.

information/experiences may distort its ability to comprehend the world. Neglecting the child and its vulnerability by letting it have experiences that it cannot yet integrate can thus amount to a violation of its dignity, too. Respecting children's dignity thus demands that we treat children as beings who are capable of encountering the world from their own perspective, but who are particularly prone to lose hold of reality and lose orientation.

Admittedly, it is not always easy to decide this matter. A case in point is the example that Richards puts at the centre of his discussion: Is it justified to withhold the information from the boy, because it will distort his activity and erode his own perspective, or should he be informed about his condition for reasons of respect for dignity? While we refrain from giving a definite answer to this question, the important point to note is that already by *asking* the question this way, an important *additional* concern is introduced into the discussion. Whether we should provide the boy with the information is no longer only a question that needs to be discussed in the light of (contested views about) his well-being or autonomy, but also with reference to the idea of dignity. Similar considerations apply to the case of lying: If we ask whether and in which cases lying to children is justified, we should not only dwell on questions about what good (or harm) is done by lying, or whether the autonomy of the child is violated. We should also ask first and foremost whether it amounts to a violation of their dignity by disregarding their specific ways of being active. Thinking about the issue in this way is, in our view, illuminating with regard to the moral discussion about this matter, and our considerations point towards a rather revisionary assessment of this common practice: if our argument is convincing, it could be argued that lying to children *always* calls for a *specific* justification that addresses concerns about their dignity.

Up to this point, we have talked only about children's ability to find orientation and get a grasp of the world. We now turn to another example that focuses on the *evaluative dimension of perspectiveness*, i.e. to the question of what it means to respect children's dignity with regard to their evaluative activity and standpoint. This dimension is not covered by Richards' account, since he is specifically concerned with providing information and with the related capacities to experience and interpret the 'state' of the world.

In general, many philosophers believe that (at least young) children cannot be respected in their evaluative activity, in their decisions and desires, because they are not yet autonomous. For example, Robert Noggle has argued that children lack a stable and temporally extended evaluative perspective,[23] and Tamar Shapiro has portrayed children as being driven by sheer impulses and having no evaluative standpoint of their own.[24] They thus challenge the claim that children have an authentic self. Such a self they regard as necessary in order for one to act or decide autonomously. Others have pointed out that children are not competent, since they cannot take a reflective stance towards their attitudes and since they cannot understand and

---

[23] Cf. Noggle (2002).
[24] Cf. Shapiro (2003).

process relevant information in order to arrive at self-determined decisions (see above).

We have already indicated that the question whether children are to be respected in their autonomy is a controversial matter. Although we cannot enter these discussions here in detail, we think that there are good reasons to question recent attempts to ascribe autonomy even to young children:[25] In our view, such views run the risk of overstretching the concept of autonomy, and thereby are in danger to lose hold of its distinctive content. We thus believe that philosophers should not rely too heavily on the concept of autonomy when it comes to young children.[26] However, the conclusion that it makes no sense to respect children's decisions or their evaluative stance can still be criticized as unjustified: similar to cases of withholding information and habitually lying to children, it can be argued that not taking children's decisions or evaluative perspective seriously amounts to a violation of their dignity.

Building upon a proposal by Agnieszka Jaworska,[27] and relating it to our idea of what it means to respect children's dignity, we want to stress that children can indeed exhibit evaluative activities and take an evaluative standpoint that demands our respect. Jaworska argues that even young children do already care about other persons or things. She thereby departs from the views of other theorists like Harry Frankfurt, David Velleman or Michael Bratman who believe that caring about something necessarily entails that a person reflectively identifies with the object of her caring. Jaworska claims that to care about something just means that a certain attitude is expressive of a person's perspective, irrespective of whether she is consciously aware of this fact or not: "It simply asserts that a child's caring always represents the child's point of view as an agent."[28] In addition to caring about something, children also exhibit evaluative activity when they, e.g., try to understand rules that are given to them, or when they form evaluative beliefs about certain matters (often implicitly).

Examples of violating children's dignity with regard to their evaluative activity are easy to find, and they seem – as in the case of habitually lying or withholding information from children – quite common: For example, it is often the case that parents only comply with the wishes and desires of their children if these accord with their view of what is good for their children. Harry Brighouse has contended, along these lines, that children's views are not authoritative for parents, but only of consultative value: they help parents to better understand what is good for their children.[29] In our view, however, respect for dignity *prima facie* demands that even if this is not the case, what children care about deserves

---

[25] Cf. e.g. Mullin (2007).

[26] This is why we have confined the group of children to those from the age between 2 and 12 years at the beginning of our paper.

[27] Cf. Jaworksa (2007).

[28] Cf. ibid.: p. 536.

[29] Cf. Brighouse (2003); for an interesting discussion that tries to reconcile the best interests of children with the child's view, see Archard and Skivenes (2009).

to be taken seriously. To do otherwise means treating children as puppets or beings with no perspectives of their own.

One instructive example of not taking seriously the fact that children can already be active with regard to what they do and what they value is the debate about the so-called 'Tiger Moms'. It goes back to a book by Chinese mother Amy Chua,[30] in which she describes her exceedingly demanding parenting style as typically Chinese and most notably superior to Western parenting styles. The book depicts how author Chua forced her two daughters to practice the violin or the piano for hours, persisting even during holidays; or how she demanded they achieve top grades at school and forbid them to watch TV, skype or chat on the internet. Chinese parents are better at raising children than Western parents, Chua claims, because applying the demanding Eastern parenting model empowers children to display their talents, to endure suffering and to ultimately succeed in life. The permissive Western style, in contrast, indulges children and eventually discourages them since children have not experienced true mastery, or so Chua argues.

The book created a huge public dispute about parenting styles and the aims of education. The opponents of the book blamed the author for being an obsessively controlling and unloving mother, citing revealing passages such as when Chua threatened to burn her older daughter's stuffed animals if the child didn't improve her piano playing, or when she refused to let her child leave the piano to use the bathroom or even slapped her for playing poorly. It goes without saying that, from a moral point of view, such educational methods cannot be approved by any means: parents are strictly forbidden to beat their children or to chastise them by prohibiting the use of the toilet. Welfarists would criticize these methods as would proponents of autonomy-based accounts.[31]

In contrast to our former examples of withholding information from children or lying to them, the notion of dignity thus does not seem to be required in order to morally condemn these educational practices. What we want to stress, however, is that framing this discussion in the light of concerns about dignity helps to shed a different, and in our view more adequate, perspective on this discussion. We have argued so far that a child needs to be encouraged to find a perspective of her own, meaning to understand herself as distinct from the world and as an individual person who cares about things and persons she values dearly. Only through this double sense of perspectiveness will a child remain active and confident that she can influence the world and unfold trustfully. But perspectiveness is essentially about finding a standpoint and setting goals of one's own. By contrast, Amy Chua sets the goals for her daughters, and she contends that she regards her daughter as deficient because she prefers tennis to the violin. In our view, the problem with success-obsessed parents is, first and foremost, that they define what success is: it is not about having a lot of friends, training on the skate board or reading Harry Potter, but about well-respected hobbies and being accepted to attend highly ranked schools.

---

[30] Chua (2011).

[31] Even Chua herself conceded later that she exaggerated. Cf. e.g. Chang (2013).

The point we want to draw from this example is that although children are also violated in their well-being or their (future) autonomy by some educational practices, what seems crucial is that raising children in such a way means to treat them as puppets, as beings who are not active and who do not already possess and strive for a perspective of their own. When Amy Chua writes: "What Chinese parents understand is that nothing is fun until you're good at it", she is mistaken for several reasons: Nothing is fun until you *engage* with it, until you become a part of the activity you care about.[32] More importantly, even if children, such as Amy Chua's daughter, approve of their upbringing retrospectively, this does not constitute a sound justification for these practices. By raising children in such a way, they are not given due respect *as children*, who are already active and strive to develop their own perspective.

Again, we do not want to claim that it always constitutes a violation of children's dignity to disregard some of their decisions or to guide them away from certain things that they care about. In this connection, the approval with which some reacted to Amy Chua's book is instructive. Some pointed to the fact that what Chua called the Western style of parenting involves mainly a 'laissez faire' which is indulging instead of empowering, and that most children in Western societies simply waste their talents because their parents shirk responsibility, out of an ill-conceived idea of respect. In our view, it is important to guide children in their evaluative activity, because – as with regard to getting a grasp on the world – they are vulnerable to lose hold and to become distorted in their very activity.

However, the justification that is provided in such cases should take into account concerns about children's dignity, and are not exhausted by reasons of well-being or (future) autonomy. They should be about respecting and securing children's ability of being active, and about helping children to find a stable evaluative standpoint.[33] By including such considerations, a rather basic moral aspect of the situation is brought into focus that is surprisingly often neglected.

9.4 Filial Dignity and the Dignity of Persons

The central aim of this paper was to introduce the notion of human dignity into the debate on the ethics of childhood and to show that adding the concept of dignity enriches these debates in an important way. By analyzing some possible reasons why the notion of dignity has been mostly absent from the ethics of childhood so far, and why dignity theorists have neglected the children as a group up to now, we have formulated several challenges that must be met by any conception of filial dignity: On the one hand, such a conception has to give the notion of dignity a distinct

---

[32] Cf. Marano (2008).

[33] For a comprehensive account of what it means for children to remain active and for parents to foster their children's activity by motivating them to engage in projects of their own, see Betzler (2011).

content, provide it with a sound justification and relate it to a general and plausible idea of human dignity; on the other hand, it has to be shown that such a conception captures something important with regard to children that cannot already be adequately covered by other concepts such as welfare or autonomy.

We have then suggested that the most promising and plausible accounts of human dignity, namely personhood accounts, can and should be modified and expanded in a way that makes room for children. Our argument has taken the following form: the basic idea underlying all personhood accounts is that human beings are active rather than passive and possess a perspective of their own. Being a person therefore means experiencing oneself as being actively involved in the world by adopting a perspective. It is precisely these features which demand that we do not treat persons and also children as puppets or things. By asking for and identifying the specific ways in which children are active rather than passive and aim at finding orientation and a perspective of their own, it is possible to identify what constitutes violations of their dignity. The argument opens up interesting perspectives about practices such as withholding information from children, habitually lying to them, being overly protective towards children, or raising children according to very strict and entirely future-oriented life plans and rules.

While we have not tried to provide definite answers to the complex questions about the moral permissibility of these practices, we have stressed that concerns about dignity are both distinct from concerns about well-being and autonomy, and they are practically relevant: If we ask whether respect is given to the ways in which children are active, we pay attention to an important moral aspect of the situation that is not captured by welfarist or autonomy accounts yet. At least with regard to the examples given in the paper, expressing worries about withholding information, lying to children or raising them like tiger-mom Amy Chau seem to be more adequately captured by drawing upon the notion of filial dignity that we have developed throughout the paper, than drawing upon the notions of welfare or autonomy.

In conclusion, we finally want to take a step back from the debate about the ethics of childhood, and to briefly consider what lessons can be learnt from taking children as a group into consideration when thinking about the notion of human dignity. As we have emphasized at several points, personhood accounts do not only exclude children, but also demented and disabled persons from having dignity. This is a problematic shortcoming. The account we put forward in this paper builds upon the basic idea of personhood accounts – that dignity is related to the idea of humans beings as active rather than passive – but emphasizes the specific ways in which persons are active. This allows for also including persons who are, e.g., not fully autonomous or do not possess self-consciousness yet. Children as well as demented or disabled persons are also active and have a perspective of their own, and these demand our respect.[34]

---

[34] One could argue that our account of human dignity still excludes children born with anencephaly from having dignity, and that this exclusion seems rather counterintuitive. It is true that even though the concept of human dignity put forward in this paper is more inclusive than previous personhood accounts, it does not include human beings who are not considered as persons. But this

One advantage of our account and the above argumentation is precisely that it facilitates and clarifies discussions about what it means to respect demented or disabled persons. While these persons are (like children) not able to govern themselves autonomously, to stand up for their rights or to provide justifications for their conduct, they are (again, like children) beings who are in specific ways active and who have a perspective of their own. When it comes to the question of how to treat such persons, we thus propose that it is necessary and productive to consider whether, and in what ways, their ways of being active can be respected and fostered. Instead of regarding demented persons as beings who have lost their dignity because they no longer have certain agential capacities, and instead of treating them as beings who only need to be taken care of, respect for dignity demands that we are attentive to their ways of being active and encourage them to remain active rather than passive.[35]

References

Archard, D., & Skivenes, M. (2009). Balancing a child's best interests and a child's views. *International Journal of Children's Rights, 17*, 1–21.

Betzler, M. (2011). Erziehung zur Autonomie als Elternpflicht. *Deutsche Zeitschrift für Philosophie, 59*, 1–17.

Brighouse, H. (2003). How should children be heard? *Arizona Law Review, 45*(3), 691–711.

Chang, E. (2013). Amy Chua's 'Battle Hymn of the Tiger Mother'. Washington Post 7.11.2011. http://www.washingtonpost.com/wp-dyn/content/article/2011/01/07/AR2011010702516.html. Accessed 15 Apr 2013.

Chua, A. (2011). *Battle hymn of the tiger mother*. New York: Penguin.

Dworkin, R. (1994). *Life's dominion. An argument about abortion, euthanasia, and individual freedom*. New York: Knopf.

Feinberg, J. (1970). The nature and value of rights. *Journal of Value Inquiry, 4*, 263–267.

Forst, R. (2009). Der Grund der Kritik. Zum Begriff der Menschenwürde in sozialen Rechtfertigungsordnungen. In R. Jaeggi & Th. Wesche (Eds.), *Was ist Kritik?* (pp. 150–164). Frankfurt a.M.: Suhrkamp.

George, S. (2009). *Too young for respect? Realising respect for young children in their everyday environments: A cross-cultural analysis*. http://www.bernardvanleer.org/Too_young_for_respect_Realising_respect_for_young_children_in_their_everyday_environments_A_cross_cultural_analysis. Accessed 15 Apr 2013.

Giesinger, J. (2012). Respect in education. *Journal of Philosophy of Education, 46*, 100–112.

Griffin, J. (1998). *On human rights*. Oxford: Oxford University Press.

---

is exactly what characterizes personhood accounts: they link the normatively relevant features of a human person to human dignity. But this is by no means to say that beings suffering from anencephaly do not count morally. Of course, there are ways of treating such beings that are morally wrong and should not be inflicted upon them. But to label every moral wrong inflicted upon others as a violation of dignity leads to an overexpansion of the concept of dignity and undermines its conceptual strength in the end. (Thanks for this critical remark to Alexander Bagattini und Colin Macleod.)

[35] For helpful comments, thanks to Andreas Maier, Sebastian Muders, Peter Schaber, and, especially, to the editors of the volume, Alexander Bagattini and Colin Macleod.

Heyman, G., Hsu, A. S., Fu, G., Lee, K. (2012). Instrumental lying by parents in the US and China. *International Journal of Psychology*, 1–9, ifirst.
Jaworska, A. (2007). Caring and internality. *Philosophy and Phenomenological Research, LXXIV*(3), 529–568.
Kass, L. (2002). *Life, liberty and the defense of dignity.* San Francisco: Encounter Books.
Macklin, R. (2003). Dignity is a useless concept. *British Medical Journal, 327*, 1419–1420.
Marano, H. E. (2008). *A nation of wimps. The high cost of invasive parenting.* New York: Crown Archetype.
Margalit, A. (1996). *The decent society.* Cambridge: Harvard University Press.
Melton, G. (1991). Preserving the dignity of children around the world: The U.N. convention on the rights of the child. *Child Abuse and Neglect: The International Journal, 15*(4), 343–350.
Mullin, A. (2007). Children, autonomy, and care. *Journal of Philosophy, 38*(4), 536–553.
Noggle, R. (2002). Special agents: Children's autonomy and parental authority. In D. Archard & C. M. Macleod (Eds.), *The moral and political status of children* (pp. 97–117). Oxford: Oxford University Press.
Pinker, S. (2008). The stupidity of dignity. *The New Republic* May 28, 2008, online: http://www.tnr.com/article/the-stupidity-dignity. Accessed 15 Apr 2013.
Reed, P., Smith, P., Fletcher, M., & Bradding, A. (2003). Promoting the dignity of the child in hospital. *Nursing Ethics, 10*, 67–76.
Richards, N. (2011). What shall we tell the children? (unpublished manuscript).
Schaber, P. (2010). *Menschenwürde und Instrumentalisierung.* Paderborn: Mentis.
Shapiro, T. (2003). Childhood and personhood. *Arizona Law Review, 45*(3), 575–594.
Stoecker, R. (2003). Menschenwürde und das Paradox der Entwürdigung. In R. Stoecker (Ed.), *Menschenwürde. Annäherung an einen Begriff* (pp. 133–151). Wien: öbv&hpt.
Stoecker, R. (2010). Three crucial turns on the road to an adequate understanding of human dignity. In P. Kaufmann, H. Kuch, C. Neuhäuser, & E. Webster (Eds.), *Humiliation, degradation, dehumanization: Human dignity violated* (pp. 7–19). Dordrecht: Springer.
United Nations General Assembly. (1989). Text of the UN convention on the rights of the child. http://www.ohchr.org/en/professionalinterest/pages/crc.aspx
Waldron, J. (2012). *Dignity, rank, and rights.* Oxford: University Press.

Chapter 10
Who Decides?

James G. Dwyer

10.1 Introduction

Child rearing has been a focus of attention for many political theorists in recent decades. Their specific preoccupation has been with situations in which religious beliefs lead parents to make child rearing decisions that the state deems contrary to children's well-being. Such conflicts between parents and the state over child rearing practices and choices raise the basic question: "Who decides?" – that is, whose view of children's welfare should control? Relatedly, who should hold ultimate power to determine important aspects of children's lives such as whether and how they will be schooled or whether and what kind of medical care they will receive? Discussion of this fundamental question of ultimate authority over children's lives has been severely limited, however, in several ways that I endeavor to correct in this Chapter.

First, there are the mundane deficiencies of oversight and over-simplification. Many people who stake a position in academic and popular debates over parent-state conflicts do not recognize or care to address the question of who should have ultimate decision making authority. Others raise the question only to answer it with unhelpful rhetoric like "children are not their parents' property," "parents know best," or "the child is not the mere creature of the state," or with bald assertions about natural law.

Second, many who wade further into the debate limit their attention to ideological differences between religious parents and the secular (or secularist, in the view of some) state as to specific aspects of children's governance and care. They do not recognize that the question actually arises in every context in which the state

J.G. Dwyer (✉)
Admission Office, William & Mary Law School,
P.O. Box 8795, Williamsburg, VA 23187-8795, USA
e-mail: jgdwye@wm.edu

(or anyone, really) disapproves of a parent's (or any other person's, really) treatment of or choices regarding a child. Other such contexts include the more common run-of-the-mill child abuse and neglect; one could ask also as to, for example, parents who because of drug addiction do not feed their children: "Who should have ultimate authority to determine whether not feeding a child is acceptable?" Indeed, the question also arises in connection with the prior question of who will be a child's legal parents and custodians. Thoughtful examination of the question "Who decides?" should begin with a more complete view of child rearing issues, one that encompasses decision making as to parentage and as to child rearing situations in which conflict arises from parental incapacity or indifference rather than religious conviction.

Third, scholarly and popular debate generally acknowledges, at least with respect to younger children, only the state and a child's parent(s) as candidates for the position of holding ultimate decision making power. In fact, there are innumerable other possible holders of such power – for example, other members of a child's biological family, a private child welfare agency, or children themselves.

To launch a broader and more rigorous examination of this crucial question, I begin with the earliest point in time at which a new human life form acquires sufficient moral status for the moral community to attribute moral considerability equal to that of the standard object of political theory. Call it "personhood" if you like. For present purposes, it does not matter what the criteria are for affixing that label nor whether it typically vests sometime before birth or at the time of birth. It only matters in what follows that it happens before a child begins to make and communicate conscious decisions, which is consistent with prevailing views of moral status (Dwyer 2011: 1–3). How should we think about who decides important matters for babies? I will start by discussing prevailing norms and practices regarding ultimate authority over the lives of autonomous persons, and then consider whether and how the principles underlying those could be extended to the case of young children.

10.2 Decision Making Authority Regarding the Lives of Autonomous Persons

Traditionally, moral and political theory has focused on only autonomous persons, who constitute a substantial fraction of all persons but not nearly all. Theorizing posits some bedrock first principle, such as self-ownership, autonomy, or personal integrity, that has as one of its implications that autonomous persons have ultimate authority over their own lives to a substantial degree – that is, that there are some aspects of such a person's life that, as a matter of fundamental human right, he or she is morally entitled to control regardless of what anyone else thinks or desires (Sobel 2012; Galston 2006: 826–27). Determining what all those aspects are is the project of much philosophical work, but some widely accepted examples are one's intimate relationships and one's thoughts. Whether one agrees to form a family relationship with another person and what one believes are matters that can affect others, but their effect on others is either too insubstantial or indirect or it is outweighed by the great importance the decision has for the well-being of the individual or by the centrality it has in the individual's personhood. Specifying the precise scope or even providing a general description of this category of life aspects is unnecessary here. What is significant for present purposes:

(1) Some such aspects of life can exist also for babies (e.g., whether they enter into a family relationship with particular other persons) yet there are no aspects of a baby's life as to which we can sensibly assign to them ultimate authority, because babies cannot make and communicate decisions about such things;
(2) As to older children, as well, there are aspects of life as to which autonomous adults ordinarily would have ultimate authority but with respect to which there is a consensus that the children themselves should not hold ultimate authority – for example, a 5 year-old's attending school; and
(3) There are no central aspects of the lives of autonomous persons[1] as to which anyone today believes ultimate decision making power should reside in some other private individual.[2]

An implication of (1) and (2) is that as to some central aspects of children's lives, someone other than the children must have ultimate decision making power. To elaborate on (3): As to aspects of autonomous persons' lives regarding which many believe they should *not* have ultimate decision making authority, such as how they drive or whether they keep promises, the alternative ultimate decision maker people generally look to is the moral community as a whole, for which the state is an agent that creates and enforces legal rules based on the community's moral judgments. If the question arises what should be the standards for my driving, no one would say I should have the authority to decide that for myself, nor that my wife or any other private party should have such ultimate authority. Rather, the only sensible position is that the moral community collectively decides whether I am constrained by the safety interests of others, environmental concerns, or other competing values, and the state properly implements that moral conclusion with specific laws. When two or more individuals have conflicting interests tied to their self-determination, the moral community collectively assumes ultimate decision making authority and resolves the conflict by imposing a regulatory regime authorizing some conduct and prohibiting other conduct.

---

[1] By "central aspects" I mean choices lying within the realms of self-determination and bodily integrity for any individual. I mean to exclude conduct directed at other persons or aspects of one's life that necessarily involve agreement with others. Choice of career to pursue is a central aspect of my life, but whether I get a particular job properly depends on someone else's decision.

[2] I say "today" because there are potential historical counter-examples – namely, slavery and the authority husbands were ascribed with respect to their wives under the coverture regime. And I say "potential" because one might plausibly argue that the state actually retained ultimate decision making authority with respect to slaves and wives, but we need not settle that here.

The foregoing are merely observations of our collective practices and shared moral and political views. From these observations I will construct a coherentist account of what we should think about decision making authority in relation to children's lives. A coherentist account aims to make our normative views consistent with each other, by discerning the basic principles undergirding certain convictions and determining how those principles would extend to other contexts sufficiently similar that one might expect consistency of principles across contexts. The exercise is especially effective when the convictions with which one begins have held up for a long time under rigorous scrutiny, as seems to be true of the division of authority over autonomous persons lives described above, and when the other contexts to which the underlying principles might be extended have not yet received much rigorous attention, as is true of many aspects of children's lives.

10.3 Extending to Child Rearing

The consensus view is that human beings possess moral status, meaning they matter morally in their own right and their welfare and integrity must factor into moral and political decision making, at least from the time of birth. However, when they first acquire such moral considerability they are incapable of effectuating or communicating decisions, let alone self-determining decisions that merit deference from others. Typically many autonomous persons individually and the larger community collectively take an interest in the well-being of infants and other dependent persons, for both self-interested and altruistic reasons. In fact, there is a consensus that babies' moral status entails positive duties on the part of other individuals and the community collectively to care for them in some way.

As to almost any baby in developed western societies, there are actually more adults who would like to take custody of and raise the child than could feasibly do so; usually birth parents wish to and in addition the demand for newborn adoption currently far surpasses supply. Further, a society collectively is affected by the survival and upbringing of children; that is why schooling, for example, is deemed a public good. On the other hand, there are some biological parents who do not wish to care for a baby before or after birth, yet a biological parent's care could be essential to a baby's survival at certain points – in particular, the physical retention of a non-viable fetus by a pregnant woman. How are the potentially conflicting interests of baby, biological parents, would-be custodians, and society to be addressed? By what decision making process should a baby have one fate rather than another?

We might first ask whether any of the pertinent decisions that need to be made as to babies are matters that, for any involved individuals, fall within the category posited above of life aspects over which autonomous persons ordinarily are deemed to have ultimate authority. If we characterize those aspects of life at a particular level of generality, then with respect to all involved persons *other than the babies*, the answer is clearly and almost uniformly "no." Neither 'having custody of another person' nor 'making decisions about another person's education or medical care' can plausibly be characterized as a matter of self-ownership, autonomy (i.e., *self-determination*), or personal integrity. The single exception among decisions relating to babies is the abortion decision; it is a matter of perennial debate precisely because it impacts not only the baby's survival but also the biological mother's control over her own body. Both survival and control over one's body are matters at the core of an individual's life, so central that the law reposes decision making about them as much as possible with the individual. But apart from that context and that interest of biological mothers, custody and care of babies does not implicate any aspect of any adult's life that lies within the realm of self-ownership, autonomy, or personal integrity. In contrast, it does implicate some such aspects of the lives of persons who are presently babies.

10.3.1 Custody of Children

With respect to custody of a baby, which we generally tie to a legal parent-child relationship, what is involved is entry into a social family relationship, and thus an intimate association, with another person. Though we do not ordinarily do so, it is useful to distinguish conceptually two components of intimate association. One component for autonomous persons is choosing to make oneself available for such association with another person. The other is actually forming an intimate relationship. The first we deem among those decisions as to which an autonomous individual should have ultimate authority, which entails that every autonomous person has a fundamental human right against forced intimate association. The second, in contrast, in the context of association between two autonomous persons, depends crucially on another person similarly choosing to be available for that association. The basic right to ultimate authority over one's own availability for a family relationship, and therefore the right to refuse any particular intimate association, is shared equally by all autonomous persons. Whether some particular other person will actually enter with me into an intimate relationship that I desire is not a matter of my self-ownership, autonomy, or personal integrity, and so it is not something I am morally entitled to decide; it is not something over which I should have ultimate authority, even though it might be of profound subjective importance to me.

We can extend this set of propositions to parenthood and to custody of newborns with minor adjustment. Doing so means, first, that any adult, including a biological parent, should have ultimate authority to decide whether he or she is available for an intimate association with a particular child. This is, in fact, the case in modern western society; the legal system does not compel biological parents to associate with their offspring (it only imposes an obligation of financial support). However, it also means that no adult, not even a biological parent, should have ultimate and unilateral authority to decide whether the association actually occurs; there would have to be a reciprocal choice that the baby is also available for that association.

Some adjustment to the rules or procedures for relationship formation is needed, obviously, because babies cannot make that reciprocal choice themselves. There are several possible alternative places to repose ultimate authority over the baby's availability for the relationship:

1. Assign it to the adult who wishes to become a legal parent and custodian, to exercise in a self-interested manner.
2. Assign it to some other private individual, to be exercised however that individual wishes.
3. Assign it to society collectively, to be exercised in a manner aimed at serving collective interests.
4. Assign it to some entity that acts as a proxy and fiduciary for the baby.

One obvious practical problem with Alternative 1 is that there could be any number of adults who choose to make themselves available for a relationship with a particular child, and it would be unworkable to give them all authority to decide that this child will enter into an intimate association with them. That problem might be solved by limiting application of this alternative to some subset of all persons seeking parenthood of a particular child, such as biological parents, but there would need to be some reason why those particular persons are favored in the process of removing the numerosity problem, in addition to the need to justify Alternative 1 rather than Alternatives 2, 3, or 4.

I will bracket the questions of whether and when biological parents should be favored under Alternative 1 and turn to an additional problem with that alternative, which it shares with alternatives 2 and 3 – namely, that 1–3 appear to jettison altogether principles of self-ownership and personal integrity with respect to infants. They give no heed to the fact that the matter at hand is one at the core of a child's life, one determinative of a child's most fundamental interests. They treat the child the same way they might treat a car. Yet we believe a child has a moral status quite different from that of a car, and in fact much like that of an autonomous adult human. And there is presumably more at stake for a baby in connection with formation of the parent-child relationship than there is for any adult in connection with forming an adult intimate partnership, because of babies' life-determining developmental needs. Alternatives 1–3 implicitly presuppose that if some persons cannot make decisions for themselves about core aspects of their lives, then their separate moral personhood becomes irrelevant and they can be treated the same as non-persons and even inanimate objects. But no plausible view of moral status and its implications is consistent with that result (Dwyer 2011: 95–117). We must rule out any solution to the conundrum of decision making incapacity that pays no heed to the equal personhood, self-ownership, personal integrity, and fundamental interests of a person lacking capacity.

Significantly, prevailing attitudes and practices concerning incompetent adult humans rule out the first three of the above possibilities for assigning ultimate decision making authority regarding their intimate associations, and in particular their custody. We do not say, as to any incompetent adult Y, that any other particular private individuals have a fundamental right, and therefore ultimate authority, to decide in a self-interested or arbitrary manner whether they or some other private party will occupy the guardian role as to Y. Instead, other persons decide whether they will make themselves available for the custodial relationship and then the state exercises ultimate authority over whether the relationship will actually occur, by means of individualized court appointment of a guardian. Moreover, we do not permit the state, in exercising that authority, to make collective interests the basis for decision. Instead, the fourth possible resolution to incapacity listed above is the one we have adopted for making as to incompetent adults a decision analogous to the parentage and custody decision that must be made with respect to children. Governing legal rules for personal guardianship of incompetent adults implicitly make courts proxies or agents for those adults, requiring that judges make the guardianship decision and do so on the basis of either an advance directive executed by the person when competent or the incompetent adult's best interests and known values (Dwyer 2009: 775–79). A judge substitutes for the non-autonomous individual and, in order to respect the distinct personhood of that individual, aims to exercise its surrogate authority in the way the individual presumably would do if able – that is, as he or she previously directed or, absent such directive, in a way most consistent with his or her well-being or previously-manifested values. And if we were to ask why a court rather than some private individual acts as the proxy, the answer is that we assume this disinterested state institution with expertise in taking and weighing evidence and reaching factual determinations is, though certainly not a perfect proxy, the best available proxy – that is, the proxy most likely consistently to reach the same conclusion that the incompetent individual would reach if competent (i.e., if contemplating future incompetence).

This now-settled way of treating non-autonomous adult humans reflects several assumptions about incapacity: (1) Incompetence does not eviscerate moral status; (2) Incompetence does not render impossible assignment of ultimate decision making authority in a way that respects such a person's self-ownership or human dignity; (3) Incompetence does not justify allowing any other private entity or the state to exercise ultimate decision making authority for its own sake; (4) the morally most appropriate response to incompetence is to repose ultimate decision making authority as to central aspects of those persons' lives in an agent acting as fiduciary; and (5) a state actor is the most reliable such agent.

The foregoing creates a strong presumption, as a matter of rational consistency, that the appropriate response to babies' inability to make their own family formation decisions is for the state to act as proxy for each newborn, to exercise in behalf of babies ultimate authority as to who will be their parents and custodians, and to do so on the basis of the babies' best interests. This response most closely resembles the way we assign ultimate decision making authority as to intimate associations for autonomous adults, and it is nearly identical to the way we deal with incompetence in adult humans (the significant differences being the possibility of an advance directive and previously-manifested personal values with incompetent adults). The crucial question is then whether there is any basis for rebutting that presumption.

This is of practical importance because although it is the case that the state in every society does exercise ultimate authority over parentage, by legislating default assignments of newborn children to parents and having courts adjudicate exceptions, no society's default assignment or individualized adjudications rests solely on what is best for the child. The universal default rule predicates initial legal motherhood simply on biological maternity and initial legal fatherhood on biological relationship to child, social or legal relationship to mother, or some combination of those things. The prevailing exception requires a waiver of entitlement. Significantly, there is no legal basis for denying initial legal parent status to biological parents who are grossly unfit, let alone to biological parents who are simply not the best available parents for a child all things considered (Dwyer 2012: 24–45). As a result of this legal regime, the state condemns a significant percentage of children to maltreatment and permanent damage despite the state's awareness of birth parents' unfitness at the time of the children's birth, as evidenced, for example, by government records of past child abuse or violent crimes or by medical tests showing serious drug addiction or mental illness. There is the possibility of later divesting unfit biological parents of their legal parent status, in a termination of parental rights proceeding, but that generally occurs only after substantial damage has been done a child, and even then it is not a sufficient condition for that occurrence that the child would be better off not being in that relationship (Dwyer 2012: 641–57).

A likely place to find a rational basis for rebutting the presumption of state proxy decision making for children is in any assertions or arguments people make either for alternatives 1–3 above or for some proxy decision maker other than the state. I am not aware of any significant support for alternative 3; no one argues the state should assign children to custodians based on its judgment of how best to serve collective interests. As to alternative 2, a few legal scholars have taken the position that birth mothers should have legal power to decide who else, if anyone, will occupy a parental role with their children (e.g., Baker 2004). Some who take that position might hint at a basic moral entitlement of birth mothers to have that power, perhaps arising from the effort they expend in sustaining the child before and after birth. However, they also assert that reposing such legal power in birth mothers would, in general, be best for children, and that assertion is what really gives their position moral purchase. They likely would not condone, for example, birth mothers' selling parent status to the highest bidder and being compensated that way. Their view is therefore really best interpreted as an instance of alternative 4, with a private proxy for children rather than a state proxy. Moreover, unless they were to go further and insist that the state could never override birth mothers' choices – even if, for example, a birth mother chooses a drug-addicted sexual predator as a co-parent, in actuality they would be presupposing that the state holds ultimate decision making authority and their position would amount to saying simply that the state should provisionally delegate its proxy role to birth mothers. Assuming that to be the case, then I am also unaware of anyone endorsing alternative 4 with some private person or group as the proxy for children rather than the state.

That leaves alternative 1, which many people do appear to endorse. The apparent endorsement is strictly limited, though, to instances in which the person wishing to be a legal parent is a biological parent of the child. No one takes the position that applicants for adoption should have ultimate authority to decide whether they will form a family with a particular child – that is, that their preference is the proper substitute for the autonomous choice of the baby. Adoption applicants are not viewed as having a fundamental right, superior to the power of the state, to decide for a child that he or she will be in an intimate association with them. Rather, the approach taken with adoption is the same as that with adult guardianship – namely, alternative 4, with the state acting as a proxy for the child and applying a best-interests standard of decision making.

It is only with respect to biological parents that some people, including some judges, speak of a fundamental right of an adult to be in a family relationship with a newborn child.[3] Typically people who make this assertion do not present any normative argument for it, and it would be exceedingly difficult to mount any such argument regarding biological fathers per se, whose physical contribution to creation of the child is necessary but typically not burdensome. Additionally, those who speak of biological parents' fundamental or natural right to raise their offspring also do not delve into detail sufficiently to determine whether they really are endorsing Alternative 1, rather than Alternative 4 with a strong state-created default rule in favor of parents. In particular, they do not address the problem of demonstrably and chronically unfit parents.[4] If pressed, probably most would waver in their devotion to the biologically-based fundamental right notion when considering a birth mother who has horribly abused several prior children and refused all rehabilitation services offered. Certainly they would concede that the state may properly take into custody a newborn child who is at immediate risk of harm if sent home with the birth mother; this is a common practice in the western world. And they would concede that the state may terminate the parental status of a birth mother if it is or becomes clear that the baby could not safely be placed in her custody in the foreseeable future; termination of parental rights (TPR) proceedings are also common and accepted.

It is just a short conceptual step from those concessions to accepting that the state could properly deny legal parent status in the first instance to birth mothers or fathers who are manifestly unfit at the time of a child's birth to care for the child when there is no reasonable prospect of their becoming fit within the foreseeable future. Indeed, given that a TPR amounts to a state decision that from time T forward biological parent P will not be in a family relationship with baby B, it would be difficult to reconcile (a) acceptance of the propriety of such a state decision at some T after legal parent status has already been invested in P (but no custody of the child was ever permitted) with (b) rejection of the propriety of such a state decision at the moment of birth and before the state has conferred on P legal parent status as to B. The practical effect for the biological parent would, in many instances, be precisely the same (Dwyer 2009: 824–26).

It seems unlikely, then, that any thoughtful person would actually endorse Alternative 1 even for biological parents. Everyone accepts that the state may properly prevent intimate association between a biological parent and a baby when that

---

[3] See, e.g., Adoptive Couple v. Baby Girl, 133 S.Ct. 2552 (2013) (Scalia, J., dissenting).
[4] A generally overlooked implicit assumption in U.S. Supreme Court decisions attributing to biological fathers a constitutional right to serve as legal parent is that the biological father in question is not unfit. *See* Dwyer (2009: 815).

association seriously threatens the baby's very survival. And accepting that is implicitly to accept that it is the state that exercises ultimate authority over the decision whether a non-autonomous person is available for an intimate association with any particular autonomous person who has chosen to be available for that association. What is subject to reasonable debate is just the specific content of the legal standard by which state actors make that judgment – for example, should it be high risk of imminent death or best-interests or something else. In other words, even if one believes (despite the difficulties of explaining why) that biological parents possess some fundamental moral right to raise their offspring, one is likely to concede that the right is not absolute and that the state, in the form of legislatures and courts, must determine when the right exists and controls and when it does not – that is, when it must give way to other values, such as the welfare of the child. And that is to concede that the state must ultimately decide who will be a child's legal parents and custodians.

Importantly, the debate about the content of the legal standard must be shaped by an assumption as to what the state's role is in deciding for which intimate associations a newborn is available. Alternative 3 above represents a "police power" role in which the state aims to serve collective interests. Within that role, the state could treat newborns as a distributable good, like jobs or treasury funds, and allocate them in such a way as to reward, ingratiate, or punish people. Or it could treat newborns as a public good and assign them in such a way as to maximize their future productivity, fill gaps in the employment market, or prepare them for military service. Treating newborn persons as commodities or public goods is obviously not consistent with respect for their moral status, their dignity as persons, their fundamental right of self-ownership, or the way we treat non-autonomous adults. The *parens patriae* role that Alternative 4 embodies, in contrast, is consistent with these commitments, and thus is the best candidate for an alternative to autonomous decision making by children with respect to their parentage and custody.

As to who, among those wishing to occupy a parental role with respect to any child, will actually do so, we should therefore conclude that attributing to the state ultimate decision making authority, as a proxy for the child, is most consistent with respect for the moral status of children. It is the legal resolution that most closely resembles the legal regime governing autonomous adults' formation of intimate family relationships with each other. With children, the state simply steps in as a proxy for a child, to exercise his or her right to decide in accordance with his or her best interests. That proxy, fiduciary consent by the state for the child should be a necessary condition for formation of any parent-child relationship. Current state practices concerning parentage are subject to criticism insofar as they depart from this fiduciary model.

10.3.2 Child Rearing Decisions

How does the analysis change, if at all, once the state has conferred legal parent status and decisions must be made about specific aspects of a child's life such as nutrition, medical care, and education? Like entry into an intimate relationship, these are things mostly within the ambit of an autonomous person's self-ownership, self-determination, and personal integrity and therefore as to which autonomous persons possess ultimate authority. Assuming that they are practically available to me, I decide whether I will receive certain medical treatment or schooling. The state exerts some quality control over what providers make available, and providers retain some discretion as to what they will make available to which individuals (e.g., doctors to avoid addiction, universities to secure the best students) but otherwise neither the state nor any other private party can interfere with my decision that I will or will not take certain medicines, undergo certain procedures, enroll in particular classes, or eat certain foods. Some other private parties might believe they know better than I what is good for me, but their belief is of no moral or legal significance. They certainly can claim no moral entitlement to have their judgments be legally effective. What I do with my body or mind is certainly not a matter of their self-ownership, their personal integrity or dignity, their autonomy, the core of their lives, or their fundamental right.

Again we should ask whether and how this moral framework for decision making as to the life of an autonomous person carries over to the case of non-autonomous persons. One possible answer is that it is irrelevant to child rearing, because it is conceptually impossible or inappropriate to try to extend or modify it to address such aspects of non-autonomous persons' lives. But if we again look to prevailing moral views and laws regarding non-autonomous adults, that answer appears implausible. With respect to incompetent adults, we find again that ultimate decision making authority as to such things as their medical care and training rests with the state, acting as fiduciary or agent for the individual. The state holds and exercises ultimate authority, with state actors making some choices for non-autonomous adults and state-created laws establishing boundaries of permissible decision making by any private caretaker, such as a guardian. Neither prevailing moral beliefs nor legal rules repose in any other private individual or in state actors' *ultimate* authority to decide such things about the life of a non-autonomous adult in such a way as to serve the aims and interests of the decision maker or of anyone else besides the incompetent adult whose care or training is at issue.

The legal system does commonly authorize private parties, such as guardians or next of kin, to make some decisions regarding basic aspects of the lives of incompetent adults. However, it does not do so based on any assumption about the private parties' entitlement nor for the purpose of gratifying their desires, regardless of what role a particular private party might occupy or previously have occupied in the life of the incompetent adult. Rather, a court will confer such authority based on the incompetent person's previously (while competent) having appointed a particular private party to act as a proxy, or based on a decision as to which decision maker would best promote the incompetent adult's welfare *as the state sees it*. And the law then imposes a fiduciary obligation on the private decision maker, requiring that that private party make decisions consistent with the incompetent adult's best interests as the state sees it, prohibiting certain forms of treatment, and standing prepared to take back the delegated authority should the appointed person deviate substantially from what the state views as in the incompetent adult's best interests. The state grants guardians and other caretakers some discretion, but as a matter of privilege rather than entitlement and within state-imposed limits.

Thus, if someone (e.g., a family member or doctor) challenges a guardian's decision concerning a ward's medical care, a court would override the guardian's decision if it determined that the decision was contrary to the ward's welfare. In doing so, the court would not deem the guardian entitled to any deference or to substitute his or her own values or religious beliefs for the secular criteria of well-being that the state applies. Again, this is true regardless of what role the guardian might have occupied in the incompetent adult's life, and regardless of whether the guardian regards it as "an essential element of expressive liberty" (Galston 2002: 102), "as important as any other expression of conscience" (Callan 1997: 143), or otherwise of vital personal importance to decide how the ward's life will go. If, for example, a parent-guardian for a mentally disabled adult joined a religious group who preached that disability is the mark of the devil and that giving medical care to disabled persons defies divine command, the judgment of the moral community, expressed through state institutions, would be that the guardian has no right whatsoever to make decisions for the ward on the basis of those beliefs and that, in fact, a court should consider appointment of someone else as guardian. The state thus holds ultimate decision making authority and simply delegates authority to some degree and always subject to oversight and recall. The state, not the guardian and not any political theorist, determines the bounds of decision making and treatment. I am unaware of anyone who believes that inappropriate.

Notably, no aspect of the just-described legal regime governing custody and care of incompetent adults rests on an assumption of state infallibility or on a denial that family members typically care and know more about those persons than do any state actors. As is true with its policies and practices relating to children, the state sometimes blunders in its decisions and actions relating to incompetent adults, because of ignorance, indifference, inefficiency, or some other defect. Incompetence is a predicament, because there is no especially good alternative to competent self-determination (which is itself quite fallible). Our society has developed this legal regime respecting incompetent adults based on a judgment that it better serves them than would any alternative regime, considering that dangers would also inhere in giving private parties ultimate authority over the lives of those incompetent persons, and considering that state decision making and activity are relatively visible and susceptible to legal challenge.

So, if we list the possible alternative holders of ultimate authority to decide central aspects of non-autonomous persons' lives, as we did regarding custody, we would have to include as one possibility: "some entity that acts as a proxy and fiduciary for the non-autonomous person." And in fact, settled convictions about self-determining decisions by autonomous persons and about decision making authority over the lives of incompetent adults would seem to create a strong presumption, as a matter of rational consistency, that *ultimate* authority over central aspects of children's lives, such as their medical care, education, and discipline, ought to reside with the state as fiduciary for children – that is, with the state acting in a *parens patriae* role, as a proxy for persons unable, because of youth, to decide these things for themselves. The state should decide whether to mandate certain services for children and whether to leave some things to a private caretaker's discretion, all on the basis of what legal regime best serves children's welfare *as the state sees it*, taking into account the relative expertise and motivation of alternative decision makers. To the extent the state delegates some decision making authority to private parties such as parents, it should charge those private parties with a fiduciary obligation to exercise that authority in a manner conducive to the child's welfare as the state sees it, and it should stand ready to override particular decisions of private caretakers or to withdraw authority from them when, in the state's judgment, the private caretakers are acting so contrary to the child's well-being as to warrant the disruption of the child's life that this intervention will entail.

Thus, for example, the state should limit parents' choices for a child's education to only those schools that demonstrably provide a good secular, autonomy-promoting education (though they might also provide religious instruction) and do not treat children in ways the state deems harmful (e.g., sexist teaching and treatment). Parents would have no right to make religious beliefs or illiberal values the basis for choosing a child's school (Dwyer 1998). But within the range of schools the state approves, parents should be free to select the one they deem most consistent with their child's abilities, temperament, and learning style, with the family's values, and with their financial circumstances and priorities. Indeed, the state should be free to support financially whatever choice parents make within the range it sets, even if they choose a religious school (Dwyer 2002a, b).

Consistent with this moral framework, we should view private parties to whom the state delegates some power over children's lives as possessing no moral *entitlement* to direct children's lives however they wish or to insist that whatever ideological beliefs or values they happen to hold should be the ultimate standard of decision making rather than the state's views about what is best for children. Anyone who insists that legal parents themselves have such a basic moral right, and therefore should have a trumping legal right, to control a child's life as they wish, bears the burden of demonstrating why treatment of decision making about children's lives should diverge conceptually from treatment of the lives of autonomous persons and of non-autonomous adults.

In fact, though, one would be hard pressed to find any serious scholar who takes the position that parental control over children's lives should not be subject to state-imposed limitation. Even those who view themselves as defenders of strong parental rights concede that there must be constraints on parental freedom, typically characterizing such constraints in vague terms such as "reasonable," without elaboration (Galston 2002: 102; Gilles 1996: 945, 986). They most readily concede this when the topic is run-of-the-mill, non-ideological child maltreatment. Even those who defend corporal punishment recognize that some entity other than parents themselves must ultimately determine the bounds of acceptable violence toward children, and they generally assume that this will be the state acting in a *parens patriae* capacity. And even those who insist that parents are generally the most competent and motivated carers for children acknowledge that there must be some check on parents who would starve their children or leave them unsupervised in dangerous surroundings. Indeed, even in the context of ideological divergence between parents and the state, defenders of parental authority are careful to point out that deference to parental values can go too far, that some ideologically-driven parental choices might be "unreasonable."[5]

Moreover, although such scholars sometimes write as if they themselves should have ultimate authority to define the bounds of reasonableness, undoubtedly all would concede, if pressed, that it actually must be the state, reflecting the moral and empirical judgments of the community, that properly holds that ultimate authority. Their position thus really amounts to a claim that the state should delegate more rather than less control over children's lives to parents. And their strongest arguments for doing so are in terms of what is best for children as a general matter, claiming that parents are the most knowledgeable and caring decision makers and invoking such interests of children as having parents who feel secure and valued in their role, sharing a normative outlook with those who raise them and live with them on a daily basis, and having a foundation for moral decision making that the state itself is not well-positioned to supply (Gallston 2002: 105; Callan 1997: 138–39; Schoeman 1980: 15; Gilles 1996: 953).

These sorts of arguments are consistent with viewing both the state and parents as fiduciaries rather than right holders, and would in fact be more conceptually coherent and therefore more persuasive if expressed in terms of children's rights rather than parents' rights (Dwyer 1994: 1429). One could plausibly speculate that a given child would, if counter-factually capable of deciding who should hold what degree of control over his or her life, endorse this rough division of labor and discretion between state and parent, whereby the state establishes bounds of "reasonableness" and confers power on parents to act within those bounds to govern children's daily lives. Or, perhaps less conceptually awkward, one could analogize to a situation in which a competent adult anticipates becoming child-like again, as a result of accident or disease, with the potential to develop again toward autonomy and independence, and executes an advance directive concerning ultimate decision making authority over his or her life in that child-like condition. A survey study would likely reveal that the vast majority of competent adults would say that if they become child-like in that sense again, they would want certain private parties to possess

---

[5] Galston, for example, argues that ideological communities should possess some sovereignty of their own, on an equal par with the civil state, and so that parents within such communities should be entitled to dictate the cognitive development and value formation of their children, but accepts "a substantial degree of legitimate governmental regulation of families' educational decisions". Galston (2006: 827), though he would endorse much less regulation than American courts do and not for child welfare reasons. Galston (2002: 18–20, 114–22). Gilles takes the position that "the *Pierce* reasonableness standard should be interpreted to require states to show that the parental educational choices with which they would coercively interfere are plainly unreasonable." Gilles (1996: at 944). Gilles also suggests as a standard "consensus that [particular parents'] aims or methods are in fact destructive of [their] children's well-being," which appears to concede ultimate authority to the state and simply require super-majoritarian votes in favor of particular restrictions on parental freedom, while also suggesting another vague and undefined substantive standard – namely, "destructive of well-being").

presumptive decision making authority but would also want the state to hold *ultimate* authority over their lives – that is, to establish some limits for decision making and treatment by the private caretakers, as a backstop against harmful decisions or actions. And they would not deem the freedom that private caretakers enjoy within those limits a matter of the caretakers' fundamental right, but rather simply conducive to their own best interests. This is also not a perfect heuristic, because a competent adult would already have values they are likely to want to have reflected in the rules for their care, and they are likely to designate persons known to them as potential caretakers. But the example suffices to show that it is rational for an individual contemplating incapacity to endorse a legal regime in which the state holds ultimate decision making authority over their lives, as imperfect as that regime is as a substitute for self-determination.

What rejoinders are left to those who insist that parental entitlement occupies some moral space in child rearing and that parents' must have ultimate authority to some degree? They might insist that there must be some scope of parental liberty, regardless of any state judgments about children's welfare, and that this is so as a matter of parental fundamental right. Even if the state must set the bounds, it must set them in such a way that meaningful freedom is left to parents and that parents' religious beliefs receive some deference. This is so not because it conduces to children's well-being (e.g., because it makes parents happier caregivers); that consideration can be fully and more sensibly expressed in terms of children's rights. Rather, it is because, the claim would have to be, parents are morally entitled to it regardless of whether it conduces to children's well-being. This would be different from saying that parents have a right to freedom absent "harm" or "serious harm" to a child, which would require the state to define what is harmful and so to exercise ultimate authority comprehensively. It would instead be to say that the state may not pass judgment on parental choices or conduct within some range. But how is that range to be specified other than by a state judgment as to which choices or conduct present an intolerable danger of harm to children? Are parents themselves to determine what that range is with respect to their particular child? Or are the scholars who defend the concept of parental entitlement to make that determination themselves, as some purport to do?

In addition to such practical and conceptual problems with the idea of parents having ultimate authority over some aspects of children's lives, there is the very serious problem of justification. Scholarly analysis of this issue tends to be distressingly *sui generis*, devoid of appeal to general principles or attempt to reconcile assertions about care of children with beliefs about care of other non-autonomous persons. What moral basis could there possibly be for claiming that one person has a fundamental right to ultimate authority and control over the life of another person, or even some limited part of it? If there is such a basis, would it also apply to persons other than children whom some people want to control? If the major premise of the moral argument is "One has a fundamental right to control the life of a person whom one creates,"[6] then do adoptive parents not possess that fundamental right

---

[6] See, e.g., Narveson (2002: 267), Gilles (1996: 961).

with their adopted children whereas parents of adult mentally disabled persons do? If the major premise is "One has a fundamental right to control the life of a person for whom one has cared,"[7] then we have to ask whether settled convictions and legal rules concerning guardians for incompetent adults are mistaken, why any parents would lose their right to control when their offspring reach the age of majority, and whether a husband's caring for a wife during a period of severe illness would generate a fundamental right on his part to ultimate authority over her life or some part of it. And if the major premise is "One has a fundamental right to control the life of another person when doing so is a matter of supreme importance or central to one's conception of the good and life plan or a matter of expressive liberty," as it seems to be for some of the most well-known defenders of parental entitlement,[8] then we are all in danger of some others claiming a right to ultimate authority over some aspect of our lives. Why is it that only in connection with decision making about children's lives the law should ensure "maximum feasible scope for different ways of life to find expression in the choices of [caretakers] and civil associations"? (Galston 2011). Notably, no proponent of that view has ever addressed the analogy to incompetent adults – that is, has answered the question whether a guardian for an incompetent adult similarly has a fundamental moral right to direct the ward's life in accordance with the guardian's religious beliefs if that is of great importance and morally mandatory in the guardian's mind.

A related question is whether and why the autonomy of a person whose life is at issue is relevant to what authority others possess? If no one would ever claim that ultimate authority over the education or medical care of an autonomous person should be reposed in another private individual as a matter of that other individual's fundamental right, then what is it about the lack of autonomy in a child (or incompetent adult) that changes the moral analysis so dramatically? The attribution of a fundamental right to one person to possess ultimate authority over the life of another person undeniably treats the latter instrumentally, or conflates the identify of other person with that of the supposed right-holder, given that any defense of authority based on the welfare or dignity of the other individual as a distinct person could and should be expressed in terms of that person's right. So does lack of autonomy make it appropriate for the moral community to treat a person instrumentally or as devoid of separate personhood? Defenders of so-called fundamental rights of parents have never engaged these questions.

---

[7] Callan suggests this compensatory view of parental entitlement. *See* Callan (1997: at 143) ("the reward we seek from the work (of child rearing) is perhaps opaque in its deepest aspects, but much of it surely has to do with the gradual realization in the life of the child of those educational ends that give content to our understanding of success in child-rearing").

[8] See, e.g., Galston (2002: 102) (treating parental control over children's education as "an essential element of expressive liberty"); Callan (1997: 143) (resting parental entitlement on the supposition that directing a child's life in accordance with one's religious beliefs is "as important as any other expression of conscience"); Gilles (1996: 960 (asserting that parental educational authority "is central to the human flourishing of parents and children alike") and 996 (characterizing "conscious familial reproduction" as "a basic human need")).

As with parentage and custody, therefore, there seems no way around a conclusion that ultimate authority regarding the entirety of the lives of non-autonomous persons, including children, must rest with the state. The state holds some authority in its police power role over both autonomous and non-autonomous person, but as to aspects of non-autonomous persons' lives over which autonomous people typically have ultimate authority, such as whether they will receive available medical care or education, the state holds ultimate authority as a proxy for the non-autonomous persons, making decisions (including decisions to delegate some authority to private custodians) as a fiduciary and with the sole aim of trying to replicate what the non-autonomous persons would decide for themselves if able.

This analysis does not purport to resolve all specific conflicts the state might have with parents over child rearing. What it does establish is some normative ground rules for argument and disposition – in particular, ruling out claims by parents and their defenders to ultimate decision making authority as a matter of fundamental right. The state must hold ultimate authority, and parents should be directed to express their objections to specific regulations or interferences in terms the state can accept in its role as fiduciary for the child – namely, in terms of children's temporal well-being. That does not mean parents should never win; state actors certainly sometimes disserve children even when they view themselves as fiduciaries for children, and parents are well-positioned to challenge them. Moreover, parents can assert all the empirical claims typically made in defense of parental freedom, such as the importance of the parent-child bond and the potential threat to that which particular forms of state interference with childrearing might constitute. What is morally essential is simply that the focus remain on the well-being of the child and that any court adjudicating such a dispute recognize that it is operating as fiduciary for the child, constrained always to aim for the result the child would choose if able, in light of all relevant facts.

Before closing, it bears mention that some scholars have actually endorsed a third possibility for ultimate decision making authority, at least with respect to children's education. Liberal statist proponents of "democratic education" have implicitly adopted something like Alternative 3 in the list set forth in Section II(a) above – that is, authority reposed in society collectively, to be exercised in a manner aimed at serving collective interests. They contend that adult citizens have a collective right to prescribe certain aspects of children's education in order to serve whatever aims they happen to have for society (Callan 1997: 9; Guttmann 1989: 14). These scholars presuppose that a majority of adults have attractive aims such as preserving democratic values and producing productive future citizens, but they do not make their valorization of democratic control dependent on the majority's having a particular set of values; otherwise, their views would not rest as they suppose on a collective right or on respect for democratic decision making, but rather on some perfectionist vision of their own. For Guttmann, for example, there is a basic "right" of current adult citizens to engage in "conscious social reproduction" and to use children's education to do so.

The instrumental treatment of children that this entails does not trouble these theorists, perhaps because they do not recognize it. But they do treat children instrumentally, to a degree and in a way they likely would not do with any adults, autonomous or non-autonomous. We can imagine state policies regarding the education of competent adults or training decisions regarding mentally disabled or mentally ill adults that aim principally to serve collective ends or embody a majority's "conscious social reproduction." For example, it might serve collective interests to have the state choose college students' course of study for them based on the state's forecast of future employment needs. Or a majority of competent adults might decide that it wants to channel able-bodied adults with particular mental illnesses into certain military roles – for example, certain conditions might make some individuals great candidates for suicide missions. Or to force mentally disabled adults to dress in red, white, and blue and process in patriotic parades because the majority supposes this will promote national pride. Liberal statists engaged in the debate over children's education, like defenders of parental entitlement, unreflectively rest their case on *sui generis* ruminations about children's lives. Their views lose all plausibility when their implicit major premises are generalized to cover other groups of people.[9]

10.4 Conclusion

As to both custody and control of children, the answer to the question "Who decides?" must be that the state holds ultimate decision making authority, and that any power over children's lives private parties properly possess they must have by delegation from the state, subject to child-centered limits the state imposes, and as a matter of privilege rather than entitlement. This normative conclusion is conceptually compatible with a legal regime conferring on parents extensive power to control children's lives, and with interference by local state actors only in rare circumstances. But whether that sort of regime is the right one must ultimately be decided by the state, based on the best available empirical evidence about what is, in general, most conducive to children's welfare as the state sees it.

References

Baker, K. K. (2004). Bargaining or biology? The history and future of paternity law and parental status. *Cornell Journal of Law & Public Policy, 14*, 1–69.
Callan, E. (1997). *Creating citizens: Political education and liberal democracy*. Oxford: Clarendon.
Dwyer, J. G. (1994). Parents' religion and children's welfare: Debunking the doctrine of parents' rights. *California Law Review, 82*, 1371.
Dwyer, J. G. (1998). *Religious schools v. children's rights*. Ithaca: Cornell University Press.
Dwyer, J. G. (2002a). Changing the conversation about children's education. In S. Macedo & Y. Tamir (Eds.), *NOMOS XLIII: Moral and political education*. New York: NYU Press.

---

[9] For fuller response to liberal statist views, see Dwyer (2002a, b).

Dwyer, J. G. (2002b). *Vouchers within reason: A child-centered approach to education reform.* Ithaca: Cornell University Press.

Dwyer, J. G. (2009). A constitutional birthright: The state, parentage, and the rights of newborn persons. *UCLA Law Review, 56,* 755.

Dwyer, J. G. (2011). *Moral status and human life: The case for children's superiority.* New York: Cambridge University Press.

Dwyer, J. G. (2012). *Family law: Theoretical, comparative, and social science perspectives.* New York: Aspen Publishers.

Galston, W. A. (2002). *Liberal pluralism: The implications of value pluralism for political theory and practice.* Cambridge UK: Cambridge University Press.

Galston, W. A. (2006). Families, associations, and political pluralism. *Fordham Law Review, 75,* 815.

Galston, W. A. (2011). Parents, government, and children: Authority over education in a pluralist liberal democracy. *Law & Ethics Human Rights, 5,* 284.

Gilles, S. G. (1996). On educating children: A parentalist manifesto. *University of Chicago Law Review, 63,* 937–940.

Guttmann, A. (1989). *Democratic education.* Princeton: Princeton University Press.

Narveson, J. (2002). *Respecting persons in theory and practice.* Lanham: Rowman & Littlefield.

Schoeman, F. (1980). Rights of children, rights of parents, and the moral basis of the family. *Ethics, 91,* 6–19.

Sobel, D. (2012). Backing away from libertarian self-ownership. *Ethics, 123,* 32–60.

Part III
Children's Well-Being and Policy

Chapter 11
The Concept of Best Interests in Clinical Practice

Jürg C. Streuli

11.1 Introduction

> The role of staff members in acting in a child's best interest is similar to that of the parents, but the opinions of professionals have greater weight. (Hallström and Elander 2005)

> The most frequent theme (in 89.1 % of all interviews) was "doing right by my child," conveying parents' desire to make decisions in the child's best interest (…) in an unselfish manner. (Hinds et al. 2009)

> Estimating an individual's best interests indirectly demands placing a value on that life. It seems that we are prepared to place less moral value on a human life just born than one that has begun to develop attachments. (Armstrong et al. 2011)

> The real question is not so much about identifying which medical alternative represents the best interests of the child, but rather about identifying a harm threshold below which parental decisions will not be tolerated. (Diekema 2004)

> (…) due to the variability demonstrated above, the BIS is neither internally nor externally consistent. (Salter 2012)

The Best Interests Standard is a difficult and controversial concept, and its implementation in clinical practice faces substantial concerns from conceptual and linguistic points of view.

Within this chapter, I aim to present of how a concept of best interests of the child could be applied in clinical practice in a consistent manner. I do not defend or question the "best"-language itself, which is under critique mainly because of its rhetorical power based on inconsistent or normatively weak arguments (Holm and Edgar 2008; Salter 2012). Nevertheless I would contest a rash discard of the concept of "best interests". The herein presented approach is essentially shaped by my own

J.C. Streuli (✉)
University Children's Hospital Zürich, Steinwiesstrasse 75,
8032 Zürich, Switzerland
e-mail: streuli@ethik.uzh.ch

daily work as a medical doctor in pediatrics and it is informed by excerpts from semi-structured interviews with health care professionals conducted from 2008 to 2012 including a comprehensive review on medical literature regarding the use of best interests (Streuli 2011; Streuli et al. 2014). Although I hope to advance the efforts of promoting the well-being of the child, I'm well aware of the limits of the applied methods, which do neither have the normative strength to confirm nor to discard the best interests standard as a leading concept in pediatrics. But my intention is a different one. Much more I will argue for a less normative but nevertheless comprehensive idea of the concept of best interests. Thereby speaking of "best interests" does not imply a normative principle but rather a motive to sharpen our perspective for a continuing attempt to understand what we use to call "children", what we think is "best" for them and to what "principles" we should adhere to in our efforts to respect the child and its family.

11.2 Premises on What Is in the Best Interests of a Child in Clinical Practice

Recommendations concerning the best interests of the child tend to contain vague and sometimes conflicting interpretations. In clinical practice, however, best interests are applied on a regular basis and normative statements in a particular situation usually are ready-to-hand (Streuli et al. 2011). As indicated by the opening quotes there are some variability in talking about best interests, which sometimes lead to the conclusion that the concept of best interests "is neither internally nor externally consistent" (Salter 2012). To have an idea of differing interpretations, which may lead to inconsistency, I will start with presenting some important underlying assumptions and premises, which I repeatedly found in interviews and daily practice.

11.2.1 The Child as a Subject Subjected to Parental Authority

Parents are widely seen responsible for their minor children, including decision-making concerning their child's development and health. The associated authority is either based on the assumption that parents do qualify best to respect their child's needs or on the overarching value of the family and the underlying assumption of an "intimate relationship" (Downie and Randall 1997). According to the first perspective parental authority is an implication of the best interests of the child, according to the second perspective best interests of the child is an implication of the value of a family. In clinical practice both perspectives are important. Therefore, parents do hold the authority to act in ways that are *not* necessarily for the child's good (e.g. change of residence of a family due to personal but not financially compelling reasons) but at the same time do have responsibilities concerning the needs of an individual child, independent of efforts to preserve and enhance the family as a hole (e.g. the prohibition of child-labour for increasing the family income). In short, there is much, but not endless room for parental authority.

Of particular interest for pediatric ethics is the notion that parental authority not only includes the power to make decisions on behalf of the minor child but also the decision of how much participation parents like to share with their minor offspring. The question about the point, where a child receives authority in decision-making hence depends on one hand on the child's competence to make a decision but on the other hand largely on the parents' concept of participation, education, and what for them seems best for the child. The increasing awareness of the burdens among children with cancer who are not sufficiently informed might have changed the relationship between medical professionals, parents and the child during the last years. But current literature still gives little guidance about the implication of parental authority in clinical practice. However, from a clinician's point of view the question of parental authority also implies the question of how parents can be supported in applying authority in difficult situations. Using the example of differences (or disorders) of sex development (DSD), also called intersex, we are just starting to learn how important it is to strengthen the parents' competence in talking about difficult issues with their minor children and exert authority in complex clinical situations (Streuli et al. 2013).

11.2.2 The Child and Its Family as a Relational Unit

As mentioned above the intimate family can be a justification for parental authority. At the same time the assumption that the parents and the child are a relational unit with significant influences on the development and well-being of children is a cornerstone of the concept of best interests (Coleman 2002). It is a common and central claim that the patient's family and the health care team must work cooperatively with each other and communicate effectively to provide the best patient care (Committee on Bioethics 2007). Based on early research concerning the impact of bonding, pediatricians see the child's outcome regarding physical and emotional health, including cognitive and social functioning, strongly related to the (patchwork) family's functioning as a unit (American Academy of Pediatrics 2003). A significant inability of providing certain conditions for an effective bonding between the parent and the child can lead to protective measures against parental authority. An example could be seen in a single parent with severe depression and repeated hospitalizations, who has not been able to give sufficient love and attendance to the child without support from a foster family. In another example of an unconscious dying child with acute worsening conditions the premise of relational units may be used for balancing the parents' need for having some more time with their dying child against the inclination not to prolong distress by invasive procedures like intubation for mechanical ventilation.

Moreover, the values within a relational unit also provide guidance in situations, where the harm principle as a base for child protection measures, as proposed by Diekema, might not be sufficient (Diekema 2004). In the example of a depressive single parent, the need of the child for emotional warmth and security may demand certain supportive measures independent of the mere quantification of resulting harm, because harm in this particular situation may be of rather hypothetical consequence. In my experience the act of fostering the relationship to a continuing (professional or personal) person of trust usually cannot be done by a court but needs a long-term relationship to the child and its environment (e.g. school teacher, psychologist, social worker etc.). In the second example of a severely ill and unconscious child the principle of do-no-harm is also of great significance but not the sole argument. Although one could certainly argue that parents prima facie do not have the right to demand invasive, potentially harmful and medically not indicated treatments, there are other normative aspects than solely the harm principle. Moreover, the harm principle itself is a multifaceted concept as shown below.

11.2.3 The Child as a Vulnerable Person

It is a frequently heard premise that children are characterized by their exceptional vulnerability. Its source can be grouped into primary and secondary origins. Primary origins of the vulnerability of the child are related to the absolute or relative child-like weakness, frailty, and immaturity, which objectively make the child dependent on others in particular situations. Vulnerability in pediatric hospital settings, however, is not just bound to primary biological and psychological constitutions of the child but also to the imbalance of power between adults' and minors' concepts, spaces, and bodies. Drawing a line between adulthood and childhood involves the danger of a certain "adultism", which is associated with a conscious or unconscious control of children by demanding obedience and conformity, independent of evolving capacities to participate in a process of decision-making (Bricher 2000). This may lead to the denial of rights and, subsequently, to the accentuation of vulnerability.

An extreme form of such secondary origins of vulnerability was proposed in 1964 by Solnit and Green under the name of the "vulnerable child syndrome", observed in families which experience the premature death of a close person, recovery from a nearly missed death in infant- or childhood, or burdening situations during pregnancy. In the absence of a biomedical or psychological disorder in the child, the authors reported overemphasized and secondarily enforced vulnerability associated with pathologic separation problems, overuse of medical care services, and overprotectiveness (Green and Solnit 1964).

11.2.4 The Child as a Participating Person with Evolving Capacities

As children develop and acquire enhanced competencies, there is a continuously reduced need for direction, and consecutively a greater capacity to take responsibility for decisions affecting their lives. Speaking of best interests, there is always a need to balance the understanding of children as active agents in their own lives, with their own understanding of value and happiness, entitled to be listened to, respected, and granted increasing autonomy in the exercise of rights, while they are also entitled to protection in accordance with their relative immaturity and youth. The concept of evolving capacities, introduced in Article 5 of the Convention on the Rights of the Child, provides the basis for an appropriate respect for children's agency, without exposing them prematurely to the full responsibilities normally associated with adulthood (Committee on the Rights of Children 1989; Lansdown 2005). There is little literature about the relation between the best interests of the child and autonomy, but they are sometimes believed to be oppositional, as the risks resulting from autonomous choice could be contrary to the child's best interests (Buchanan and Brock 1989; Partridge 2010). Other authors do not share these concerns and draw a strong link between the ability to understand, communicate, and value certain choices and the ability to cope with the burdens of illness and its treatments (Alderson 1992). Both perspectives, however, do have in common that they perceive the acknowledgment and support of evolving capacities as a delicate and important issue, while an all-or-nothing discussion between the autonomous versus the vulnerable child would hardly reflect reality. For example, in clinical practice there is a widespread awareness of the importance of play and toys in a child-friendly clinical environment, acknowledging the value of childhood itself. At the same time plays and toys, including children's book are frequently used to explain concepts and obtain opinions of topics such as chemotherapy, side effects, suffering or death – topics, which often are reserved for the adult world. However, we always must be aware that autonomy and evolving capacities are concepts coined by an adult understanding of competence and decision-making. Nevertheless there are a myriad of specific competences of a child to discover, to respect and to build on. On one hand this draws a connecting line to a particular form of vulnerability and the problem of "adultism" mentioned above, on the other hand it leads us to the last premise of the child and the prospect of its future state.

11.2.5 The Child and the Prospective Future Person

Normative statements based on adult concepts may conflict with a value system of a child. While children in some aspects do have the capacity and the right for having their very own value system, the common adult perspective (above introduced as "adultism") typically argues that children only have an incomplete value systems closely related to still evolving capacities and limited life experiences. A value system, according to this perspective, is perceived as mature as soon it coincides with a value system and the underlying capacities of a "fully developed" adult. As so often, when two extremes are opposed, both do have at least some weight: While professionals try to respect the child's own perspective and values, it is also necessary to consider in some regards the future person with different phases of life. This happens by caring for the child's health and education based on principles such as protection and provision (Streuli et al. 2011). While the children's rights approach combines the principles of protection and provision with the demand for participation, thereby including the respect of evolving capacities, Feinberg's well-known account of the child's right to an open future focuses almost exclusively on the preservation of prospective opportunities in later life, with the aim of "[sending the child] out into the adult world with as many open opportunities as possible, thus maximizing his chances for self-fulfillment" (Feinberg 1980; Salter 2012). While Feinberg's perspective certainly is compatible with the respect of evolving capacities, as far as open opportunities also depend on capacities learned earlier in childhood, the open future account is still highly prescriptive, fully dominating opportunities in childhood by future opportunities in a hypothetical state of adulthood.[1] There is, however, another aspect of the child and its prospective phases of life, which is less intrusive but equally powerful for clinical practice: the perspective of evidence-based medicine, which urges professionals to collect and implement data and insights from mid- and long-term results. A particularly difficult example can be found again in the treatment of children with disorders of differences of sex development, where recent studies shed a critical light on the outcome of surgical sex assignment and the absence of follow-up data for many years (Köhler et al. 2012). Therefore, returning to interpretations of best interests, I would argue, that the collection and consideration of data regarding long-term outcome after childhood is an essential part of the best interests of a child.

11.3 The Triad of Best Interests in Clinical Practice

The short and probably incomplete summary of five premises suggests that inconsistencies are not primarily part of an inconsistent concept but the (inevitable) consequence of tensions between different values and perspectives in clinical practice. Medical indication is bound to a medical professional's opinion. However, daily care and choice reach far beyond medically indicated therapy or support. Professionalism in clinical practice embraces innovative approaches of planning, delivery and the evaluation of health care grounded in a mutually beneficial

---

[1] Feinberg's approach fails to show why the open future argument is applicable on children (e.g. desires and whishes in childhood should be sacrificed for the opportunities of an adult person in her 30s) but not on adults (e.g. desires and whishes of a person in her 20s should be sacrificed for the opportunities of an adult person in her 60s).

partnership among patients, families, and providers that recognize the child's needs, the child's evolving capacities, and the importance of the family in the child's life (Committee on Hospital Care and Institute for Patient- and Family-Centered Care 2012; Lansdown 2005). In a nutshell, this is what the best interests of the child in clinical practice are aiming for: a well-considered implementation of multifaceted needs, aims and conditions.

The here presented concept has strong similarities with the theoretical concept of Loretta Kopelman (Kopelman 1997). Kopelman defines the Best Interests Standard as an umbrella term, by identifying its employment, first, as a threshold for intervention and judgment (as in child abuse and neglect rulings), second, as an ideal to establish policies or prima facie duties, and, third, as a standard of reasonableness. In my opinion Kopelman's concept of a triad is capturing the needs and requirements regarding interactions with children and their families best. In practice, the best interests of the child are not limited to a punctual approach of solving conflicts and averting harm, but deeply related with a comprehensive understanding of the child's need to develop within a functional system of caregivers and heteronomous as well autonomous capacities. In the following three paragraphs I will show a way, which captures the best interests of the child best, from an empirical and philosophical perspective. The here presented triad slightly differs from what Kopelman earlier proposed. The following approach embraces and modifies also the classic definition of Brock and Buchanan, which conceives the best interests standard literally as a maximal best solution, as well as a proposal by Diekema, who argues for interventions against parental authority exclusively based on the harm standard (Buchanan and Brock 1989; Diekema 2011; Salter 2012). After presenting central premises, on which discussions regarding the best interests of the child are based, I will next present three different but complementary discourses from which statements regarding the best interests and based on the proposed premises arise.

11.3.1 *The Optimum*

The main discourse from a clinical point of view could also be called a standard of optimum care and choice. Finding an optimum is a process, which takes place within a continuously changing field of multiple choices and different forms of care. The discourse about the optimum is characterized by changing perspectives, needs, and capacities of a child and its environment, including its family and a particular health care system. The idea of an optimum is based on the observation that decisions in clinical practice often refer to a level of effort that strives to maximize the benefit for a particular child over a long time period without significantly decreasing the ability of the family or its environment to support the continuation of a certain level of care and choice. Although a particular patient might be the center of considerations, the optimum care and choice is based on the premise of the family as a unit and therefore takes all family members into account. The optimum typically corresponds to an effort level somewhere between the maximally best solution mentioned by Brock and Buchanan and the "good-enough parenting" mentioned by Winnicott (Buchanan and Brock 1989; Winnicott 1965). Most health care professionals I interviewed were in accordance that "just" good-enough or suboptimal care or choices would not be in the best interests of the child and should be encountered by prevention or additional support. Nevertheless, the standard of optimum care and choice reigns on the important role of parents in deciding on behalf of a child, which is not yet or no longer capable of deciding for itself. Whether a certain care or choice is rather "good-enough" or "maximally the best" therefore depends on the mutually beneficial partnership among patients, families, and providers formed by a dynamic process within the triangle of the patient, the parents, and the responsible professionals.

11.3.2 The Threshold Value

Statements considering a threshold value refer to situations where a certain stakeholder loses its significance in favor of interdisciplinary, democratically legitimated expert groups (e.g. child protections services, ethics committees and/or courts). Threshold values of best interests are primarily based on the principle of non-maleficence and distinguish acceptable from unacceptable courses of action or consequences. While the best interests as an ideal or an optimum are represented by a multitude of differing principles, the threshold value is primarily guided by a negative definition of best interests focusing on the prevention and/or protection from harm. As a consequence, the effect of threshold values is limited to situations where significant and obvious harm occurs or very likely will occur. Therefore every optimum is surrounded by certain boarders, which demarcate an area, where parents, in relation with the minor patient and the supporting professionals do have a certain freedom to act in regard of their child's need and capacities.

Health care professionals typically are well aware of the difficulty of defining such threshold values and the nuances involved. Whether the harm principle should be the leading argument or just one argument inter alia, will not be discussed here. However, contrary to individual and close partnerships within the area of optimum care and choice, the threshold values should be based on well-considered resolutions by transdisciplinary working groups, ethic committees, courts, and other democratically enacted authorities. Although the threshold value as a part of the best interests of the child governs the limits of parental consent, parents have an important role in determining what a threshold value is. As a consequence, a threshold value is closely associated with the assisted search for an optimum. By defining threshold values based on children's rights and modern child protection services, it became clear that harm to a child can not simply be seen as a sum of threshold crossings but also as a problem requiring knowledge about coping strategies and the resilience of a child's environment to identify the underlying causes of harmful behaviors or conditions. For example, the best interests of a child living within a family of Jehovah's Witness would be insufficiently covered by only discussing the limits of parents' authority in deciding about life-saving transfusion in an emergency situation (threshold discourse). By making a substantiated decision against the parents' and/or the child's will, the best interests of the child are not yet fully considered. Dependent on particular situations professionals should strive for an optimum in how parents and the child can be prepared, informed and supported in advance and after a potential transfusion. This brings me to a third discourse on which the best interests of the child rely.

11.3.3 The Discourse of Ideology

Ideology is the most private and individual but also most controversial aspect of the best interests of a child. Ideology is based on particular ideas of what makes life and decisions good and right, independent of democratically legitimated, well-argued, or evidence-based resolutions within the discourse of thresholds. Similar to its origin in the platonic idea, the ideologies exist as archetypes of which only shadows or certain excerpts become visible for the observer. Considering the best interests of a child implies a process of perception, comprehension and translation, and of underlying ideologies in families; but also in health care. Medical professionals should always bear in mind that definitions of what is health and healthy are nevertheless bound to particular perspectives and ideologies. There is however no reason to end up in multicultural relativism. Other than the critically reflected optimum and threshold discourses the discourse of ideology is not necessarily subject of normative statements and judgment. To implement personal and sometimes controversial ideologies is mainly a way to show respect for someone. Moreover it facilitates planning and delivering optimal care and a choice. Therefore, the best interests of the child demand a consideration of the families' ideologies as a starting point for further reflection on the optimum and certain threshold values. This statement is sufficiently vague so that its value mainly can be seen in reducing child/parent/professional conflict.

11.4 Implications

If there is a simple message about best interests in clinical practice, then certainly that best interests are not simple. They are multifaceted, dynamic and sophisticated. However, in contrast to a widely held belief the concept of best interests does not itself balance principles, rights and needs of children and parents but describe and integrate them on several levels or discourses (Ainsworth and Hansen 2011).

Basically it ensures a well-considered implementation of the multifaceted needs, aims and conditions. Table 11.1 offers a matrix, which has to be filled with relevant data, necessary to incorporate these needs, aims and conditions. The concept of best interests thereby does neither represent a particular argument, principle or philosophy nor does it come to use only for situations where the child has no competence at all. For using "best interests" as a meaningful concept it is necessary to differentiate between the discourses of ideology, optimum and threshold based on different perspectives resulting from premises such as parental authority and the evolving capacities of the child. In practical terms this means that a decision on a threshold value made by a child protection service, for instance against the preference of religious parents who reject blood transfusions, cannot be claimed as being in the best interests of the child without aiming at the same time to install a relationship between the child, the parents, and the professionals. Then, and maybe only then, it is possible to learn about the underlying ideology and to offer at least the possibility of sincere reflection on the optimum based on different options (such as overriding parental authority, mechanical blood cell-saver with support by a religious advisor or a step-wise transition to a less fundamental interpretation of religious commands). Under true time pressure, a treatment can be rightly enforced based on a (provisional) juridical decree but the claim of the concept of best interests doesn't end there. The child has a right to be the subject of a comprehensive assessment, which requires considerations not only of a single time point of a particular intervention or a single principle, but also of subsequent questions and problems regarding the consequences of a certain decision.

As a consequence, there should be no use of the term before trying, firstly, to understand underlying ideologies, secondly, to delineate a particular area of optimum care and choice, and, thirdly, to learn about established or needed thresholds. If only one of these three considerations is missing we should either conceive the concept of "best interests" as a mandate to complete these considerations or refrain from using it.

Table 11.1 A matrix of "best interests"

	Ideology	Optimum	Threshold
Experts	(…)[a]	(…)[b,c]	(…)[d]
Parents	(…)[a]	(…)[b,c]	(…)[d]
Children	(…)[a]	(…)[b,c]	(…)[d]
Future person	(…)[a]	(…)[b,c]	(…)[d]

[a]Assess, communicate and respect individual values and opinions
[b]Consider content, such as development, feeling of security, quality of life, bodily integrity
[c]Discuss inter- and transdisciplinary
[d]Elaborate thresholds with transparent and democratically legitimated working groups, commissions, and courts

References

Ainsworth, F., & Hansen, P. (2011). The experience of parents of children in care: The human rights issue. *Child & Youth Services, 32*(1), 9–18.

Alderson, P. (1992). In the genes or in the stars? Children's competence to consent. *Journal of Medical Ethics, 18*(3), 119–124.

American Academy of Pediatrics. (2003). Family pediatrics: Report of the task force on the family. *Pediatrics, 111*(6), 1541–1571.

Armstrong, K., Ryan, C. A., Hawkes, C. P., Janvier, A., & Dempsey, E. M. (2011). Life and death decisions for incompetent patients: determining best interests – The Irish perspective. *Acta Paediatrica, 100*(4), 519–523.

Bricher, G. (2000). Children in the hospital: Issues of power and vulnerability. *Pediatric Nursing, 26*(3), 277–282.

Buchanan, A. E., & Brock, D. W. (1989). *Deciding for others: The ethics of surrogate decision making*. Cambridge: Cambridge University Press.

Coleman, W. (2002). Family-focused pediatrics: A primary care family systems approach to psychosocial problems. *Current Problems in Pediatric and Adolescent Health Care, 32*(8), 260–305.

Committee on Bioethics. (2007). Professionalism in pediatrics: Statement of principles. *Pediatrics, 120*(4), 895–897.

Committee on Hospital Care and Institute for Patient- and Family-Centered Care. (2012). Patient- and family-centered care and the pediatrician's role. *Pediatrics, 129*(2), 394–404.

Committee on the Rights of Children. (1989). *Convention on the rights of the child*. United Nations Office of the High Commissioner for Human Rights.

Diekema, D. (2004). Parental refusals of medical treatment: The harm principle as threshold for state intervention. *Theoretical Medicine and Bioethics, 25*(4), 243–264.

Diekema, D. S. (2011). Revisiting the best interest standard: Uses and misuses. *The Journal of Clinical Ethics, 22*(2), 128–133.

Downie, R. S., & Randall, F. (1997). Parenting and the best interests of minors. *Journal of Medicine and Philosophy, 22*(3), 219–231.

Feinberg, J. (1980). The child's right to an open future. In W. Aiken & H. Lafollette (Eds.), *Whose child? Children's rights, parental authority, and state power* (pp. 76–97). Totowa: Rowman & Littlefield.

Green, M., & Solnit, A. J. (1964). Reactions to the threatened loss of a child: a vulnerable child syndrome. Pediatric management of the dying child. *Pediatrics, 34*, 58–66.

Hallström, I., & Elander, G. (2005). Decision making in paediatric care: An overview with reference to nursing care. *Nursing Ethics, 12*(3), 223–238.

Hinds, P. S., Oakes, L. L., Hicks, J., Powell, B., Srivastava, D. K., Spunt, S. L., Harper, J., Baker, J. N., West, N. K., & Furman, W. L. (2009). "Trying to be a good parent" as defined by interviews with parents who made phase I, terminal care, and resuscitation decisions for their children. *Journal of Clinical Oncology, 27*(35), 5979–5985.

Holm, S., & Edgar, A. (2008). Best interest: A philosophical critique. *Health Care Analysis, 16*(3), 197–207.

Köhler, B., Kleinemeier, E., Lux, A., Hiort, O., Grüters, A., & Thyen, U. (2012). Satisfaction with genital surgery and sexual life of adults with XY disorders of sex development: Results from the German clinical evaluation study. *The Journal of Clinical Endocrinology and Metabolism, 97*(2), 577–588.

Kopelman, L. M. (1997). The best-interests standard as threshold, ideal, and standard of reasonableness. *Journal of Medicine and Philosophy, 22*(3), 271–289.

Lansdown, G. (2005). *The evolving capacities of the child*. Florence: UNICEF.

Partridge, B. C. (2010). Adolescent psychological development, parenting styles, and pediatric decision making. *Journal of Medicine and Philosophy, 35*(5), 518–525.

Salter, E. K. (2012). Deciding for a child: A comprehensive analysis of the best interest standard. *Theoretical Medicine and Bioethics, 33*(3), 179–198.

Streuli, J. C. (2011). *Ethical Decision Making in Pediatrics – An empirical study on the relationship between "Kindeswohl" and "Best interests" and a proposal to their implementation* [in German]. Unpublished, School of Social Work, University of Applied Sciences and Arts Northwestern Switzerland.

Streuli, J. C., Michel, M., & Vayena, E. (2011). Children's rights in pediatrics. *European Journal of Pediatrics, 170*(1), 9–14.

Streuli, J. C., Vayena, E., Cavicchia-Balmer, Y., & Huber, J. (2013). Shaping parents: impact of contrasting professional counseling on parents' decision making for children with disorders of sex development. *Journal of Sexual Medicine, 10*(8), 1953–1960.

Streuli, J. C., Staubli, G., Pfändler-Poletti, M., Baumann-Hölzle, R., & Ersch, J. (2014). Five-year experience of clinical ethics consultations in a pediatric teaching hospital. *European Journal of Pediatrics, 173*(5), 629–636.

Winnicott, D. W. (1965). *The maturational process and the facilitative environment.* New York: International University Press.

Chapter 12
Children's Well-Being and the Family-Dilemma

Alexander Bagattini

12.1 Introduction

Physicians have to take care of the health of their patients as well as to respect their autonomy. This can lead to conflicts of duty for the physician when her medical opinion concerning the health of a person deviates from what the person herself thinks about that matter. Consider a case when a physician has to attend a person that denies vital medical help. On the one hand her profession as a physician requires her to save the life of the person. On the other hand she cannot do this without ignoring the patient's consent. Since there is a strong claim for autonomy in liberal societies, the duty to respect the consent of their patients is here overriding by default. Only if there are good reasons for the physician to believe that the relevant capacities for autonomy are in some way limited or lost, this might change.

Things change *in principle* when physicians treat children as their patients. Children typically count as 'incompetents' lacking the relevant capacities for autonomy (Buchannan and Brock 1990). Parents are standardly considered the right persons to make decisions on behalf of their children. This is called parental autonomy (Archard 2004; Macleod 1997) and entails the right of the parents to judge on what serves, in medical contexts, the interests of their children. Hence, when physicians treat children as their patients, they have firstly to ask for the parents' proxy-consent. However, according to most Western legal systems, parental autonomy is not unconditional. It has its limits when the well-being of

---

I want to thank Colin Macleod and Felicitas Kraemer for their helpful comments on this paper and the Fritz Thyssen-Foundation for the funding of my research-stay at the University of Victoria, BC (Canada).

A. Bagattini (✉)
Department of Philosophy, University of Düsseldorf, Germany
e-mail: bagattini@phil.hhu.de

the child is endangered. This entails at least that the vital interests of the child must be protected. David Archard calls this the *liberal standard* (Archard 2004), which entails basically a claim about the relation of parents, children and the state: parents have a default-right to child-rearing. This right is, however, restricted by the state because children's interests are of public concern. This, in turn, entails that children's interests must be protected by the state. (The liberal standard will be addressed in more detail in the next section).

The liberal standard is certainly a high achievement of liberal society, as it helps to protect the vital interests of children. However, it leads to a very unpalatable situation for physicians when they suspect that parents maltreat their children. In this case the physician is confronted with two conflicting duties: on the one hand she has to care for the health-related well-being of the child, and hence has to report to the responsible public institution when parents have maltreated their child. We may call this the duty to report (DR). On the other hand she has to respect parental autonomy and the privacy of the family, and has, therefore, a duty to keep medical information confidential. This duty is well-known as professional confidentiality (PC).

While DR protects the interests of children, PC protects the interests of the parents (or of the family) in the first place. Because both duties are mutually exclusive, the physician can end up in the following situation: she has to decide if specific evidence for child-maltreatment is sufficient to justify a report to the responsible public institution. This situation is particularly awkward in legal contexts, as the physician is liable to legal consequences when she neglects either DR or PC. In the first case she runs the risk to be charged because she has violated the child's interests, while in the second case the parents might charge the physician for slander (Fangerau et al. 2010). Hence all elements of a moral dilemma are given: two duties that contain legal and moral values that can conflict with each other. Because the question concerns the legitimate interference with family-decisions concerning child-rearing I call such situations cases of *family-dilemma* for physicians.

The family-dilemma arises for physicians because the law protects both: children's and parental interests. The liberal standard is the normative framework within which both sides are balanced against each other. My main question in this paper is if the law should implement the liberal standard. I will presuppose, rather than argue for, an egalitarian framework of justice according to which all basic interests matter equally. Consequently, I will endorse the view that all interests of all members of a community matter equally.[1]

Hence, a normative standard should be implemented in law that fits this task. If the liberal-standard leads to the family-dilemma, there is, however, good reason to be sceptical that it is the right candidate to be implemented in the legal system, because the family-dilemma is a substantial obstacle for physicians to protect children's interests. Furthermore, I will point out that the liberal-standard is unjustly biased towards the interests of parents. This leads to the question for an alternative normative standard that protects children's interests properly and prevents physicians from falling prey to the family-dilemma. I will argue that the implementation

---

[1] Making this point I follow authors like R. Dworkin (1983) and Macleod (1997).

of such a standard in law is accompanied by costs for the parents. The structure of the paper is as follows:

Sections 12.2 and 12.3 are dealing with the normative background of the family-dilemma. Section 12.2 points out that, according to the liberal standard, physicians must only report to public institutions when they have sufficient evidence that parents have maltreated their children. Section 12.3 discusses how this normative requirement leads to the family dilemma for physicians by analysing the concerned duties, PC and DR, in more detail. Section 12.4 deals with a possible solution of the family-dilemma for physicians by introducing a revised version of the liberal standard. The upshot of this discussion will be that such a solution will not come without considerable social and economic costs on the side of society and parents.

12.2 Parental Autonomy and the Liberal Standard

It has been pointed out by several authors that parental autonomy (the right of the parents to decide what is in the interest of their children) has its limits where the well-being or the interests of the child are violated (Archard 2004; Macleod 1997; Bagattini 2013). In his book "Children. Rights and Childhood" David Archard calls this the *liberal standard* (LS) because it is the default state and generally recognized in liberal societies (Archard 2004). According to Archard, LS entails three elements: (i) It serves the interests of children and parents if children are raised by their parents. This entails the right to parental autonomy and privacy of the family for the parents. (ii) Parents lose their right to parental autonomy and privacy when they expose their child to serious harm. (iii) In such cases the state will act to protect the interests of the child. In extreme cases the custody will pass from the parents to the state (Archard 2004).

Archard discusses LS at some length. In this paper I will focus on some specific aspects of LS, foremost the normative relation between (i) and (ii). In terms of justification this relation can be expressed as follows: in the default case parents have a right to parental autonomy and privacy of the family. This right can, however, be defeated in cases when the parents do not promote the interests of their children.

An example of the implementation of LS in the legal system is the concept of *custody* in German law. In §§ 1626 and 1666 of the German Civil Code we find a clear expression of LS:

§1626: Parents have the duty and the right to care for the well-being of their child.

§1666: If the physical, mental or psychological well-being of the child is endangered and if the parents are not willing or not able to prevent the danger, the family court has to impose those sanctions as being necessary for the prevention of danger. (My translation, author)

In §1626 the value of parental autonomy is implemented which, according to the sixth paragraph of the German constitution, is accompanied by the concept of the privacy of the family. In §1666 we find the implementation of the value of the *child's well-being*. Hence, German law protects, on the one hand, the privacy of the family and parental autonomy and on the other hand the well-being of children.

Here is an important terminological point: While Archard uses the concept of the interest of a child, in §1666 the concept of children's well-being (German: *Kindeswohl*) is introduced. What does this contrast mean? A well-known definition of the concept of children's well-being is in terms of children's interests. Interests are, contrary to preferences, not a purely subjective matter. A child might have a strong preference for a chocolate 'diet' while eating chocolate all day is certainly not in the child's interest. In this way the normative force of the concept of children's well-being is to protect children's interests.

In light of this clarification we can summarize LS as follows: In the default case parents have the right to parental autonomy and to privacy of the family. This entails that child-rearing practices happen at large parts without public recognition. The state and the public have to respect the way parents raise their children. Only if clear evidence for the endangerment of a child's well-being is given, a claim against the custody of the parents is justified.

In other words: *For any claim that parents endanger or violate the well-being of their children the burden of proof is on the side of the claimant and not on the side of the parents.*

Note now that physicians can be in the role of the person expressing such a claim against the parents. This is the case when they, in the course of medical check-ups, find evidence that parents have maltreated their children. Yet if the physician reports to the responsible institution, she has to violate PC and risks to be charged for slander. In other words: if LS is implemented as a legal standard, physicians have to be cautious about DR. However, as a consequence many cases of child-maltreatment stay undetected or are considered past the statute of limitations. In this vein LS leads to the family-dilemma for physicians and is responsible for the violation of children's interests. The next section will point out in more detail how LS leads to the family-dilemma for physicians. For the moment I want to press the point that LS has its serious shortcomings because it helps to create a space within which children cannot be properly protected (for example against abusive parents).

12.3 The Physician in the Family-Dilemma

In order to analyse the family-dilemma it will be helpful to firstly consider PC and DR in more detail. Afterwards we can proceed by pointing out where the points of conflict between both duties lie and why in some cases they even create a dilemmatic situation for the physician.

12.3.1 Professional Confidentiality (PC), Privacy of the Family, and Parental Autonomy

Being part of the Hippocratic tradition, PC is related to medicine as we know it right from its early beginnings. In recent medical ethics PC has been justified in a variety of ways.[2] In the first place it has been pointed out that PC is constitutive for patients having *trust* in physicians. Trust is important because most people take their health-state as something private that must not be reported to other persons without the patient's consent (Beauchamp and Childress 2013). Furthermore, it has been pointed out that there is a societal interest in PC, as it promotes preventive medicine that in turn keeps the costs of the health system low. If people fear that physicians might publish information about their health, they would be less inclined to medical visits (Allen 2011). In what follows I will focus on two goods that are promoted by PC: *privacy* and *autonomy*.

Autonomy is certainly one of the key-values in liberal societies. In fact, some philosophers hold autonomy as an intrinsic value of liberal societies (Rössler 2004). Consider decisions of people concerning their health. Not only do people dislike others to decide on their behalf if they should undergo any medical treatment and if so, which one it should be. When it comes, for example, to rather controversial medical decisions like IVF (in-vitro-fertilization) or abortion, people want those decisions to be kept secret, primarily because they want to make their own decisions and they want to be in control of what people know and talk about them (Feinberg 1983). In this context, privacy theorists like Beate Rössler highlight the relevance of privacy for autonomy. According to Rössler, privacy is at least instrumentally important for autonomy (Rössler 2004). It is hard to imagine that autonomy could be developed in an Orwellian 1984-type society in which privacy is largely not given. This is especially true for medical decision-making. Furthermore, privacy is of utter importance especially in medical contexts because health problems are often correlated with shame. If people are not sure that their medical problems will remain within their private sphere, they might be less inclined to consider medical help at all.

To sum up: PC protects core values of liberal society in medical contexts. This does not mean that PC is a perfect duty in the Kantian sense that does not allow for any exemptions. Rather, there might be good reasons to break with PC, for example when the patient is a serious threat to the public. However, as fundamental liberal values such as autonomy and privacy are concerned, there must be good reasons for such exemptions.

How do children as patients fit in this scheme? At first children do not seem to fit in standard moral theory at all (Schrag 1977). At least very young children usually do not count as autonomous in the sense that they lack the relevant capacities to promote their own interests. If we endorse LS, we accept parental autonomy: that parents are the

---

[2] In my presentation concerning the relation of trust and PC I follow Allen (2011).

right persons to make decisions concerning the interests of their children. However, the interests of children limit parental decision-making. Nonetheless, as long as the interests of children are not violated, parents enjoy a default-right to decide on behalf of their children. This is especially true in medical contexts.

In this vein it is helpful to distinguish between medical treatment that is *medically necessary* and medical treatment that is *medically desirable*. According to LS, parents have no right to decide for or against medical treatment for their children if it is medically necessary because then the vital interests of the child are concerned. Parents have, however, a right to decide for or against medical treatment when it is medically not necessary. This allows parents, for example, to reject Ritalin treatment for their children. It is controversial if Ritalin is still medicine or already enhancement. In the latter case there are good reasons for parents to reject the use of Ritalin for their child – for example to protect their child against too much pressure at school. This point illustrates intuitively the merits of parental autonomy. Sometimes parents might have a different opinion concerning certain treatment such as Ritalin than physicians have, and in some cases they might indeed be right in having it.

In the same way privacy is an important aspect of the relationship between parents and physicians. In the first place it preserves a good that is constitutionally protected in most liberal societies: the privacy of the *family*. The idea of the family might change, but people have a strong affective inclination to live in families (Macleod 2002). Protecting the privacy of the family means protecting a space within which intimate and intense relationships can be lived – without intrusions by the public or the state. It might even be constitutive for the family that it is private, because relationships like romantic relationships or the relationship between parents and children can only occur in their specific form if they remain private.

There are at least three good reasons to accept and protect parental autonomy and the privacy of the family: First and most important, there is evidence from developmental psychology that an intimate and undisturbed relationship between parents and their children is vital for the development of the child (Bowlby 1988).[3] Second, parental autonomy and privacy of the family are generally appreciated by parents. Many authors claim, therefore, that parents have a right to privacy and parental autonomy (compare Brighouse and Swift 2006). Third, in families many goods such as positive identity formation, basic resource provision, specific needs identification and reciprocity of care are provided, for which otherwise expensive state institutions would be necessary (Macleod 2002). While the first reason is a moral reason per se (insofar as children have a right to proper development), the second and the third reason are at least prudential reasons for the endorsement of parental autonomy and the privacy of the family.[4] Hence these are good reasons to endorse institutions that promote parental autonomy and the privacy of the

---

[3] Attachment theory is not as uncontroversial as it is often held to be. Yet in this paper I will assume that a strong attachment to their parents is in the interest of the child.

[4] A consequentialist might, for example, argue that the frustration of basic parental interests is per se a moral reason because it diminishes overall well-being in society.

family – like PC. However, this does not mean that parental autonomy and the privacy of the family are unconditional. If children's interests count equally, parental autonomy and the privacy of the family should in principle be confined to where children's interests are concerned. I will come back to this point later.

To sum up: First, PC is a duty that protects intrinsic and instrumental goods of liberal society (like autonomy, privacy of the family and trust). Second, PC extends to parental autonomy and the privacy of the family. Third, therefore parental autonomy and the privacy of the family should be protected. It is important to stress this point as much as possible. PC protects moral goods (privacy of the family and parental autonomy). Any state intervention with PC is therefore in need of justification. This is why there is such a strong claim for LS in liberal societies.

12.3.2 *Duty to Report (DR) and the Public Role of the Physician*

Physicians have specific duties qua being physicians. When a person needs medical help, the physician has a duty to help the person. In contrast, professional medical help cannot be expected from a passer-by in the street who has no medical background. This is at least what we have to conclude when accepting the ethical principle "ought implies can". In one way the duty to provide medical help if necessary is a definitional part of medicine. Furthermore it is implemented in most legal systems. If a physician does not help a person in need she runs the risk to face legal consequences.

Parents have specific duties qua being parents. In general, parents have the duty to care for the well-being of their children. As already been mentioned in Sect. 12.2, this means that parents have to promote the interests of their children. Sometimes parents miss this duty. As the state treats children as persons, it is obliged to protect their interests. If the parents of a child violate its interests in way that might endanger the well-being of the child, the state acquires the right to interfere with parental autonomy and the privacy of the family. Physicians can notoriously get in the situation to decide if this is the case, namely if parents in some way endanger the well-being of their children. This is because physicians have to care for a vital part of a child's well-being, namely its health. In our role as members of society we all have the duty to help persons in need and we can be charged if we miss this duty. On top of their duty as citizens, physicians, in their role as medical professionals, are experts concerning the health-related well-being of the child. Both claims together – the expert-status of the physician and her role as a citizen – constitute the duty to report cases of child-maltreatment at the responsible political institution. In most cases this will be the youth-welfare office. But in extreme cases a direct charge at the investigative authority in charge might be required.

The concept of child-maltreatment is a difficult one (Cicchetti 1989). I will confine my analysis to cases proper to medical contexts, i.e. to cases of physical, psychological and sexual maltreatment. It is unquestionable in such cases that the well-being of children is endangered. If there is evidence for the physician that a child has been physically, psychologically or sexually maltreated by its parents, this would deliver a straightforward justification to report to the institution in charge. The problem is that it is not always easy to decide if there is sufficient evidence to justify such a claim against the parents. Imagine you are a parent of a child that practises some physically demanding sport like rugby or hockey. Would it be desirable that every minor hematoma resulting from this would be reported to the youth welfare office?[5] It is part of the goods protected by PC that not every minor injury of your child is a matter of public interest. Furthermore, parents have a right to defend themselves against unjustified suspicions. In severe cases this might even lead to trials. There have, for example, been cases when physicians made reports concerning an alleged physical or psychological maltreatment of children for which parents charged the physician for slander (Fangerau et al. 2010). Hence, for the physician the situation is precarious. She has to balance the evidence responsibly before reporting to a public institution.

Two facets of the justification of the physician's claim are important: first, for DR it is sufficient that the physician's claim is *evidentially* justified. However, complete certainty or knowledge is not necessary for DR. What is required is rather that adequate evidence is given that parents have maltreated their child. If the vital interests of the child are indeed concerned, the physician has to report. Second, physicians have to deal with *specific medical evidence*. I am not concerned with medical evidence in general but with evidence in the case of medical routine-checks. Medicine is primarily the science of health, or strictly speaking, of the absence of health. The concept of health is of course a rather controversial matter in medical ethics.[6] But even most constructivists would not deny that medical evidence is statistical evidence at least to some extent. When physicians talk about the well-being of a person, what they have in mind is that this person's physical properties are approximately close to normalized measurements of physical functions. For example, the normal blood pressure of an adult is about 120/80 mmHg. For young children the normal blood pressure is about 90/60 mmHg.

The essential criterion for the question whether evidence is sufficient to justify reporting to a public institution is that the child's well-being is endangered or that the child's vital interests are at stake and that the parents of the child are susceptible of being the cause of this. There are three possible situations for physicians:

(a) The child's well-being is safe according to the medical standard values.
(b) There is clear evidence that the child's well-being is at risk because of parental child-maltreatment.
(c) There is no clear evidence, but a well-grounded suspicion from the side of the physician that the child's well-being is at risk.

---

[5] In such cases, physicians might already report while, from the parental point of view, this would mean a loss of trust.
[6] Boorse (1977); Conrad (2007).

In cases of type (a) no report is justified as no evidence at all is given. If the physician is confronted with a 'normal' child (according to medical standard values) she will not have to even think about her professional confidentiality.

In cases of type (b) the physician must report because both conditions for DR are fulfilled: the child's well-being is at risk, and the parents of the child are the cause of the endangerment of children's well-being. Examples of sufficient evidence in this context are distinct symptoms for physical or sexual abuse, like broken limbs or traumatized sexual organs.

But what about cases of type (c)? Consider, for example, the battered child syndrome. The battered child syndrome is caused by severe shaking of a child's body, leading to dangerous life-threatening conditions like concussions, spinal cord hematoma or even sudden infant death (Kempe and Helfer 1974). In the paradigmatic case of a concussion parents might tell the physician the classical story of their child having fallen down the stairs. The physician might believe the story or not. Her problem remains the same, though: does she have to make a report or not? It is important to recognize another practical issue: physicians are notoriously short on time. This means that not only physicians are confronted with epistemically vague cases (in terms of given evidence), but also that the physician has to make her judgment in a rather short period of time. This is no minor problem for the physician because she is faced with serious legal consequences in both cases: to report or not to. This is what I have called the family-dilemma. It should be clear so far that the family-dilemma for physicians arises only in epistemically vague cases of type (c).

12.3.3 The Normative Structure of the Family-Dilemma

The family-dilemma arises because LS forces the physician to decide if her specific medical evidence justifies the claim that parents have maltreated their children. Yet there are cases in which it is not really clear for the physician which duty she has to follow. The important question for now is this: Is this uncertainty grounded in *epistemic* or in *normative* reasons? On the face of it, the uncertainty is grounded in epistemic reasons like not always having completely reliable indicative methods at hand and having limited time to decide. Would improving the epistemic standards be enough for solving the family-dilemma? Two reasons speak against it:

1. Empirically speaking, it is extremely implausible to assume that medical indicative methods will one day be reliable enough to cast out any doubts. For sure, there is steady progress in medical science. Consider the battered child syndrome again. Since the early days of diagnosis of Kempe and Helfer the indicative methods concerning the battered child syndrome have improved at a large scale.[7] While up until the 1980s of the last century diagnostic methods were insufficient, contemporary methods like medical imaging have improved to such

---

[7] See Kempe and Helfer (1974).

a degree that much more refined medical examinations have become possible. In 2012 a study by Edelbauer et al. showed that spinal subdural effusion can be reliably traced back to the battered child syndrome and that other causes cannot cause this typical condition (Edelbauer et al. 2012). Such new methods can be of great help for the physician when she has to decide if the evidence is sufficient for DR. Medical imaging provides physicians with specific medical evidence. This evidence clearly indicates injuries that can be considered in relation to certain plausible causes. Hence, this medical evidence shifts the burden of proof to the parents. They have to explain what has happened to their child.

It is, however, important to notice that even a clear indication for the battered child syndrome or, to give another example, multiple fractures are not as reliable indicators for child-maltreatment as one might wish. Other physical injuries like lacerated ears or hematoma could be caused by other children. These examples make clear that the physician is confronted with a vast limbo of possible cases when she works out if the evidence at hands is sufficient for DR. Some might argue that the frequency of a child's injuries counts as well. If a child suffers from the same injuries again and again, even minor injuries can be a reliable indicator for child-maltreatment by the parents. This is an important point. But it does not help with solving the family-dilemma. This is because there is still enough space for uncertainty, for example when the physician is confronted with a child she sees for the first time. As long as uncertainty is part of medical indicative practise (in contexts of child protection), and as long as the burden of proof is on the side of the physician, in unclear cases of child-maltreatment the family-dilemma will endure. Yet in this situation the epistemic reasons for the physician to follow PC only count as legitimate reasons because of the normative background assumption given by LS, according to which the burden of proof is always on the side of the physician.

In other words: *the family-dilemma is a normative dilemma that applies on the level of corresponding duties (DR and PC) because of the burden of proof-entailment in LS.* Endorsing this entailment means that physicians not only have to deliver the evidence against the parents, furthermore they are forced to withhold their report until they are certain enough to prevent severe legal consequences due to a negligence of PC. Yet if the law protects children's and parental interests alike, there should be no substantial obstacles for physicians to report suspicious cases.[8]

Hence, the question is at least on the table if, in the above mentioned epistemic vague cases, the burden of proof should be on the side of the parents. If this was the case, the family-dilemma could be solved. Accordingly, physicians would be

---

[8] In many cases LS makes it difficult for physicians to protect the vital interests of children. Therefore, LS has to be questioned from the moral point of view. To put it in more specific terms: When children have a right that their vital interests are protected, this right includes the necessity to widen the scope of action for physicians to actually protect those children against abusive and maltreating parents. From this perspective, LS puts things in the wrong order. LS entails serious obstacles for the protection of children's rights.

provided with better tools to protect the interests of children. However, at this point liberals as well as conservatives notoriously claim that a system in which parents have to prove that they treat their children in the right way is no liberal system. And indeed: that parents do not have to justify their way of upbringing their children by default is exactly what is protected by LS. Yet, as will be pointed out in the next section, it is not true that shifting the burden of proof to the parents entails giving up on the idea of a liberal standard in child-rearing.

2. The second reason for calling the family-dilemma a normative dilemma concerns the concept of children's well-being which is a normative notion. Even if we had perfectly reliable indicative methods in medicine, it is still another question which actions should count as a violation of a child's well-being. Let us, for the moment, assume that such reliable indicative methods are indeed available. Why should we accept their authority for an evaluation of children's well-being? An affirmative answer would be that medical reasons are belief-independent reasons when we try to figure out what is in a child's best interest. By 'belief-independent' I mean that medical reasons, unlike religious or aesthetic reasons, do not depend on personal opinions. That a person suffers from a specific disease or that a person's condition deviates from medical standard values is a fact that can be measured.[9] Given this and given that, at least in western societies, the well-being of children is progressively a public matter, it is no wonder that medical reasons count more and more when disputes concerning the well-being of children occur. This can be called the process of medicalizing children's well-being. The concept of medicalization means in this context that the well-being of children is defined in medical terms (Conrad 2007). Medicalization per se is not good or bad. It is certainly a good thing that in many cases medical reasons defeat personal parental opinions about medical treatment of their children. Yet there is reason for caution as well. This is because there is a tendency in the process of medicalization of understanding the well-being of children strictly in medical terms. And this is certainly a problem for liberal society. Consider the notorious debate concerning male circumcision. Following the medical status quo, male circumcision is medically not necessary (at least in countries where running water is accessible). In a strictly medicalized vision of children's well-being this would already be a sufficient reason for calling male circumcision a violation of a child's well-being. But consider the correction of sticky-out ears which is normally medically not necessary as well. What this example shows on an intuitive level is that other values than brute medical necessity are relevant for the evaluation of a child's well-being. I will come back to this point in the next section. For the moment it should be clear that the normative components of the concept of children's well-being forbid a completely medicalized notion of children's well-being. This is, in turn, an obstacle for a solution of the family-dilemma for physicians.

---

[9] I take the term 'measure' in a rather broad sense to include realist and constructivist positions.

12.4 The Liberal Standard Revisited

12.4.1 Shifting the Burden of Proof?

It is important to keep in mind how the family-dilemma is related to LS: because LS protects parental interests, the physician has to respect parental autonomy and the privacy of the family. However, some parents maltreat their children, and in some families vital interests of children are violated. In this vein the family-dilemma is related to the notorious liberal conflict between freedom and safety. A solution of the family-dilemma, and by that token the warranty of safety for all children, seems to be only within reach if parents lose at least some of their liberties as parents. One does not have to call for the general licensing of parents, as some authors do.[10] In our context, it would be enough to oblige parents to take their children to routine medical check-ups. In Germany, for example, a system of such routine check-ups already exists. At least in some German counties like Baden Württemberg parents have to bring their children to routine medical check-ups. Yet what we can learn from the current situation in Germany is that a mere obligation of the parents to take their children to regular medical check-ups does not suffice for solving the family-dilemma for physicians. As long as the burden of proof-entailment of LS sustains, the situation would remain dangerous for the physician when it comes to type-(c)-cases.

A way out of the family-dilemma for physicians would be to shift the burden of proof to the parents by default in epistemically vague cases of type (c). This is exactly what has happened in the Netherlands quite recently. The Dutch Ministry of Health, Welfare and Sports has suggested a law that does not only advise that medical check-ups for children are carried out. Rather, a mandatory report code should be implemented in law. It should encourage physicians to report even minor injuries of the child to the youth-welfare office. Thereby, the burden of proof would be turned to the parents. It is important to note that the Dutch model would not implement a duty for the physician to report *all* suspicions. However, it provides a formal procedure to take action and to make other authorities aware of suspicions, and therefore alleviates the moral burden of responsibility of the individual doctor. In this vein, the Dutch model is a first step in helping to solve the family-dilemma for physicians, because DR is encouraged and formalized. As a consequence, at least from a medical point of view, children can be much better protected against abusive parents.[11]

---

[10] In his seminal paper "Licensing Parents" Hugh Laffollette considers a radical version of this position. He claims that parents should be licensed because parenting entails two necessary conditions why we license activities in general: first, that the relevant activity is hazardous for innocents and second, that the activity is sufficiently complex. (Compare Laffollette 1980)

[11] The so called "reporting code" consists of a formal procedure for cases of alleged domestic violence and sexual abuse of children. While there would be no duty for the physician to report all cases, the code is meant as a formal procedure that makes it easier for the physician to report suspicious cases to the relevant institution. (MHWS 2012)

Nonetheless, two interrelated points cause worries: The first worry concerns an alleged slippery slope in liberal values like parental autonomy and the privacy of the family. The second worry is that a more dominant role of physicians concerning the evaluation of children's well-being can easily lead to over-medicalized standards of children's well-being in society. Both worries will now be considered in turn.

Shifting the burden of proof by default to the parents means that, in many cases, parents will have to justify their actions *as parents*. However, this seems to be incompatible with the idea that parents are autonomous in their child-rearing if we understand autonomy, as it is usually understood, in terms of self-ownership. Yet parental autonomy is a very specific field of autonomy, as it concerns parental interests and children's interests alike. If children's interests count, we cannot understand parental autonomy as a mere extension of the Lockean idea of self-ownership (Archard 2004). In his paper "Conceptions of Parental Autonomy" Colin Macleod distinguishes three conceptions of parental autonomy: the conservative, the democratic and the liberal conception of parental autonomy. The conservative and the democratic conception of parental autonomy are very similar. Both claim that parents have full authority in educational questions as long as the minimum standard for children's well-being is guaranteed.[12]

The background justification is delivered by the *epistemic access argument* (Macleod 1997). According to this argument, parents have a specific epistemic access to the needs of their children which in turn justifies granting them a broad authority in educational questions. Yet, as Macleod points out, both conceptions are self-defeating as strategies indebted to the minimum standard of children's well-being that takes account of children's immediate interest in the fulfilment of their basic needs and in becoming autonomous persons. This is because both conceptions are compatible with cases when children are brought up in value systems where autonomy has no central role. In contrast, the liberal conception of parental autonomy is, contrary to the conservative and democratic conception, sceptical towards any fundamental or all-comprising conception of the good. The liberal demands, therefore, that children have to be brought up according to the sceptical standards of fallibilism. According to the liberal conception, parents have the right to impose their values on their children as long as they secure that they acquire the critical capacities to question those values or to compare them with competing values. The worries of liberals and conservatives/democrats can be put as follows: the conservative/democrat takes strong and intimate familial bonds as being vital for a child's development. Meanwhile, the liberal suspects those bonds as the main culprits for a lack of at least one specific aspect of child's development – namely the development into an autonomous person.[13]

---

[12] The difference between the democratic and the conservative conception of parental autonomy is that the former requires an introduction in key democratic values, like respect and tolerance of diversity, while the latter does not. For the sake of brevity I will not discuss this difference in the context of this paper. (Compare Macleod 1997)

[13] Compare Matthew Clayton's distinction between autonomy as an end-state and autonomy as a precondition. Clayton doesn't only argue against forms of education that harm the child's

Macleod accepts that both sides have a point and suggests a *refined liberal conception of parental autonomy*. The problem is to make parental autonomy compatible with the child's development into an autonomous person without destabilizing the family with its shared projects (Macleod 1997). To do so, Macleod distinguishes between two dimensions of the refined conception of parental autonomy: Within the family, parents should have the right to confer their preferred values on their children. Outside the family, however, (in the community-sphere) children have to be able to take part in pluralistic discourse. For instance, children raised in a certain religious faith system by their parents must be allowed to leave this system while attending school, to take part in all sorts of communication and activities of non-religious peers. This means, their parents must grant their children to have a chance to openly consider the value system imposed on them at home and to question it.

The restriction on parental autonomy in the first dimension (within the family) must therefore be that it must not disable children in becoming skilled in the outer dimension as autonomous beings. The above mentioned worry was that we risk a slippery slope in the concept of parental autonomy when accepting restrictions of parenting, like forcing parents to take their children to medical routine check-ups. However, if we apply Macleod's differentiation in the concept of parental autonomy, we can see that this is not necessarily the case. Some restrictions of parental liberties, like public schooling and public health-care, are compatible with the liberal idea of parental autonomy. Yet, there is still reason for caution, first because physicians and official persons can abuse or exceed their competencies. Here it is of utter importance to install a system of checks and balances where single persons are limited in their actions. Second, more public attention for the well-being of children in general and – more specific in the health context – will not come without social and economic costs. The economic costs concern factors like new institutions, staff, and research. The social costs concern society's basic values. For example, an increasing public attention towards children means a less intimate relation of parents and their offspring. Because there are empirical and normative reasons (like the attachment between children and parents and values like parental autonomy and the privacy of the family) for supporting such a relation, a call for more public attention has to be balanced against those reasons. Yet, and this is the main focus of this paper, the classical liberal standard does not do justice to the situation of many children. The above explained revised version of the liberal standard is an attempt to meet our basic intuitions and values about upbringing while coming to grips with the requirement to improve the situation for children.

---

development but as well against what he calls 'comprehensive enrolment'. That means he argues against forms of education that don't take account of the interests of the person the child might become Clayton (2006). Similar (but less provoking) ideas are developed in Feinberg (1992) and in Noggle (2002).

12.4.2 Over-Medicalizing Children's Well-Being?

The second worry concerns the predominance of physicians in the evaluation of children's well-being that inevitably happens when DR gains priority. This is what can be called the 'thread of over-medicalization'.[14] As pointed out above, more obligatory medical check-ups for children are not sufficient for overcoming the family-dilemma for physicians. This holds at least when physicians are not equipped with the relevant competences that allow them to easily report dubious cases. However, mandatory regular medical check-ups at least allow physicians to report problematic cases of child-development or of assumed child-maltreatment relatively early. As a consequence, better standards of child-protection seem to be at hand.

Yet we must not forget that the physician's perspective on the well-being of children is usually confined to the medical perspective. Physicians consider whether children are healthy and evaluate the children's health related well-being in relation to certain medical standard-values.[15] The problem is that those medical values can conflict with values of the parents – religious or aesthetical values for example. In the case of risky medical procedures (e.g. aesthetic surgery) the medical perspective should always have priority. But even with an empirical science like medicine there are trends, and the very concept of health itself entails values. What might have been considered a normal child 20 years ago can today easily count as a hyperactive child (Conrad 2007).

From a medical point of view, Ritalin might in some cases be the best solution to overcome the child's hyperactivity. Yet some parents might be sceptical that their child should be treated with a drug that works on the level of the cognitive system. If, however, physicians have a duty to report all medically conspicuous cases, this can easily lead to a situation when the parents are suspected of child-neglect because they refuse Ritalin treatment for their children. This example demonstrates that just calling for more competences of physicians can in itself lead to problematic consequences – even if the family-dilemma gets solved by this. One way of avoiding the problem of an over-medicalized concept of children's well-being is to set general institutional standards for check-ups for children that encompass children's education and well-being as a whole. In this set of institutional standards, medical check-ups should be part of a wider system where all relevant capabilities of children for proper development are checked on a regular basis, not only their physical condition. For example social skills, emotional development, language development, etc. should be checked as well. In such a system physicians would have to deal with

---

[14] I use the term 'over-medicalization' to point out that I don't consider medicalization *per se* as something negative. I endorse the idea that the medical point of view is indeed relevant for the evaluation of children's well-being. Yet it is still another thing to claim that medicine has the authority when it comes to controversial claims about the well-being of children.

[15] This is not to say that physicians do not at all consider other factors, like social and environmental conditions. Yet the physician's specific perspective is the medical perspective that is statistical and empirical in the first play.

social workers, psychologists, and educational scientists before reporting. The important point is to avoid any single-minded medical perspective in the general evaluation of children's well-being.

12.5 Conclusion

This paper started out from the assumption that children's interests have to be protected as well as parental interests. Most western legal systems implement the liberal standard as a legal instrument for child-protection. That means they have a conservative attitude towards values like the privacy of the family and parental autonomy: the government normally may not interfere with parental rights and may not violate a family's privacy. One of the problems caused by the liberal standard is that it can lead to the family-dilemma for physicians. The family-dilemma for physicians arises because they have contradictory duties: on the one hand, the duty to report cases of suspected maltreatment of children (DR), and on the other hand they have to keep professional confidentiality (PC). The dilemma occurs in epistemically unclear cases where the physician is not sure if her evidence is sufficient for reporting to the authority in charge. In these cases a law guided by the liberal standard protects even abusive parents. The burden of proof is on the side of the physician and the authorities: they must provide evidence for the child's actual maltreatment by the parents.

However, this is not compatible with the assumption that the interests of children should primarily be protected by the state's law (Dwyer 2006). In order to better protect children's well-being, it would be wise to shift the burden of proof to the parents. In practice, this would mean that whenever a physician has good reason to suspect that a child has been maltreated or neglected by its parents, the parents would have to prove their innocence.

Meanwhile, the protection of values like the privacy of the family and of parental autonomy is an important part of the liberal tradition and is normally not violated. This is why the burden of proof concerning proper child-rearing is usually not shifted to the parents. Rather, it usually remains on the side of the physician – even in specific cases when a child's well-being is at risk.

In order to ease the tension between a protection of children's well-being while and, at the same time, of parental autonomy, this paper suggested a way in which the burden of proof can be shifted to the parents. The suggestion still remains within an acceptable liberal framework that boils down to a concept of refined liberalism: In a pluralist society, different contexts in which a child spends her time can function as checks and balances that correct extreme parental value judgments and actions that endanger the well-being of the child. Here, Colin McLeod's idea of a fallibilist variety of liberalism is applied and fleshed out. While the liberal concept of parental autonomy is maintained by and large by this approach, it warrants that parents do not interfere with their children's exposure to other values and norms. In this vein, the government has to ensure that parents make it possible for their children to be under the influence of diverse groups that correct and relativize their parental value judgments and control their actions. For instance, attending a public school will ideally help revealing whether a child is maltreated or neglected by her parents, since the teachers will recognize certain symptoms. By the child spending time in different contexts, the burden of proof is automatically indirectly shifted towards the parents: parents who do not allow their children's exposure to a variety of values may be regarded and treated as problematic parents. Their child's physical and mental well-being will ideally be more closely monitored, and they have to justify their way of educating a child on a regular basis, for instance by forced visits by the authorities.

Hence there is a justification for an introduction of a more refined version of the liberal standard derived from children's interests. Yet it is important to note that even in this refined version of the liberal standard the family-dilemma for physicians will not be completely solved. As long as we endorse values like the privacy of the family and of parental autonomy, there will have to be limits for physician's competences concerning the evaluation of children's well-being. This is why the question of overmedicalization arises. The pluralism of liberal society does not only concern parents but physicians as well. Any society that is liberal concerning so called conceptions of the good cannot legitimately evaluate children's well-being by the authority of medical conceptions of well-being alone. This means that there must be limits for physician's authority when it comes to the evaluation of children's well-being. For instance, parents should have a right to interfere with any quick decision to give their child Ritalin. Yet, and this is the upshot of this paper, those limits must not prevent physicians from taking care of the well-being of children when necessary.

References

Allen, A. (2011). Privacy and medicine. In *Stanford encyclopedia of philosophy*. http://plato.stanford.edu/entries/privacy-medicine/. Accessed 20 Aug 2013.
Archard, D. (2004). *Children. Rights and childhood* (2nd ed.). London: Routledge.
Bagattini, A. (2013). Das Kindeswohl im Spannungsfeld liberaler Werte und behördlicher Maßnahmen. In *Ethik in der öffentlichen Verwaltung* (pp. 91–115). Bd. 4.
Beauchamp, T. L., & Childress, J. F. (2013). *Principles of biomedical ethics* (7th ed.). Oxford: Oxford University Press.
Boorse, C. (1977). Health as a theoretical concept. *Philosophy of Science, 44*, 542–573.
Bowlby, J. (1988). *A secure base*. London: Basic Books.
Brighouse, H., & Swift, A. (2006) Parents' rights and the value of the family. *Ethics, 117*, 80–108.
Buchanan, A., & Brock, D. W. (1990). *Deciding for others. The ethics of surrogate decision making*. Cambridge UK: Cambridge University Press.
Cicchetti, D. (Ed.). (1989). *Child maltreatment. Theory and research on the causes and consequences of child abuse and neglect*. Cambridge: Cambridge University Press.
Clayton, M. (2006). *Justice and legitimacy in upbringing*. Oxford: Oxford University Press.
Conrad, P. (2007). *The medicalization of society*. Baltimore: Johns Hopkins University Press.
Dworkin, R. (1983). In defence of equality. *Social Philosophy and Policy* 1, no 1.
Dwyer, J. G. (2006). *The relationship rights of children*. Cambridge: Cambridge University Press.

Edelbauer, M., Maurer, K., Gassner, I. (2012). Spina subdural effusion – An additional sonographic sign of child abuse. *Ultraschall in der Medizin, 33*(7).

Fangerau, H., Fegert, J., Kemper, A., & Kölch, M. (2010). Ärztliche Schweigepflicht bei Kindeswohlgefährdung. Mehr Handlungssicherheit durch die neuen Kinderschutzgesetze? *Ethik in der Medizin, 22*(1), 33–47.

Feinberg, J. (1983). Autonomy, sovereignty, and privacy: Moral ideals and the constitution. *Notre Dame Law Review, 58*(3), 445–492.

Feinberg, J. (1992). The child's right to an open future. In J. Feinberg (Ed.), *Freedom and fulfillment* (pp. 76–97). Princeton: Princeton University Press.

Kempe, C. H., & Helfer, R. E. (1974). *The battered child*. Chicago: Chicago University Press.

Lafollette, H. (1980). Licensing parents. *Philosophy and Public Affairs, 9*(2), 182–197.

Macleod, C. (1997). Conceptions of parental autonomy. *Politics and Society, 25*(1), 117–140.

Macleod, C. (2002). Liberal equality and the affective family. In D. Archard & C. Macleod (Eds.), *The moral and political status of children* (pp. 212–231). Oxford: Oxford University Press.

Ministry of Health, Welfare and Sport (MHWS). (2012). *Model reporting code – Domestic violence and child abuse*.

Noggle, R. (2002). Special agents: Children's autonomy and parental authority. In D. Archard & C. Macleod (Eds.), *The moral and political status of children* (pp. 97–117). Oxford: Oxford University Press.

Rössler, B. (2004). *The value of privacy*. London: Blackwell.

Schrag, F. (1977). The child in the moral order. *Philosophy, 52*(200), 167–177.

Chapter 13
Child Welfare and Child Protection: Medicalization and Scandalization as the New Norms in Dealing with Violence Against Children

Heiner Fangerau, Arno Görgen, and Maria Griemmert

13.1 Introduction: The History, Theory, and Ethics of Child Protection

At least since the 1950s and 1960s, the social and cultural sciences are characterized as academic fields, which particularly critically reflect social developments. Strongly influenced by the theories of Michel Foucault and Pierre Bordieu, a temporary string of social and cultural research lies in the observation of supersubjective interpretation patterns, structures of meaning, collective knowledge schemes and symbolic power relations and their implementation in social practices (Moebius 2012). For example, in Foucault's perspective, form and content of what is said determines the actions of actors. Institutionalized ways of talking then define the sayable and the thinkable.

Social functional systems strive for a distinct mode of discourse within their communication, while at the same time, they hope to extend their sphere of influence by trying to transfer their discourse to other functional systems. Especially within the historical science, the acceptance of the paradigm of a "social construction of reality" (Berger and Luckmann 1966), based on a reciprocal process of subjective interpretation of environment and their social, communicative mediation, is a central pillar in the analytical examination of knowledge-generating processes.

By using the example of child protection, which regularly suffers of uncritical perspectives of a teleological self-improving development (e.g. in Myers 2011), it can be shown that such processes of social construction are not only contingent, but also are influenced by quite power-strategic considerations which adopt to distinct contemporary developments. This can be seen for example in the German terminol-

---

H. Fangerau (✉) • A. Görgen, Ph.D. • M. Griemmert, Ph.D.
Institute for the History, Philosophy and Ethics of Medicine,
University of Ulm, 89075 Ulm, Germany
e-mail: heiner.fangerau@uni-ulm.de

ogy of "public guardian office" ("*staatliches Wächteramt*"), which not only defines a central task of the state in the institutionalized child protection, but also implies a very clear power polarization. Furthermore, child protection is so appropriate for a critical analysis of its discourses, ostensibly because a general consensus exists on the social need to protect children from maltreatment, abuse, and neglect. Child protection is a very strong moral norm. Child abuse represents one of the most serious social breaches and taboos in the private realm of modern societies (Hacking 1991). The concern for the welfare of children therefore legitimizes state sanctions in the traditionally autonomous and protected area of the family.[1]

The reason for the general recognition of the child's need for protection lies in the Western concept of childhood, which in contrast to adulthood, is a clearly defined phase of life and, unlike the latter, is characterized by innocence, dependence, and vulnerability. Child abuse is therefore also an exploitation and violation of these characteristics, as well as an undermining of the principles of justice, trust, and responsibility. The social and personal development of young people, and the full realization of their individual potential, demand protection against discrimination. Damage at this stage is considered particularly difficult to deal with or even irreversible. The abused child is deprived of his or her developmental potential (Daniel 2010). Finally, the concepts of freedom and self-determination of the child play an important role in the placement of child protection as a moral postulate.

Right at the interface of child protection, the compliance of which is ensured mostly by the family, and self-determination of the child, who cannot escape the family structure, lies the fluidity and socio-cultural uncertainty of what is considered child abuse or maltreatment (Smallbone et al. 2008: p. 2). Thus, it may sometimes make sense to remove a child from his family for protection. This decision contradicts the child's right to autonomy if the child wants to stay with its family. Here, public expectations, actions, and agents for child protection can come into conflict with one another. At the same time the decision to remove a child from his or her family is influenced by a variety of cultural factors (Rivaux et al. 2008).

Child protection is not only a moral axiom; it also offers adults the opportunity for concrete social self-assessment. This self-assessment is not selfishness. Rather, it is likely that the initiative for child protection originates from empathy for the potentially tragic fates of the children. Nevertheless, child protection, in its universal acceptance, provides orientation in a postmodern world that is otherwise mostly characterized by uncertainty. Therefore, child protection—in addition to its actual political and social necessity—can be viewed as a metaphor, the transfer of meaningful content onto a not directly connected contextual concept (Kupffer 1999). According to Kupffer, child protection in this sense enables a collaborative management contingency to view child protectors through their protective interests for the child. As a secondary feature, a clear social position of the adult towards the child follows wherein authority is ascribed to the adult and the possibility of self-determination is denied to the child. In this way, the identity of the adult can be

---

[1] Some of the following thoughts have been published in German before. See Görgen et al. (2013); Schmitz and Fangerau (2010). The English has been edited by Writescienceright.

enhanced. Another important point in the acceptance of child protection as a metaphor lies in the ability of the individual to be able to generate public outrage against child abuse, without sacrificing his or her moral integrity and without being active. For example, pressure to act can be built up in the mass media by accusations of incompetence, incapacity, or immorality directed at parties other than the accuser. For example, lawyers, doctors, youth services agents, or police can be accused without the accuser risking the loss of a moral high-ground (King 1999).

Finally, child protection due to its acknowledged necessity enables the establishment of a power monopoly of social authority. In complex post-modern societies, child protection represents one of the few fields where a hegemonic position in the discourse of education is equivalent to a massive increase in power. This results in sometimes violent battles for opinion leadership among social function systems, such as legal, religious and political institutions, health care providers, and the media. An example from the medical perspective is the pediatrician Henry Kempe, one of the main initiators of modern child protection, who recognized this struggle for *opinion leadership*, and therefore claimed: *"It is the responsibility of the medical profession to assume the leadership in this field"* (Helfer and Kempe 1968: p. 25).

Based on these considerations the aim of this contribution is to describe the origin of the normative framework for the well-being of children in most countries of the Western world (with examples in Central Europe, the USA and Australia) as the result of an interdiscourse of different social systems. Special emphasis will be put on the media representing a broader public and medicine with its specific medical conception of child well-being which seeks to describe children's welfare in terms of the normal, the pathological, diagnoses and therapies. Subsequently, from a historical and cultural scientific perspective, after some theoretical remarks, medicine and the media with their approach to child well-being and their mutual usage to promote their view on children's welfare shall be considered. These two systems are structure-building in child protection, interactive, and both respectively and collectively struggle for opinion leadership in child protection. After an overview of the medicalization of child protection, the focus will be on the scandalization of medicalized child protection in the media and on the norm building interactions between the two systems. In particular, the respective self-motivation of the two systems to bring about political change and new norms in child protection through media attention and "media hype" will be a topic of particular interest.

13.2 Child Protection and Discourse

According to the discourse theory based on Michel Foucault's work, the thinking and actions of operators is determined by the form and content of what is communicated and known (Foucault 2003: pp. 392f.). One consequence of this model is the insight, that institutionalized ways of speaking define what can be said and what is feasible, and conversely, what is unspeakable or taboo. On one hand, within social functional systems, attempts are made to produce coherent discourse and profiling. On the other hand, the transfer of these system-specific discourses to other systems is sought to increase their own influence. In child protection, socially influenced constructs and concepts arise which are subsumed under the terms of childhood, child, abuse, and maltreatment. Following Luhmann's system theory these constructs, which are subject to historical change, are characterized by systemic rivalries, which according to their origin are perceived as medicalization (expanding medical discourses and systems), commercialization (market expansion), or judicialization (extension of the law) of the discourse and manifest, for example, in the development or restriction of governmental or social welfare work.[2] According to Habermas, the communicative exchange in the public arena allows functional systems to differentiate themselves and disseminate their specific conceptions of childhood in recourse to changing social realities (Habermas 1998: p. 427). This is a constantly occurring process that has been enabled primarily by the use of media.

In the early modern age, moralization of public debates related to child protection has already been established with cases of infringement of children's well-being. In this process, questions of morality were coupled with questions about social welfare, religious charity, the law, and medicine. These debates were brought into the (semi-) public space as print media evolved (Pollock 1983). For example, in 1787, a surgeon elaborated on the *"outrageous cruelty of a mother"* and the necropsy findings of a 9-year-old girl who died of abuse in the *Journal für Deutschland* (Journal for Germany). The inhumanity and "devilish wickedness" of the case led him to want to continue his descriptions as more precise circumstances of the offense, beyond the medical findings and legal judgments, became available (Jaßy 1787). Two years later, another more thorough description of the case followed in the *Annalen der Gesetzgebung und Rechtsgelehrsamkeit* (Annals of legislation and jurisprudence). Therein, the doctor came to the conclusion that the mother, who had already been punished more severely than demanded by the prosecution, had been treated too leniently in the sentencing (Anonymous 1789). Thus, transgressing his disciplinary borders he expanded his medical perspective to the judicial discourse.

Later, as an example of an interaction between child protection discourses and social and cultural change, the European and American child protection movement in the nineteenth and early twentieth centuries was both heavily influenced by social Puritanism as well as by the emerging women's movement. In the nineteenth century, violence against children was seen as a problem of "moral immaturity" and attributed to the violence and drinking habits of men and therefore, *ex negativo*, the child protectors and the social environment of the upper classes postulated themselves as morally integrous and superior.[3] Conversely, from the 1920s onward, an environmental scientific basis of child protection became important with the professionalization of social work. The focus of attention shifted to child neglect. Neglect was

---

[2] On the autonomy of systems and intersystemic conflicts/rivalries see e.g. Luhmann (1998: pp. 776ff.), Schimank (2006). For medicalization as a model for the expansion of a system's influence see for example Peter Conrad (2007).

[3] A concise overview provides an interpretation of Hogarth's "Gin Lane": Rodin (1981).

considered to be primarily a female crime; and the particular "hazard potential" of single mothers was stigmatized.[4]

These historical examples demonstrate a prototype of the ritualized forms of public dealings with difficult child protection events, as they are still to this day emotionally charged subjects. A rough sketch of the ritualized course of a media processed abuse scandal goes as follows. First, the first reports of maltreatment, abuse, and neglect are followed by a wave of indignation. The issue is then taken up by social subsystems (in politics, law, medicine, etc.), recorded, and adapted to the self-interest of the systems. Usually, systems then undergo an process of instrumentalization aimed at expanding the sphere of influence of one's own system whereby one system insinuates the other systems' complicity in the events. In this way, for example, medicine can portray itself as a guarantor of the health of children and the public health system. The result is a complex cycle that begins with the generation of a public discussion through moralization in the media by journalists, politicians, scientists, economists, or even doctors.

The discursive cycle that is fueled constantly by particular debates about abuse is subject to the dilemma that while the development of child protection is desired, its contents—in particular questions about the definition of what is to count as abuse, where it begins, and what the proper treatment of children is—have not yet been clarified uniformly due to the socially constructed nature of this issue. The difficulty inherent in defining cases is almost paradigmatically evident in this discussion with questions such as: What is child protection? How is it legitimate? What processes have been subject to permanent changes in interpretation? Most significant for children to be protected is the question of the mechanisms of continuous reorientation in dealing with abused children. According to Hacking, child protection debates are always closely linked with discourses of social morality, feminism, children's rights, the judiciary, poverty, the economy, public welfare, medical care, education, social welfare, psychology, etc. (Hacking 1991).

13.3 Child Protection and Medicalization

In the past, various social subsystems have repeatedly attempted to define the complex issue of "child abuse/child molestation" with particular attention being given to medicine. Since the emergence of nation-states in the late nineteenth century and their need for efficient workers and military personnel, medical and scientific interests in the child have increased sharply. The professionalizing and differentiating medicine of the late nineteenth century increasingly recognized the differences between the protection and care of a child versus an adult. Medicine responded to the new group of potential child patients by establishing a separate pediatrics discipline, which sought to define child welfare in terms of physical and

---

[4] For a critical review of the literature on the subject of changing economic situations in child protection see Hooper (1989).

psychological well-being which could be influenced with medical measures. Although there have been treatment services and nursing facilities for children, which differed conceptually from those for adults, since early modern times, a new quality of a particular focus of medicine on children developed in the early nineteenth century (Ritzmann 2008; Shuttleworth 2010).

More and more dimensions of the child's life were transferred by physicians into medical fields by means of medically described and explained categories. This process of extending the medical definition of spheres, which in social and cultural debates is sometimes paralleled with a biologization and naturalization of social constructs, can be described accurately by the term medicalization.[5] In dealing with infants and young children, the attempt to expand medical spheres of influence meant that children's needs for optimal development were now not only examined educationally, religiously, or psychologically, but also defined medically; and parents could be more medically responsible in light of the increasingly detailed knowledge of the relationships between stages of development, nutrition, encouragement, etc. A normative framework was established which focused on medical knowledge and medical categories as a measure of children's well-being. Whereas childhood education and care had traditionally been highly intuitive, relying on instinct, common sense, and tradition, they became more and more components of a field of knowledge that had to be conveyed to parents by doctors seen as specialists (Liebel 2007: pp. 29f.). Around 1900, medical infant welfare agencies, medical checks on milk and nursing, and nutrition campaigns were state-subsidized trials in Europe and the U.S. aimed at achieving long-term reduction in infant mortality for national economic interests (Meckel 1990; Corsini and Viazzo 1997). During the course of the nineteenth century, differentiated school hygiene programs intended to protect against infectious diseases or (presumed) educational diseases such as myopia and scoliosis were established, and the field of medicine entered into this formerly purely pedagogical field.[6] This movement, closely linked to national interests, experienced its first climax in the new German Empire (Hahn 1994). The first guide for school hygiene was published in 1877 by the pediatrician Adolf Baginsky. He became involved in a pro-health organization of the educational institution, improvement of educational resources, the study of the influence of education on health, and finally school monitoring. Baginsky saw an important role for medicine in school health care, especially in the medical evaluation of physical violence against children exerted by academic institutions. School doctors described the serious health consequences of physical punishment of students by teachers, such as epileptic seizures. Medical doctors suspected a high number of unreported cases and gave educators recommendations for physical punishment that would be least harmful to long-term health. Basically, they suggested that the head or chest should never be beaten, and advised that subjecting students to prolonged standing was also dangerous and should be avoided (Baginsky and Janke 1900: pp. 175–181, 347–349).

---

[5] On the complexity of biologization and medicalization debates in modern times see the overview Wehling et al. (2007).

[6] For an exploratory v.a. transnational overview see Umehara and Halling (2006).

Head injuries, especially, were interpreted by doctors early on as signs of potential child abuse: blows to the head were cautioned from a medical perspective due to the high risk of injury not only in the school context (Al-Holou et al. 2009). At first, mainly forensic medical examiners had described cases of child abuse and sexual abuse from a medical point of view (Gries 2002: pp. 87–102). In the sixteenth century, forensic medicine had already reconstructed cases of fatal abuse of children and described the medical signs for various forms of violence against children based on medical expertise in addition to legal case reports (e.g. Höpler 1918). In the nineteenth century the French forensic pathologist Ambroise Tardieu disclosed his experience as a court expert and published several studies from 1857 to 1868 wherein he provided detailed reports of more than 1,000 cases of ill-treatment, sexual abuse, neglect, and murder of children. He described therein significant physical and psychological signs whereby maltreatment and abuse could be identified in a medical examination. To this end, he reported, among other things, anxiety, pallor, a sad appearance, multiple bruises of different ages, torn ears, burns, and multiple fractures.[7]

Tardieu's early efforts to define childhood, child development, and child abuse in the medical context drew attention, especially in the forensic and criminological environment. Commensurate with the findings of other forensic pathologist and criminologists, Tardieu's results were largely without discursive social clout. In addition to diverging views on the quality and accuracy of the evidence of abuse, there was a persistent concern that doctors may raise false accusations through misdiagnosis (Lyons 1997; Olafson et al. 1993).[8]

The same applies to the development of discourse in a psychiatric context. In particular, the appearance of "curative" child-psychiatry, together with the psychological journal *Die Kinderfehler* (*The Child Defects*; published 1896–1899) and its immediate successor *Zeitschrift für Kinderforschung* (*Journal of Child Research*; published 1900–1944), reveal a strong medical interest in the healthy physical and psychological development of the child. A special issue from 1939 showed that the physical well-being and physical child abuse became increasingly important in the field of child psychiatry (*Zeitschrift für Kinderforschung* [*Journal of Child Research*] 1939 (Jg. 47, H.2)). But this professional discourse did not achieve social significance at first.

The discourse associated with "sexual abuse" played an even lesser role amongst medical professionals. It was not considered as a potential cause for the transmission of sexually transmitted diseases (e.g. Welander 1909). For example, historian Lynn Sacco described that in the USA in the 1890s–1940s, the etiology of the child Gonorrhoea was postulated to be hygienic deficiencies rather than sexual molestation by a family member (Sacco 2002).

---

[7] For a short overview see Labbe (2005).
[8] Forensic pathologist of the nineteenth century already had this problem. In some instances they had initially interpreted injuries on corpses that had been caused by insect attack, incorrectly as signs for abuse (Benecke 2001).

Only the introduction of diagnostic methods, which enabled examining physicians to empirically and technically detect child abuse led to an initial definition of child abuse as having its own complex of symptoms. Accordingly, the issue of child abuse experienced such a medicalization push that it became recognized as a medical rather than just as a legal problem. In particular, developments in pediatric radiology after 1946 gave physicians reliable empirical evidence that could connect various injuries across different ages with abuse. The child radiologist John Caffey described unexplained bone fractures associated with subdural hematomas, followed by new fractures after being discharged home, in several children in 1946 as evidences of abuse. Radiology, as an imaging method, exposed injuries that had been hidden by previous superficial diagnoses. At the same time, x-ray imaging as a technical process evoked the feeling of independence and incorruptible objectivity, which could be juxtaposed to the relatively subjective statements of the parents (English and Grossman 1983; Evans 2004: p. 162).

The decisive step towards popularization of the "child protection" discourse complex was made possible by Henry Kempe, who recognized the lack of a clear symptom complex of victimizations in conjunction with a catchy name, and introduced the concept of the "Battered Child Syndrome" into the debate in 1962 (Lynch 1985; Williams 1983). It was not by coincidence that the diagnoses of "Battered Child Syndrome" and "Shaken Baby Syndrome" developed in a hospital context, where a sufficient critical mass of patients existed in a hospital setting to cluster cases and examine similar patterns of injuries and radiological indications. The combination of a hospital context and technical approach provided the basic conditions of diagnostic development, which in the 1960s met with a public in the midst of socio-cultural change that was sensitized by debates on violence against women, minorities, ethnic groups, and the poor and therefore receptive to this diagnosis. The term "syndrome" alone increased the willingness of physicians to recognize abuse as a medical discourse. At the same time, public willingness to finance further specialist medical research increased and the differentiation of the new syndrome as a medical discipline was realized. Thus, it became possible to diagnose child abuse commensurate with an abuse event, whereas previously often only retrospective diagnoses had been possible.

The dispersion of the medical sphere of influence, in addition to the expansion of diagnoses of child protection, at least in part was triggered by the semantic extension of the English term "child abuse". For example, in 1968, Kempe's colleague David C. Gil defined "child abuse" as a *"non-accidental physical attack or physical injury, including minimal as well as fatal injury, inflicted upon children by persons caring for them"* (Gil 1968: p. 20) but by 1975 he had revised the definition to include *"child abuse as inflicted gaps or deficits between circumstances of living which would facilitate the optimal development of children, to which they should be entitled, and their actual circumstances, irrespective of the sources or agents of the deficitn* (Gil 1975: p. 346).[9] That same year, the ambiguity of the English word "child abuse", which can mean both "misconduct" and "violence", was extended to

---

[9] See Hacking (1991: pp. 269–274).

include a third sexual dimension. Suzanne Sgroi published a major article entitled "Sexual Molestation of Children Today: The Last Frontier in Child Abuse" (Sgroi 1975). In analogy the German term for "child abuse" includes and connotes the concepts of (physical) abuse, sexual abuse, and neglect. At the same time span, the scientific perspective on child abuse focused in the 1970s on a psychodynamic model, which emphasized the role of the abuser and the abused child. On the other hand, a sociological approach tried to include socio-economical risk factors into child abuse theories. From the 1980s on, an ecological approach of child abuse broke through. This model included a multi- and interfactorial view of individual, familial and sociocultural influences in the genesis of child abuse (Sidebotham 2001: p. 102).

13.4 Scandalization in Media

Simultaneous with the medicalization of child protection, partly by mutual influence, a process of "mediatization" of child protection began. In particular, media scandals of child abuse promoted the discursive dissemination of the subject in public. In 1995 Goddard and Liddell as well as Suzanne McDevitt in 1996 described, how the increase of press coverage after child abuse cases in Australia led to a new acceptance of this topic as a public discourse. This shift enabled a policy agenda setting which enforced a reformation of the child protection laws (Goddard and Liddell 1995; McDevitt 1996: see below). Particularly from the early 1980s onwards, at least in Germany the media representation of cases of child abuse resulted in the impression that the phenomenon of abuse had been recognized only recently and that ill-treatment, abuse, and neglect incidents were increasing. Nevertheless, the abuse debate underwent a process of change in the German media as well, where it had primarily been focused on physical abuse in the 1970s, to more and more sexual-themed abuse in the 1980s, to a special "case Kevin" in 2006 whose guiding motif was neglect and a failure of child protection (Görgen and Keßler 2013).

The media played a structural role in the public debate of abuse. In doing so the media fulfilled four of their classical main tasks: informing, supporting through expression and political decision-making, and mediating a review and monitoring function (Wittkämper 1999: p. 106). Mass media provide the basic mechanism for comprehensive reporting to the public and the development of a public interest and sense of responsibility towards the issue of child abuse, particularly in the area of child protection. Media outlets recognize that they can act as an interface between government, the public, and society. Furthermore, media personnel's self-assessment as a legitimate proclaimer of public opinion leads them to take on the role of shaping public opinion according to their own requirements and interests (Critcher 2003: p 15). Through so-called "framing" (i.e. the concentration on a contextual central idea), events can be subjectified and adapted to certain opinions. This interpretation and reconstruction of facts, together with a targeted positioning of messages in the information landscape, allows for an increasing spread of mediated discourses in the public sphere and considerably influences *the policy agenda setting* commensurate with the degree of media exposure. That is, the more a subject is reported on, the more important it is in daily politics (Scheufele and Tewksbury 2007: pp. 11ff.).

The described subjectification leads in many cases of child abuse reporting to an overemphasis of some aspects of content. Thus, stereotypes are confirmed or designed and incorporated into both politics and society. This over-emphasis in combination with the quantitative media exposure of a case increases the outrage potential such that it is perceived as a mediatized scandal. A scandal is, according to Burckhardt, a narrative structure that reflects the most important moral and social codes and demands correction using the alleged detection of offenses against these norms. Since political issues are affected by media ratings, the media can influence the prioritization of political (normative) actions with the help of scandals (Burkhardt 2006). An example of this kind of *policy agenda setting* is the aforementioned example of a development in Australia: In Victoria, Australia in 1991, media campaigns caused, in the wake of a child abuse case, a reform of the child protection system, achieving in particular the introduction of medical reporting. Thus, through the media coverage of the issue a political development was enforced (Goddard 1996: p. 305).

In scandal reporting, *policy agenda setting* is enabled and reinforced by the criticism of structural violence.[10] The questioning of the functionality of child protection and power structures, as well as the criticism of pro-moral institutions, which is ultimately also directed against systems that initially created child protection norms (e.g. medicine/medical child protection systems, schools, the churches) are important fields of the substantive debate. A defining example for this mechanism of criticizing structures as deficient or maleficent, which had been initially intended to protect children, is the following famous case from Cleveland, England (Görgen 2013):

In 1987, a scandal occurred at Middlesbrough General Hospital in the former Cleveland County in Northern England that ultimately changed how British print media, as well as British politicians, report about child abuse. Two pediatricians diagnosed 121 cases of sexual child abuse. After convening an inquiry committee under Judge Butler-Sloss, 26 cases turned out to be "misdiagnosed" and a total of 96 cases were closed without judgment. For the remaining cases, further investigations occurred, resulting in the confirmation of one abuse case. Some of the parents contacted the media upon initially hearing of the allegations. The report focused mainly on a poorly applied medical examination method, the so-called "anal reflex dilatation". It had been published only 1 year earlier, in 1986, by Wynne and Hobbes as an indication of sexual abuse in the *Lancet*.[11]

In the course of the scandal, there was a reversal of the indictment. This meant that now doctors and hospital personnel had to face the accusation of abuse and the parents were presented as being a victim of a feminist crusade (one of the leading doctors was female). Some family histories, in which there had been abuse, were not reported. The inquiry committee of the case concluded that the behavior of the

---

[10] On the term "structural violence" see Galtung (1971).
[11] Compare Hobbs and Wynne (1986).

doctors was in principle acceptable according to the available knowledge at the time of the medical examination and that anal reflex dilatation was an appropriate method of investigation. The scandal was largely due to a failure in the communication structure between the hospital, pediatricians, social services, and the appropriate police authorities (Butler-Sloss 1988).

The decisive scandalization potential for the media was in the abuse of the medical examination method, as well as in the executed structural violence that included the medical doctors' quest for arbitrariness and power. Thus, a failure of the medical child protection system was implied. In the case of pediatrician Marietta Higgs, personal and system criticism were united (Critcher 2003: pp. 84ff.). To increase the degree of outrage in the audience, the media worked heavily with stereotypes and generalizations, which were derived from the contradiction of conservative gender and role images, and the biography of Higgs, who was assumed to have feminist and leftist tendencies.

On the political level, the scandal led to the Children's Act of 1989, in which the relationship of family autonomy and child protection was to be newly regulated (H: M: S: O. 1989) as well as to new guidelines from the Ministry of Health for physicians and practitioners in child protection in 1991 (Department of Health and Social Security in 1988; Department of Health 1991).

With its victimization of parents in the media, the scandal in Cleveland followed a trend of popularizing the *False Memory Syndrome* that culminated in 1993. *False Memory Syndrome* is the theory that memories of abuse can be constructed subconsciously. From the mid-1980s until the 1990s, there was a shift away from reporting on child abuse and outrage over suffering inflicted on children, towards an empathetic view of perhaps innocently accused parents. Changes in the content orientation of print media underlay the family policy critiques and distrust of the therapist, whose supposed "effeminacy" did (at least according to the analysis of Kitzinger) not fit the image of the masculine journalistic world view (Kitzinger 1996: pp. 320ff.). Also the general potential for accusation where anyone could become a victim of false accusations was included in the media argument structure and contributed to the outrage, and to the politicization and distortion of the facts.

In the Cleveland case, the media had stood on the side of the accused parents and completed a personalized campaign against the pediatrician Marietta Higgs. A similarly strong response, but with a strong contrarily focus on the perpetrator, was generated in 2008 by a scandal in Poland. In 2008, the 45-year-old Krzysztof B. was arrested after his daughter accused him of having confined and abused her since 2002. She conceived two children by him during this time. After publication of the case, a mass of scandalous and "parasitic" (i.e. professionally unethical) media coverage emerged. Every day one would read reports about the "Polish Fritzl" (Woźniak et al. 2008) (referring to an older Austrian case) and the "Monster of Podlasie" (Dudek 2008), as the father of Alicja B. was soon labeled, and the lives of the family in the Polish tabloid. A transfer of the rhetoric from the media level to the political level came quickly. This development in Poland is particularly noteworthy because of the extremely rapid transition from the media to the political discourse level. Prime Minister Donald Tusk argued, ultimately successfully, for forced castration, because, according to Tusk, "individuals, such creatures that do something like that do not deserve the name human and one should not speak of human rights here" (Donald Tusk after Rötzer 2009). The perpetrator was marginalized discursively and dehumanized. In 2009, a law calling for the forced castration of child molesters was adopted (Dudek 2008; Kazmierczak 2009).

The media (in cases like this) may direct coverage against individual actors and their immediate environments, as in the case of the "Polish Fritzl"; and it may also use previously published medical discourses relatively uncritically, without questioning their veracity or the power of medical discourse. Similarly, uncritical medical-cultural concepts were used in France in 2005, when a medically justified collective guilt was constructed in the course of legal proceedings in Angers. There, a total of 66 defendants were charged with the rape of a minor, prostitution, child abuse, and aiding and abetting the aforementioned crimes. The prosecution counted 45 victims, the youngest being only 6 months old. However, the media had reported even younger victims, without verifying the information. The crimes were committed from June 1999 to February 2002. In March 2005, the German *Frankfurter Allgemeine Sonntagszeitung* reported the following about this case:

> A life "on the edge of imbecility"
>
> Accused is another France, a France in moral decay, a France of the disadvantaged and excluded, who increasingly lead lives of their own hardly perceived by the rest of the country. Many defendants have long been unemployed and alcoholics and have a below average IQ. Some are illiterate. A lawyer in Angers spoke of a life "on the verge of imbecility". In a police report, there is talk of a "population group with deficiencies at all levels." (Braunberger)[12]

As in this article in the *Frankfurter Allgemeine Sonntagszeitung*, "the socially weak" background and profiles of the accused were also presented in other media as being responsible for the abuses. Some media presented the case as a social-pathology being the product of problems of socio-economic decay and following psychological abnormality. This framing allowed the moral conscience of the average bourgeois population to be excluded from the child abuse troubles in the report. Social structures were to blame for child abuse cases which could not be influenced by the average citizen.

13.5 Conclusion

Norms of child protection today, as in the past, are propagated and exercised mainly in public with different functional systems of society competing for discourse sovereignty (see Table 13.1).

---

[12] Original (translated by the authors): "Ein Leben 'am Rande des Schwachsinns'

Auf der Anklagebank sitzt ein anderes Frankreich; jenes moralisch im Verfall befindliche Frankreich der Benachteiligten und Ausgeschlossenen, das zunehmend ein vom Rest des Landes kaum mehr wahrgenommenes Eigenleben führt. Viele Angeklagte sind seit langer Zeit arbeitslos und alkoholkrank und weisen einen unterdurchschnittlichen Intelligenzquotienten auf. Einige sind Analphabeten. Von einem Leben 'am Rande des Schwachsinns' sprach ein Anwalt in Angers. In einem Polizeibericht ist die Rede von einer 'Bevölkerungsgruppe mit Mängeln auf allen Ebenen'".

Table 13.1 Main cycles of instrumentalization of concepts of child abuse and child protection (scandalously simplified)

	Main actors	Main objectives (with the development of child protection as a side effect)	Means
Pre-modern Era	Early legislation	Establishment of a compensation in "property crimes" (in case of damage done to the child by others)	Punishment of the perpetrator
Eighteenth century	Church	Enforcement of a "Divine Order" and religious ideas of morality	Ban of non-compliant behavior, punishment of the offender
Nineteenth century	E.g. associations for the prevention of cruelty to children	Control and regulation of "amoral" low social classes	E.g. removal of children from families with 'doubtful' way of life, etc.
Nineteenth century	Expansive political systems (e.g. Prussia)	Preservation of military capability and national strength	Early labor protection regulations, breastfeeding propaganda
Nineteenth century	Professionalizing medicine and psychology	Expansion of spheres of competence	Medicalization of the child
Twentieth century	Feminist movement	Liberation of the woman	Initiating public outrage
Twentieth century	Politicians	Electoral campaigns: moral profiling	Promise of tough action against maltreatment
Twentieth century	Mass media	Increase of press circulations	Scandalization
Twentieth century		Control	E.g. early interventions

Even conflicts over the respective roles of societal systems, such as medicine, social work, politics, and the law, in child protection will be aired in public media, especially when it comes to problematic child protection developments. Depending on the interpretation of the scientific value, authenticity, and centrality of the inherent functionality of the respective child protective professions, guilt is attributed in public in cases of child protection failures. Medicine has won certain territorial discourse fights in the middle of the twentieth century and has popularized them in the media. Accordingly, medical evidence is considered as valuable, authentic and central.

Media and medicine have played decisive roles in shaping national and international debates on child protection. However, child abuse events and the corresponding scandalous critical narratives in the media are sometimes uncoupled from each other, with core medical definitions of one case being taken up repeatedly in the next case as symbols. Thus, one can speak of a self-referentiality within the medical and media discourse of "child abuse".

As described in the introduction, both child protection and scandals can be viewed as instruments of social and moral self-assurance as well as instruments of their normative recalibration. In particular, the structures of child protection are products of discursive/media processes and, therefore, are socially constructed (and not self-evidential anthropological constants). Common to the examples presented was the fact that the scandalized reporting was intently politicized or resulted in a political development, as when a child abuse scandal catalyzed a political development in child protection norms. Two basic narratives emerged in the media: criticism of "the system" and criticism of individual offenders. However, the scandals themselves were mostly hybrid structures that simultaneously personalized the critique of institutions and focused on the structural embeddedness of individual perpetrators.

It may be noted that in the interaction between media and medicine, people in the media are concerned about their own system expansion and, therefore, occasionally develop paradoxes in their reporting. Media outlets may occasionally oppose the structural violence of medicine, in their view, only to demand the use of medical child protection structures in the next case. It would be interesting to follow how the two basic narratives influence each other in producing norm establishing opinions. One (maybe oversimplifying) hypothesis might be that the more "respectable" the accused offender is, the more the targeting criticism of the medical system increases. In contrast, it might be assumed that an "asocial" perpetrator serves as stabilizing the system and its norms in question. It was not be possible to elucidate these questions fully within the existing German and international research frameworks. Elucidation will require a closer analysis. However, what should have become clear from our perspective is that norms of child well-being are – at least in part – the result of an interdiscourse of different systems working in the field of child protection, systems that equally demand normative leadership in a highly interdisciplinary field of child protection.

References

Al-Holou, W. N., O'Hara, E. A., et al. (2009). Nonaccidental head injury in children. Historical vignette. *Journal of Neurosurgery: Pediatrics, 3*(6), 474–483.

Anonymous. (1789). Grausamkeiten einer Mutter. *Annalen der Gesetzgebung und Rechtsgelehrsamkeit, 3,* 3–65.

Baginsky, A., & Janke, O. (1900). *Handbuch der Schulhygiene zum Gebrauche für Ärzte, Sanitätsbeamte, Lehrer.* Stuttgart: Schulvorstände und Techniker.

Benecke, M. (2001). A brief history of forensic entomology. *Forensic Science International, 120*(1–2), 2–14.

Berger, P. L., & Luckmann, T. (1966). *Social construction of reality: a treatise in the sociology of knowledge.* Garden City: Anchor Books.

Braunberger, Gerald. Ich hasse meine Kinder. *Frankfurter Allgemeine Sonntagszeitung,* 24.07.2005 (29), 54.

Burkhardt, S. (2006). *Medienskandale: Zur moralischen Sprengkraft öffentlicher Diskurse.* Köln: Halem.

Butler-Sloss, E. (1988). *Report of the inquiry into child abuse in Cleveland 1987 (the butler-sloss-report).* London: H.M.S.O.

Conrad, P. (2007). *The medicalization of society: on the transformation of human conditions into treatable disorders.* Baltimore: Johns Hopkins University Press.

Corsini, C. A., & Viazzo, P. P. (Eds.). (1997). *The decline of infant and child mortality. The European Experience, 1750–1990.* Den Haag.
Critcher, C. (2003). *Moral panics and the media.* Buckingham: Open University Press.
Daniel, B. (2010). Concepts of adversity, risk, vulnerability and resilience: a discussion in the context of the child protection system. *Social Policy and Society, 9*(02), 231–241.
Department of Health. (1991). *Working Together under the Children Act 1989: A Guide to Arrangements for Inter-Agency Co-operation for the Protection of Children.* London: H.M.S.O.
Department of Health and Social Security. (1988). Diagnosis of Child Sexual Abuse: Guidance for Doctors. Child Protection Guidance for Senior Nurses, Health Visitors and Midwives. Protecting Children: A Guidance for Social Workers Undertaking a Comprehensive Assessment. Working Together: A Guide to Arrangements for Interagency Cooperation for the Protection of Children from Abuse. London: H.M.S.O.
Dudek T. (2008). Kastration im Namen des Volkes. In *Telepolis,* 25.09.2008, http://www.heise.de/tp/r4/artikel/28/28796/1.html, Zugriff: 02.02.2010.
English, P. C., & Grossman, H. (1983). Radiology and the history of child abuse. *Pediatric Annals, 12*(12), 870–874.
Evans, H. H. (2004). The medical discovery of shaken baby syndrome and child physical abuse. *Pediatric Rehabilitation, 7*(3), 161–163.
Foucault, M. (2003). In D. Defert & F. Ewald (Eds.), *Schriften in vier Bänden. Dits et Ecrits, Bd. 3: 1976–1979.* Frankfurt a.M: Suhrkamp.
Galtung, J. (1971). Gewalt, Frieden und Friedensforschung. In D. Senghaas (Ed.), *Kritische Friedensforschung.* Frankfurt a.M: Suhrkamp.
Gil, D. (1968). Incidence of child abuse and demographic characteristics of persons involved. In R. E. Helfer & C. H. Kempe (Eds.), *The battered child* (pp. 19–40). Chicago: The University of Chicago Press.
Gil, D. G. (1975). Unraveling child abuse. *American journal of Orthopsychiatry, 45*(3), 346–356.
Goddard, C. (1996). Read all about it! The news about child abuse. *Child Abuse Review, 5,* 301–309.
Goddard, C., & Liddell, M. (1995). Child abuse fatalities and the media: Lessons from a case study. *Child Abuse Review, 4*(5), 356–364.
Görgen, A. (2013). Die "Cleveland Crisis" 1987. Medikalisierung und Skandalisierung des Kinderschutzes. *Medizinhistorisches Journal, 48*(1), 67–97.
Görgen, A., & Keßler, S. (2013). Der Einfluss von wissenschaftlichen, medialen und politischen Präventionskonjunkturen auf die Frühen Hilfen. *Prävention – Zeitschrift für Gesundheitsförderung, 1,* 10–14.
Görgen, A., Griemmert, M., & Fangerau, H. (2013). Kindheit und Trauma, Medikalisierung und Skandalisierung im Umgang mit der Gewalt gegen Kinder. *Trauma & Gewalt, 7*(3), 218–229.
Gries, S. (2002). *Kindesmisshandlung in der DDR.* Münster: Lit Verlag.
H.M.S.O. (1989). *Children Act. An introduction.* London: H.M.S.O.
Habermas, J. (1998). *Faktizität und Geltung. Beiträge zur Diskurstheorie des Rechts und des demokratischen Rechtsstaats.* Frankfurt a.M: Suhrkamp.
Hacking, I. (1991). The making and molding of child abuse. *Critical Inquiry, 17*(2), 253–288.
Hahn, S. (1994). Die Schulhygiene zwischen naturwissenschaftlicher Erkenntnis, sozialer Verantwortung und vaterländischem Dienst: Das Beispiel der Myopie in der zweiten Hälfte des 19. Jahrhunderts. *Medizinhistorisches Journal, 29,* 23–38.
Helfer, R. E., & Kempe, C. H. (Eds.). (1968). *The battered child* (2nd ed.). Chicago: The University of Chicago Press.
Hobbs, C., & Wynne, J. (1986). Buggery in childhood – A common syndrome of child abuse. *The Lancet, 8510,* 792–796.
Hooper, C.-A. (1989). Rethinking the politics of child abuse. *Social History of Medicine, 2*(3), 356–364.
Höpler, E. (1918). Über Kindesmißhandlung. *Archiv für Kriminologie, 69*(3/4), 224–285.
Jaßy. (1787). Unerhörte Grausamkeit einer Mutter. In *Journal von und für Deutschland* (Vol. 4, pp. 220–225).

Kazmierczak, L. (2009). "Chemische Kastration" für Kinderschänder eingeführt. In http://www.tagesschau.de/ausland/polen180.html, Zugriff: 02.02.2010.
King, M. (1999). *Moral agendas for children's welfare*. London: Routledge.
Kitzinger, J. (1996). Media representations of sexual abuse risks. *Child Abuse Review, 5*, 319–333.
Kupffer, H. (1999). Kinderschutz als Metapher. *Zeitschrift für Soziologie der Erziehung und Sozialisation, 19*(2), 119–127.
Labbe, J. (2005). Ambroise Tardieu: the man and his work on child maltreatment a century before kempe. *Child Abuse & Neglect, 29*(4), 311–324.
Liebel, M. (2007). *Wozu Kinderrechte? Grundlagen und Perspektiven*. Weinheim: Juventa.
Luhmann, N. (1998). *Observations on modernity*. Stanford: Stanford University Press.
Lynch, M. A. (1985). Child abuse before Kempe: an historical literature review. *Child Abuse & Neglect, 9*(1), 7–15.
Lyons, J. B. (1997). Sir William Wilde's medico-legal observations. *Medical History, 41*(4), 437–54.
McDevitt, S. (1996). The impact of news media on child abuse reporting. *Child Abuse & Neglect, 20*(4), 261–274.
Meckel, R. A. (1990). *Save the babies: American public health reform and the prevention of infant mortality, 1850–1929*. Ann Arbor: University of Michigan Press.
Moebius, S. (Ed.). (2012). *Kultur: Von den Cultural Studies bis zu den Visual Studies: Eine Einführung*. Bielefeld: Transcript.
Myers, J. E. B. (2011). A short history of child protection in America. In J. E. B. Myers (Ed.), *The APSAC Handbook on child maltreatment* (3rd ed., pp. 3–15). Los Angeles: Sage.
Olafson, E., Corwin, D., et al. (1993). Modern history of child sexual abuse awareness: cycles of discovery and suppression. *Child Abuse & Neglect, 17*(1), 7–24.
Pollock, L. (1983). *Forgotten children: Parent-child relations from 1500 to 1900*. Cambridge: Cambridge University Press.
Ritzmann, I. (2008). *Sorgenkinder: Kranke und behinderte Mädchen und Jungen im 18. Jahrhundert*. Köln: Böhlau.
Rivaux, S. L., James, J., Wittenstrom, K., Baumann, D., Sheets, J., Henry, J., & Jeffries, V. (2008). The intersection of race, poverty and risk: understanding the decision to provide services to clients and to remove children. *Child Welfare, 87*(2), 151–68.
Rodin, A. E. (1981). Infants and gin mania in 18th-century London. *Journal of the American Medical Association, 245*(12), 1237–1239.
Rötzer, F. (2009). Polens Parlament verabschiedet Gesetz zur Zwangskastration verurteilter Pädophiler. In *Telepolis*, 29.09.2009, http://www.heise.de/tp/blogs/6/146021, Zugriff: 16.02.2011.
Sacco, L. (2002). Sanitized for your protection. Medical discourse and the denial of incest in the United States, 1890–1940. *Journal of Women's History, 14*(3), 80–104.
Scheufele, D. A., & Tewksbury, D. (2007). Framing, agenda setting, and psriming. The evolution of three media effect models. *Journal of Communication, 57*, 9–20.
Schimank, U. (2006). *Teilsystemische Autonomie und politische Gesellschaftssteuerung: Beiträge zur akteurzentrierten Differenzierungstheorie 2*. Wiesbaden: VS Verlag für Sozialwissenschaften.
Schmitz, M., & Fangerau, H. (2010). Geschichte, Theorie und Ethik des Kinderschutzes. In J. M. Fegert, H. Fangerau, & U. Ziegenhain (Eds.), *Problematische Kinderschutzverläufe. Mediale Skandalisierung, fachliche Fehleranalyse und Strategien zur Verbesserung des Kinderschutzes* (pp. 18–50). Weinheim: Juventa.
Sgroi, S. M. (1975). Sexual molestation the last frontier in child abuse. *Children Today, 4*, 18–21.
Shuttleworth, S. (2010). *In the mind of the child: child development in literature, science, and medicine 1840–1900*. Oxford: Oxford University Press.
Sidebotham, P. (2001). An ecological approach to child abuse: a creative use of scientific models in research and practice. *Child Abuse Review, 10*(2), 97–112.
Smallbone, S., Marshall, W. L., & Wortley, R. (2008). *Preventing child sexual abuse: evidence, policy and practice*. Cullompton: Willan Publishing.

Umehara, H., & Halling, T. (2006). Die deutsche und japanische Schulhygiene im späten 19. und frühen 20. Jahrhundert. In J. Vögele, H. Fangerau, & T. Noack (Eds.), *Geschichte der Medizin – Geschichte in der Medizin: Forschungsthemen und Perspektiven* (pp. 71–79). Münster: Lit Verlag.

Wehling, P., Viehöver, W., Keller, R., & Lau, C. (2007). Zwischen Biologisierung des Sozialen und neuer Biosozialität: Dynamiken der biopolitischen Grenzüberschreitung. *Berliner Journal für Soziologie, 4*, 547–567.

Welander, E. (1909). Über den Einfluss der venerischen Krankheiten auf die Ehe sowie ihre Übertragung auf kleine Kinder. *Zeitschrift für Kinderforschung, 14*(4), 97–113.

Williams, G. J. R. (1983). Child protection – A journey into history. *Journal of Clinical Child Psychology, 12*(3), 236–243.

Wittkämper, G. W. (1999). Steuert die Politik oder wird sie gesteuert? Politisches Handeln im Multimediazeitalter. In R. Funiok, U. F. Schmälzle, & C. H. Werth (Eds.), *Medienethik – die Frage der Verantwortung* (pp. 95–113). Bonn: Bundeszentrale für Politische Bildung.

Woźniak, A., Jakubowska, P., Matuszkiewicz, T. (2008). *Oto polski Fritzl!* Available at: http://www.se.pl/wydarzenia/kraj/oto-polski-fritzl_71122.html

Zeitschrift für Kinderforschung. Organ der Gesellschaft für Heilpädagogik und des deutschen Vereins zur Fürsorge für Jugendliche Psychopathen, *47*(2) 1939.

Chapter 14
Children's Rights, Well-Being, and Sexual Agency

Samantha Brennan and Jennifer Epp

14.1 Introduction

Talk about children and sexuality, or worse sexual children, and you are likely to provoke anxiety.[1] This is especially true when discussion strays from the need to protect children from abuse. But stray we will, right into the contested area of whether children are sexual agents in their own right, with elements of their well-being entwined with that sexual agency. This discussion is necessary both so that we do not misrepresent the lives of children, and in order to deliberate about how to treat them both now and with a view to their development into fully autonomous, flourishing adults.

In this paper we offer a review of some of the literature about childhood sexuality, draw attention to certain gaps in that conversation, and suggest directions for future research. We also provide support for the claims that sexuality may be a good of childhood, and that a self-chosen and explored sexuality can be an aspect of children's well-being. It is likely, we suggest, that children have some degree of sexual agency that ought to be supported in order to support their well-being and to fully respect them as they are in the present and not simply as future adults.

We begin by describing two sets of discourses that direct and constrain common understandings of child sexuality. Section 14.2 contrasts 'romantic' with 'knowing' children, i.e. understandings of children as either asexual innocents or little adults made so by premature exposure to sexuality. The discourse is problematic in that it makes childhood sexuality inconceivable. Section 14.3 presents two recent and

---

[1] A reaction dubbed "visceral clutch" by Masters and Johnson (Stainton Rogers and Stainton Rogers 1992: 162).

S. Brennan (✉) • J. Epp, Ph.D.
University of Western Ontario, Stevenson Hall 4127, London, ON N6A 5B8, Canada
e-mail: sbrennan@uwo.ca

conflicting discourses. One represents sexual children as 'out-of-control', while the other represents them as legitimately 'developing' their sexuality. Proponents of the former view argue that children's sexual agency ought to be strictly controlled, while those supporting the latter argue that it ought to be carefully encouraged. In this context, debates about children's sexuality focus on rights to sexuality-related health services, comprehensive sex education, and freedom from abuse. Discussion about sexuality as a good of childhood or as an aspect of child well-being finds no place in this context.

In the third section we take up three sets of worries raised by the suggestion that children may be legitimately sexual. These worries center on questions about the ability of children to legitimately consent to sexual activity, about parental rights, and about what to do in cases where children's welfare and autonomy conflict. The fourth section asks what rights follow from thinking of sexuality as something in which children have an interest.

Some important qualifications: First, throughout this paper we assume that children are appropriate bearers of, at the very least, a set of human rights.[2] We understand rights in developmental terms according to which rights first protect interests (in the case of the very young) and later protect choices (in the case of fully autonomous adults) and in the middle defend a mix of the two.[3] Second, though we focus on children's abilities to act as sexual agents we do not mean to imply that children are fully autonomous, fully mature, or that their sexuality is identical to that of adults. Children are not adults, though the boundaries of the two categories blur during adolescence. Third, 'children' is not a uniform category. Though we suggest that it is important to recognize children's sexuality without focusing solely on their development, children are in the process of maturing physically, cognitively, socially and emotionally. As a result, they will have different and expanded interests, needs, desires and abilities related to sexuality as they get older and their knowledge and skills increase, i.e. as they become more confident, informed, and competent decision-makers. Different behaviours and expressions of sexuality will be appropriate for children of different ages. Less mature children and adolescents do require protection from adults and sometimes from themselves; however, as stated above, their immaturity does not negate the degree of autonomy they do have, nor should protection be understood strictly in opposition to that autonomy.[4] Fourth, nothing that is said here should be construed as suggesting that children ought to be sexual in any particular way. We argue only that when they are, both their sexual

---

[2] For a defense of this position, not universally held, see Brennan and Noggle (1997).

[3] See Brennan (forthcoming), and Brennan (2002).

[4] As we discuss below, a person is autonomous when she has and uses the capacity to understand, deliberate between and endorse (or identify with) her desires, values, actions and so on, with the possibility of making significant choices between them. We would argue that she does not need to be self-transparent, perfectly informed, or uninfluenced by others, though she cannot be coerced in order to be autonomous. To be an autonomous agent, rather than simply an agent, is to be able to choose relatively freely rather than simply to chose. See John Christman's article on "Autonomy in Moral and Political Philosophy" in the *Stanford Encyclopedia of Philosophy*.

well-being and autonomy ought to be supported and respected. Finally, children are regularly sexually abused and those violations need to be taken very seriously. Claims about children's sexual agency or autonomy should not be used to attempt to justify sexual abuse.

14.2 Innocence and the Romantic or the Knowing Child

There was a shift, during the Enlightenment in the West, from thinking of children as "faulty small adults" tainted by "original sin," to thinking of them as asexual innocents, blank slates in need of protection and guidance as they grew into adulthood. On this later view children are innocent because they lack knowledge. They have nothing to hide because they have yet to become aware of the adult meanings of their actions. Without that knowledge they cannot do or intend to do anything wrong, much less anything sexual. This image of the "romantic child" was a highly sentimentalized picture of blissful innocence and natural purity. Such innocence is fragile. In their unknowing state children cannot protect themselves from unwitting exposure to the experiences or information that might erode their innate naivety.[5] (Irvine 2002; Ferguson 2003) Instead adults become the guardians of innocence.

The figure of the all too "knowing child" acts as a foil to that of the romantic child. Knowing children have seen things they shouldn't have: poverty, drunkenness, life on the streets, and who knows what they've done. They are portrayed as innocent victims of an uncaring society, forced to grow up too soon and morally compromised in the process. Describing this image, Christine Piper notes the Victorian connection between unlimited exposure to the world, as with urban street children, and the taint of precocious sexuality. She repeats, for instance, the 1882 Select Committee description of "girl street sellers in Liverpool" which reads "though she may carry a basket, there is very little difference between her and a prostitute" (Piper 2000: 33, note 43).

According to Piper, knowing children are those who should be but are no longer children. Their innocence, and with it their childhood, has been lost or stolen.[6] In these portraits of the romantic and knowing child Piper finds evidence for the claim that "child + sex = abuse" and "child + sex = adult" are the only socially acceptable configurations of childhood sexuality. Lost is any possibility for recognizing the existence, let alone legitimacy, of childhood sexuality or agency in the form of "child + sex = OK"[7] (Piper 2000: 28–29). Romantic and knowing children cannot

---

[5] This suggestion resonates with Rousseau's prescriptions for Emile.

[6] This image of the child in danger and in need of protection, and of the threat posed to childhood by sexuality, is explicit in Postman (1982).

[7] Daniel Monk concurs writing that "the traditional construction of the child as a non-sexual innocent" is often protected by "excluding the sexual child from the category of childhood itself" this time in using a medical model of childhood (Monk 2000: 187).

be sexual agents. In the former case they are innocent of all things sexual, and in the latter they are both adults and passive victims.[8]

Piper notes a socially accepted link between claims of innocence and claims to protection. The available configurations of "children + sex" described above leave out the possibility that children might be voluntarily sexual and yet still deserve protection from adults. On this view the innocent are defined as helpless; they are dependent on others to guide and protect them and they deserve help because they are not yet responsible for themselves. There is no room here to recognize that children may have an interest in exploring, developing, or expressing their sexuality as semi-autonomous sexual agents who can be *involved* in their own protection but who nonetheless remain children who deserve and benefit from adult help and guidance.

To support her claim that discourses of the romantic and knowing child are still major influences on our understanding of childhood Piper cites the fact that despite being unable to give legal consent to sex underage prostitutes in Britain are regularly prosecuted as offenders themselves, rather than treated as victims (Piper 2000: 27–28). Further evidence that romantic notions of childhood innocence, the dangerous role of sexual knowledge, and the adult status of knowing children are still with us can be found in all manner of places including:

- Outrage in 2011 in response to a link, posted on the US Department of Health and Human Services website, to a KidsHealth webpage that describes children as "sexual beings."[9]
- Extraordinary funding levels for abstinence only education in the United States from 1996 to 2010. For example, 2005 funding for the program was $170 million.[10]

---

[8] The knowing child was a figure that was popular during the eighteenth century and which proved especially useful to social reformers who aimed to keep children off the streets, out of the factories and back in homes and schools. The purity movement of the time in fact used such images to strictly control female sexuality and to deny female pleasure (Piper 2000). The knowing child image resurfaced again during the depression in the 1930s and circulates today in discussions aimed at curbing abuse and youth pregnancy, restricting child pornography and international sex tourism, and even in discussions that advocate for abstinence-only sex education. Our point, and Piper's, is that this definition of children desexes them so that, while it is crucial in many of these circumstances, protection comes at a price. Though in many cases protection is absolutely necessary the knowing child figure helps to solidify an image of children as victims and as passive non-agents who cannot be sexually autonomous—this is an image that can greatly limit the rights they are accorded regarding sexuality.

[9] Fox News gives an overview of the situation online (see Fox News 2011) while Krepel (2011) gives an overview of outraged responses which, it claims, "boil down to a demand that information about sexual health not be discussed by public health officials," especially in regards to children.

[10] See Collins (1999) and government information available at http://www.hhs.gov/news/press/2010pres/09/teenpregnancy_chart.html, http://www.hhs.gov/news/press/2010pres/09/teenpregnancy_abstinencegrants.html, and www.aids.gov/federal-resources/pacha/meetings/2012/may-2012-cse-resolution.pdf.

- News articles published in 2011 online with titles such as "Sex Education and the Rape of Our Children's Innocence"[11] and "A Child's Innocence is Precious. That's Why It Must Be Protected" with opening lines like "Children seem to be disappearing. They are physically present, but infant clothes, toys and street games seem to have been subsumed by a rush to adulthood"[12]
- The following public responses to a BBC news story on sex education and the pregnancy of three girls aged 12–16:

    1. Children are growing up far too early nowadays and their innocence is taken away from them.
    2. It seems to me that the answer is to stop sex education…
    3. Children were allowed to be children and didn't know about sex until it was necessary. Nowadays infants know what it is. There is too much knowledge.
    4. These children obviously knew what they were doing and if they are mature enough to make that decision to engage in a sexual relationship, then they must accept the responsibility for themselves.[13]

A number of authors have criticized the image of the romantic child. Many cite James Kincaid (1998), who argued that images of childhood innocence work together with an almost complete eroticization of children. The "cultural doublespeak" Kincaid uncovers, writes Kevin Ohi, "allows us the pleasures of imagining and perpetuating the victimization of children while praising ourselves for protecting them" (Ohi 2004: 82). At the same time eroticizing childhood innocence requires us to erase certain realities of the lives lived by actual children. In this way, we come to define children by what they don't know, need or do, rather than by examining their actual understandings, desires, needs, and activities[14] (Ohi 2004: 82–83).

David Archard identifies three dangers posed by the romantic ideal that positions children as asexual innocents. First, it obfuscates the reality of a child's actual sexual development. Second, it is an ideology that denies facts to maintain the appearance of what is wanted from the child, a "natural" innocence adults cannot have. Third, such an ideology may be dangerously sexual…attractive for being that which is not yet but can be corrupted (Archard 1998: 118–119). Together the work of Kincaid, Ohi and Archard suggests that failure to recognize child sexuality not only misrepresents but may actually undermine children's well-being.

---

[11] See Brown (2011).
[12] See The Guardian (2011).
[13] See BBC News Online (2005).
[14] This empty understanding of childhood, writes Ellis Hanson, allows us to project our fantasies of innocence and corruption onto children "to construct, watch, enjoy the erotic child without taking any responsibility for our actions" (Hanson 2004: 134).

14.3 Sexuality and the Out-of-Control or Developing Child

Humans are sexual, broadly understood, from a very young age and certainly before puberty. Children are curious about their own and other bodies, they ask about babies and sex, touch their genitals, are aware of themselves early on as gendered, they engage in pre-adolescent sex play, and they have "crushes" when they are quite young (Larsson 2001; Coleman and Roker 1998; Friedrich 2003; Ince 2004). Though young children do not understand their emotions and behaviour as adults with greater knowledge of the physical, social, and emotional aspects of sexuality do, it is reasonable to claim that their behaviours are sexual. In Canada "the proportion of teens who reported having had sexual intercourse before they were 15 years old fell from 12 % in 1996/1997 to 8 % in 2005" and approximately one-third of teens aged 15–17 years have had intercourse (again with percentages decreasing since 1996/1997)[15] (Rotermann 2008). Other non-coital yet interpersonal sexual behaviour also occurs among teens (Princeton Survey Research Associates International 2004). Given this information, insisting on the romantic innocence of childhood is unlikely to lead to an adequate understanding of children's abilities, needs or well-being in relation to sexuality.

Adults who accept evidence that children and teens are sexual usually respond in one of two ways. First, they may focus on the need to control what they perceive as premature and irresponsible sexual behaviour. Members of this group often promote abstinence sex education and highlight the dangers of precocious sexuality.[16] They often use inflammatory language, for example describing "the same frightening story…that rattled me to the core…—STDs, risky behaviors, and in younger and younger kids. Not just in the tough crowds—in all types of crowds" (Meeker 2004). Such language leads to the perception of a sexual crisis facing youths and the parents who have to deal with them. With headlines like "It's An Oral Sex Epidemic,"[17] books such as the 2004 *Epidemic: How Teen Sex is Killing Our Kids*,[18] and newspaper articles about sexting that focus on fear (for example in Ross 2013; Meeker 2005) this 'Out-Of-Control' discursive representation of teen sexuality can lead to what some describe as "moral panic" (Coleman and Roker 1998; Potter and Potter 2001).

There are legitimate reasons to be concerned about risky behaviour, but sensationalized discussions that credit teens with little or no responsible agency are unhelpful. They ignore the importance of sex education for younger children; often interrogate only female sexuality as girls risk pregnancy and are usually the ones performing oral sex; and importantly, distract from the fact that the majority of 13–17 year olds are purposefully not becoming sexually active. A 2004 poll in the United States indicates that "The vast majority (87 %) of teens aged 13–16, have not had sexual inter-

---

[15] For further information on teenage sexual behaviour in a Canadian context see McKay and Bissell (2010).

[16] For a discussion of adolescent sexuality and sex education that explicitly rejects this focus on danger see Moore and Rosenthal (1998).

[17] See The Oprah Winfrey Show (2002).

[18] Meeker (2004).

course. Most (73 %) have not been sexually intimate at all. Seventy-four percent say they have not had sex because they made a conscious decision not to. As many (75 %) have not because they believe they are too young" (PSRAI 2004).

Despite evidence of adolescent responsibility, 'out-of control' understandings of child sexuality continue to position children and teens as non-autonomous objects of adult attention rather than as potentially responsible sexual agents. Often the parents or schools of these "kids gone wrong" are seen as irresponsible, at fault by reason that they didn't teach children "any better" or restrict children's freedom. While parents and schools do have a responsibility to guide and educate children, on this view children and teens cannot be involved in protecting themselves.[19] The assumption is that, given their immaturity, lack of knowledge and potential to "go wrong," it would be dangerous for young people to enjoy their current sexuality. Sexuality is not seen as a potential source or arena of well-being on this account.

This understanding of sexual youths can also create a class based and racialized distinction between 'bad kids and good kids'. Public response to the BBC report on child pregnancy above, where the three teen mothers were black, includes regular reference to "people like these" whom the "government throws money at" and to "the country's underclass" whom the new babies are "destined to join." One respondent, Elizabeth, uses language that is racially coded saying that the teens share their mother's "'whateva' attitude to sex" (BBC News Online 2005). These attitudes are repeated in *Epidemic*, the book quoted above as an example of moral panic. The author, Meg Meeker, begins her story saying that "even the suburbs" are now infected by the diseases and teen pregnancies that used to appear only in the "mess" of the inner-city and that such problems "didn't belong in my patients," that is in white middle-class suburban kids. Without sympathy, she contrasts "multitudes of kids with countless problems" in the inner city to suburban "red-faced babies who nursed beautifully," babies of young girls who are now in danger from "inner-city" disease (Meeker 2004).

Jessica Fields' examination of the rhetoric of "children having children" confirms that images of the out-of-control sexual child are not neutral with respect to race, class, or gender. She writes that "Those advocating 'abstinence-only sexuality education' argued that their curricula would protect innocent children from others' corrupting influence; racialized language and images suggested that these 'others' were poor, African American girls" (Fields 2005: 549). It might not be an out-of-control, hyper-sexualized child's fault, but here they are still seen as "bad," dangerous to the "good kids" and potentially irredeemable. Especially in the United States, where access to public health care is limited, where eugenics has been practiced on a

---

[19] The public response to the BBC article on teen pregnancy again illustrates this point. Respondents cite children's mothers, schools and, though rarely, the older fathers of the girl's babies as responsible, rarely examining the choices girls themselves make. One person writes, for example, "This mother is entirely to blame and her children should have their children taken away to be adopted by adults ready and willing to take on the responsibility of children" (BBC News Online 2005). Of course there is still a question of whether or not these girls could be expected to choose differently given their circumstances and lack of education, but that does not mean that children of this age are naturally incapable of responsible choice.

strikingly similar basis (even in 2010),[20] and where similar "controlling images" were used to legitimate slavery and now to limit citizenship rights and deny institutional racism,[21] the effects of racialized and classed images of overly sexual, out-of-control children on children's well-being need to be interrogated.

That was one common interpretation of the fact that children are sexual. A second response comes from those who argue that children displaying sexuality are in the process of developing as competent and mature sexual agents, which they need help to do safely. This response can itself proceed in one of two ways: either with a sole focus on the need for adult guidance that once again makes children into objects of concern, or with an awareness of the complexities engendered by a need to balance children's "best interests" with their developing sexual autonomy.

Fields discusses the former move as a strategy for ensuring protection for sexually active young people in a context where being responsible and deserving of protection are taken to be mutually exclusive. She writes that "Those promoting 'comprehensive sexuality education' recast these girls as 'children having children'—innocents who needed guidance and who could not be held responsible for their missteps" (Fields 2005: 549). This image of the innocent yet sexual child differs from romantic images of child purity, but still fails to make any room for the possibility that children may be capable of some degree of autonomous sexual agency (see Tolman 2002). As Fields notes, it also preempts questions about responsible or irresponsible sexuality in boys.

Roughly, a person is autonomous when she is a competent decision maker with the ability to act, uncoerced, on the basis of her significant decisions. She is a competent decision maker when she has and uses the capacity to understand, deliberate between and endorse her desires, values, actions etc., and she need not be self-transparent, perfectly informed, or uninfluenced by and/or completely independent of others in order to do so.[22] If we recognize that sexual children often posses some degree of autonomy and are, as they should be, in the process developing that autonomy, and if autonomy depends on skills and competencies related to understanding and deliberation, then children can be well sexually only with adequate access to information about sex. They have an interest in maturing into adulthood by becoming better decision makers about sexual and other matters, which information helps them to do.[23] Since the ability to act on the degree of autonomy that one has developed is part of one's well-being, if children are already autonomous to

---

[20] See Center for Genetics and Society (2012) and Johnson (2013).

[21] Collins (1999).

[22] See Christman (2009).

[23] On this point, Corrine Packer adds "any young individual seeking information on sex and human reproduction demonstrates ipso facto a certain degree of maturity and competency to deal with the subject matter" so that children ought to be given the information they seek (Packer 2000: 169). The UN Convention on the Rights of the Child agrees, saying in article 13.1 "The child shall have the right to freedom of expression; this right shall include freedom to seek, receive and impart information and ideas of all kinds, regardless of frontiers, either orally, in writing or in print, in the form of art, or through any other media of the child's choice." See also article 17.

some significant degree then they also have an interest in deciding certain things for themselves, at least when they are relevantly competent.

Claims about children's autonomy then lead to a host of further questions. To mention only a few: Would children's well-being be better supported if they had easier access to contraception? Should girls or young women be able to choose to have an abortion in contexts that allow adult women to do so? If so, should they be required to secure parental consent? Should children have a right to privacy about their sexual lives and health? Can young people legitimately consent to and engage in sexual activity, and if so what kind, with whom?

14.4 Consent, Parental Rights, and Autonomy/Welfare Conflicts

Three sets of worries arise from the suggestion that children may be legitimately sexual, worries hinted at by the questions in the previous section. They are: first, about children's ability to legitimately consent to sexual behaviour and to make sexual related health care decisions; second, about potential conflicts between parental and children's rights and interests; and third, about conflict between children's own decisions and their "best interests," that is, between their autonomy and welfare. We will discuss each in turn.

Questions about consent: What must obtain for a child to be able to give consent to sexual activity? Do those requirements change depending on her age, her partner, or the activity in question? What is at stake when asking about a child's right to consent?[24] We will use David Archard's discussion of child sexual consent to sketch the terrain here.

First, in order for a child to have the ability to consent that child must be relevantly competent. As described above, competence obtains when a person has and can use the set of skills, abilities, character traits and knowledge relevant to making a given decision. We cannot give an exhaustive list of everything required for competence in this case; however one might be expected to know and understand the significance of the physical, emotional, social, and possibly moral risks involved. As David Archard puts it, one ought to have "a certain level of cognitive development—that is, an ability to understand the relevant facts, a certain degree of acquired knowledge" and the maturity to appreciate those facts and to act based on that appreciation[25] (Archard 1998: 124). In other words, young people require more than information about the risks and mechanics of sexual activity to be competent as "information alone does not allow teenagers to take control of emotions and relationships" (Rees et al. 1998: 140). They also require social skills and character traits

---

[24] We do not address her ability to consent to sexual health care, though perhaps there are similarities between this and the case of sexual activity.

[25] Note the similarity here to the Gillick test to determine a child's competence to give medical consent (Downs and Whittle 2000: 202–203).

including, but not limited to: the ability to resist peer pressure; a sense of self-worth and self-trust; an ability to evaluate the trustworthiness of potential partners; the ability to acquire and insist on using protection; understanding of their motivations and values; knowledge of and the ability to set limits regarding the activity they are comfortable with; and so on (see Moore and Rosenthal 1998). Archard also notes that physical maturity is relevant and adds that we ought to attend to the ages at which most kids actually are choosing to engage in a particular behaviour when considering where to set the age of majority for such acts (Archard 1998: 126).

Second, it seems reasonable to posit that a child's level of competence does not need to be as high to consent to lower risk activity, such as kissing or genital touching with a peer, as it does for higher risk activity, such as intercourse. People have different standards of what counts as higher and lower risk activity. Some argue, based on homophobic premises, that the age of consent for same-sex activity ought to be higher than for the same behaviour when heterosexual. We leave Archard and others to argue against that proposal though we believe it to be discriminatory and flawed. We add, however, that it is not clear what a bisexual young person should do here. Such a proposal appears to contradict itself since it will have to say that a bisexual person both is and is not legally ready to have sex.

Third, Archard argues that in order for a child's consent to be legitimate it must not be coerced or negated by a significant power imbalance with a potential partner, where that imbalance may occur either because of age difference or because of a "special relationship" between the parties. The question of consent between an older and younger partner has been hotly debated both because of apparently unfair prosecution of boys who are consensually partnered with slightly younger girls and because of claims about "harmless" intergenerational sex or pedophilia.

The question of prosecution of boys or young men who are close in age to younger but consensual partners is complex. We offer considerations here, rather than answers. To begin with, in some places the age of consent for girls was set higher than for boys, so that a boy might be prosecuted for sex with a girl of a given age when the same would not be true had she been the older and he the younger partner (Archard 1998: 121–122). We can find no good defense for this imbalance, especially as girls begin puberty earlier and mature more quickly than boys. Likewise it seems unreasonable to prosecute a young person for something that his partner wants to engage in. However even differences of only 3 years are significant between partners of, say, 13 and 16. In many places these teens are still in different schools (the difference between middle and high school) and the 16 year old is likely to have the benefit of knowledge, experience, skills, and social status (as a highschooler) that his partner lacks. Aware of these considerations, Archard provides a strong defense of a young person's right to consent if she has the competence to do so. To legally discount her consent and her sexual wishes, to say she does not have the right to make sexual choices for herself, is to define her as asexual. Doing so makes her chosen actions criminal and positions her as confused, misguided or naive. As a result her sense of being an agent and a competent chooser may be undermined, thereby limiting her autonomy (Archard 1998: 120).

Proponents of pedophilia or intergenerational sex use evidence of children's autonomy and competence to claim that such involvement is harmless when it is apparently consensual. They may also argue that young children give legitimate consent if they appear to enjoy the interaction and that even children at a young age can know what they want sexually (Archard 1998: 127). They may even argue that they are caring for or beneficently teaching children by engaging with them sexually. Archard is quick to note the obvious inconsistency in claiming that a child can know what she wants and likes in order to consent to it, and at the same time positioning oneself as a teacher of what the child does not yet know (Archard 1998: 127). Archard objects to imposing adult sexual needs on children, and he relates the position of feminist and gay critics of pedophilia that "Fundamentally, there are issues of disparity of experience, needs, desires, physical potentialities, emotional resources, sense of responsibility, awareness of consequences of one's actions, and, above all, power between adults and children" (Archard 1998: 127). He is correct to assert that those imbalances negate consent. Though some may disagree, where one cannot reasonably say no, certainly one cannot say yes. For similar reasons certain "special relationships" involving an imbalance in authority, for example between teachers and students, likely do not allow for legitimate consent. These consent issues are closely tied to claims about a child's right to protection from harm and abuse as well as to her right to make her own decisions.

Questions about parental rights and balancing autonomy and welfare: Mention of conflict between parental and children's rights usually arises around discussions about state-mandated sex education when parents wish to withdraw their children for moral or religious reasons. Parents may also act in ways that violate a child's "human rights," i.e. rights that are not dependent on her autonomy or ability to take up various social roles. Those possibilities aside, a semi-autonomous young person may very well wish to make decisions that her parents do not approve of. She may wish to have an abortion for instance. When she is a minor, but seems to appreciate the potential consequences of her decision, should she require her parent's permission to do so? Does she have a right to privacy in this case or the right to make her own moral, medical and life-affecting decisions? Or do her parents have a right to know, and to guide her choices for her own good, especially if she is not fully mature? (see Rodman et al. 1984).

Parental, or rather paternal, rights were originally understood as a kind of property right to one's children and to the income generated from their labour. Samantha Brennan and Robert Noggle argue instead that parental rights should be understood as stewardship rights. They justify this position by arguing that children are immature and require physical, mental, and emotional care and guidance. Someone must protect, care and advocate for them and, given their probable emotional ties to and personal investment in their children, parents are often best suited for the job. Stewardship rights come with thresholds, i.e. they can be infringed if a child is being harmed, if her needs are not being met, or if her parents violate her basic rights. As stewards, parents have a duty to further their children's development and promote their interests, but this is an imperfect duty so that there is "a great deal of leeway" in how parents may decide to do so (Brennan and Noggle 1997: 13). Likewise, a child's rights may be infringed but only when there is a great deal at stake—perhaps, suggest Brennan and Noggle, her future ability to exercise her rights—and her rights do not cease to exist when they are over-ridden and must be considered in the process (Brennan and Noggle 1997: 16–17).

Since a parent's stewardship rights "exist only insofar as the parent is indeed promoting the interests of the child" questions about what those interests are become crucial (Brennan and Noggle 1997: 13). Certainly it is in a child's interest to learn how to exercise autonomy through competent decision making. Respecting and guiding her actual decisions will help her to learn this ability. Parents must balance this interest with the child's other interests, some of which might be endangered if she is allowed to make her own decisions. We return here to questions of risk and best interests. The concern is that too much leeway in parental determination of best interests may not, in fact, be in a child's best interest nor respect her sexual rights. Some parents, for example, may hold that a child's interests are best served by demonstrating concern for the welfare of her moral character and perhaps the state of her soul. In that case, as demonstrated above, they may well interfere with a child's decision to access information about, say, contraception or HIV. Community standards, wider public debate, objective considerations about potential harms (here of unwanted pregnancy and possible death), and the affect on other rights the child may have (such as the right to health) will all need to be weighed when considering whether or not parents really are acting in a child's best interest by balancing her need for protection and respect for her sexual rights.

Things get more complicated when older children and teens become competent enough to be semi-autonomous. In that situation a child may have rights to make decisions for herself when she is able to do so. That is, she now becomes not only an object of adult concern but a fellow subject. The issue now is about respecting the rights she does have, not the abilities she is developing. There are two questions here: first, "what does it mean to be semi-autonomous?" and second, "Is there a relevant difference between a competent young person and an adult such that when both decide to engage in high risk behaviour, using acceptable decision procedures, the child's right to chose may be infringed while the adult's may not?"

Reference to "semi-autonomy" indicates that a child is not fully competent, or is competent in some areas and not others. In the former case parents ought to respect the competence she does have and consider her intended decisions but may violate them given sufficient risk to her other rights, interests, and abilities. In the later case parents should respect a child's decisions in the areas in which she is competent, though perhaps that competence will not itself be complete without competence in other areas. The issue of what constitutes risk and best interests arises again here, and must be addressed on a decision by decision basis with serious consideration given to the child's stated preferences, and to the degree of autonomy she does have. As we suggested when discussing consent, significant leeway should be given to semi-competent children making lower risk decisions. Questions to ask here are "What happens to a child's rights when he is partially autonomous?;" "Does she thereby gain more than basic or 'human rights?;'" "Do her basic rights require that we respect the autonomy she does have?;" "When can that autonomy be infringed?;"

"Are there reasons to hold that respecting her autonomy is the best way to further her interests?;" "How do we decide what her interests are?;" and "Are there special considerations if her decisions are sexual in nature?"

We cannot fully address the second question, regarding a fully competent minor's right to make a bad decision using a good decision procedure. Some have proposed that the quality of the decision making method teens use is more important than the actual choices they make, so that it is better for them to be autonomous choosers than good choosers.[26] This would mean that if they have considered all their options, realize the risks involved, believe it actually could happen to them, and so on, that they might legitimately choose to have intercourse without protection and it would be better for them to do so and contract an STD than to have others interfere with their decision. Though we will not repeat their discussion here John Rees et al. argue that this position is clearly mistaken.

Nevertheless choosing badly is part of what we protect with rights that protect our choices. The right to act in a way that sets back our well-being is part of what it means to have one's actions protected by rights. An older teenager making sexual choices may well make mistakes. Some of these mistakes will be part of the learning process. Some of them will be part of the process of sexual experimentation that seems to be associated with teen sex. We try to protect our children from bad choices by educating them about options available—safer sex, for example—but ultimately at some point the choices are theirs to make. At this point, when acting within their rights, it's our sense that we would do better focusing on good sex and fostering well-being than on harms, bads and wrongs. A sex education program that focused positively on good sex and how to get it is far more likely to engage and influence teenagers than one which points only to dangers and counsels sexual abstinence. Abstinence-only education may even lead to rather than prevent risky behaviour and bad decision making. A teen who believes that choosing to have sex is terribly wrong may not acquire or use condoms, for example, because to do so would indicate the premeditated choice to have sex—an action perceived as blatantly rebellious and morally worse than being "swept away in the moment."

In any case, questions to ask here include, to repeat, "What is the relevant difference between competent minors and adults that would allow the later and not the former to make high risk bad decisions?;" "Are fully competent minors young people or adults?;" "Can good decision procedures actually lead to bad decisions?;" "What kind of bad choices, if any, is it alright to allow minors to make?;" once again "Are there special considerations if her decisions are sexual in nature?" and so on. Notice that a child's right to make her own decisions may, or may not, include the right to pursue her own pleasure and to engage in certain levels of consensual sexual activity. Most authors do not discuss this possibility.

---

[26] See Rees et al. (1998).

14.5 Expanding the Conversation

While authors often state that sexuality does not consist solely of intercourse, or other forms of physical sexual activity, their awareness has not led to broader discussions of childhood sexuality. Debate instead centers on children's rights to sex education, pre- and post-natal health care and contraception, freedom from abuse (including debate about pedophilia) and on their ability to give consent (see Ekman Ladd 1996, for a useful discussion of these topics). These discussions are absolutely essential; however they should not completely distract us from other significant topics. Discussions that focus on protection, physical health and sex education leave at least two kinds of gaps in understanding child sexuality: they ignore questions about whether sexuality is a present rather than future good for children; and they may mistakenly oppose autonomy and protection.

Almost all of the discussion about children's sexuality is forward looking; it focuses on the child's right to develop into a sexual being, not on her right to express or enjoy her current sexuality. Nor does it treat pleasure as valuable in itself, or as something that is good for children now, within limits, and not only in adulthood. When authors do discuss a right to sexual expression they do so mostly through the lens of potential harms. We need to ask why sexual pleasure is seen as an adult and not a child good, and whether certain forms of sexual activity really are harmful for children. While intercourse and other personally and physically intimate behaviours may pose physical, emotional, and social risks for children it is unreasonable to think that all sexual behaviour does so. There is evidence to suggest, for example, that masturbation increases self-esteem and contributes to physical, emotional, and sexual health (Knowles 2002).

A few authors have begun to take the importance of sexual pleasure for children seriously.[27] Jon Ince discusses "erotophobia" and the importance of pleasure in a chapter titled "Attacking Youthful Lust," though he is not writing for a philosophical or academic audience (Ince 2004). And in *Harmful to Minors* Judith Levine argues that sex is not, in and of itself, harmful to young people (Levine 2002). She also insists on the value of recognizing pleasure in sex education.[28] This is the morally loaded claim that sexual pleasure is valuable and that children are entitled to experience it at their own pace; i.e. that they are entitled to relate sexually to their own bodies as they choose, when they are capable of so choosing.

A number of authors have recently investigated whether there are such things as intrinsic goods of childhood, that is, things that are good for a person, not because of how they instrumentally tie to leading a good adult life but because they are valuable

---

[27] See McCreery (2004) for a review of work by three such authors, including Judith Levine.
[28] Her book resulted in what some have called "a culture-war" and threats of action against her publisher. See Bronski (2002).

for their own sake.²⁹ Some of these goods—certain kinds of play, for example—might only be attainable during childhood. We think it might be the same for the goods of early explorations of sexuality. The delight of a first orgasm, the surprise of feeling another person's touch for the first time, the ability to be curious about unfamiliar body parts, the simple pleasure of holding hands and thinking that someone might "like" you with no thought at all of dating or sex, these firsts and childhood experiences are likely valuable and are no longer attainable in the same way for sexually experienced adults.

Further, some versions of adult goods are likely also good, in their own way, for children. Learning, self-knowledge, pleasure, comfort in one's own body, a sense of belonging to oneself, the ability to be and the experience of being intimately connected with oneself and others, all these are goods that can be gained in relation to sexuality. We see, for example, no reason to say that a child, feeling comfortable with and unashamed of her own body while experimenting on her own with her own sexual sensations, is experiencing something that is not now but would have been a good had she been older. So rather than counsel, "don't do it but if you do, don't get hurt," we actually think there may be goods associated with childhood and teen sexuality that the best sort of life ought to contain. Likewise, certain kinds of bodily exploration and self-pleasure are essential stepping stones to healthy sexuality but are also valuable for their own sake. They have both instrumental and intrinsic aspects to their good when they occur in childhood. There are a number of different kinds of contributions to well-being that childhood sexuality can make, from improvements in self-esteem and self-trust to physical and emotional well-being.

The teen years also offer an opportunity to play with gender and sexual identities and we would do well to foster and protect an environment in which teens can view their identities as fluid without feeling the pressure to reach conclusions (see Coyle 1998).³⁰ If it is right that there are certain sexual goods associated with life stages earlier than adulthood, then we should not wish that children and teens put off all sexual activity. In doing so, one misses out on an important life good. Current sex education for teenagers is negative or at best neutral about the role sex plays in life. Very rarely if at all is pleasure even mentioned. We think that a comprehensive sex education program for teenagers ought to move beyond discussions consent, safe sex, and birth control and include material about sexual pleasure, preferences, and the role of sex in healthy relationships. Such discussions might also include a much wider range of sexual and gender orientations than is currently taught in school. For example, few young people are taught about asexuality even though asexuality is a legitimate sexual orientation. The asexual person might do well to learn of the name for his orientation rather than feel so out of place in our culture.

---

²⁹ See, for example, Anca Ghaeus, "The intrinsic goods of childhood and the good society," in this volume. Also Brennan (forthcoming).

³⁰ At the 9th International Conference on Bisexuality held in Toronto in June 2006 the Focus on Youth Issues panel was presented by a group of older teenagers and young adults from a group called "Fluid." All members of the panel had felt pressure to identify as gay/lesbian/transgendered and reported wishing they had more scope for exploring these identities earlier and reported wanting more information about the range of possibilities at a much earlier age.

Heather Corrina's advice regarding the "10 of the Best Things You Can Do for Your Sexual Self (at Any Age)" (Corrina 2003) is an excellent place to start when thinking about childhood sexual well-being. Her recommendations would be an excellent starting point for a positive sex education program. She writes: Choose yourself as your first partner, learn to talk about sex, be honest with yourself and others, avoid drama, make decisions based on research and clear thinking, appreciate your own body, honor your feelings, don't make your sexual identity (whatever it is) your whole identity, learn as much as you can by reading about sex from a wide variety of sources, and last but not least, have fun. We won't elaborate here on issues of developing sexual self-esteem and the wide variety of choices one can make but we do want to ask one further question. Corrina's advice claims to be good "at any age" but we want to ask whether there might be age appropriate goods in the area of sexual well-being. Very young children are unable to do the kind of research Corrina suggests. Perhaps her advice that children be their own first partners is the most appropriate here.

One interest that follows from sexuality as a childhood good is access to sexually explicit material, such as that widely available on the internet. Although it is controversial we think that children's well-being can be enhanced through access to some kinds of sexually explicit material. It's not as if in most households they lack access now. A frank discussion with emerging adolescents about pornography and media literacy should acknowledge that it is normal to want to view this material and should give children critical tools for viewing, criticizing, and asking questions. Ideally, though this is a long stretch from where we are now, there would be material available for teenagers that was designed and produced for that audience. The alternative is that many young people will stumble across material that may be problematic (misogynistic, not representative of real bodies or real sex, etc.) with little guidance and few opportunities to process their experiences by talking to others.

Though controversial, these questions about pleasure and children's pleasure deserve further philosophical consideration. Rethinking childhood sexuality this way may change the rights we accord to children, the way we understand their well-being, or the behaviours that we accept as appropriate for them.

In addition to ignoring the possibility that sexuality might be a present good for children there is sometimes a tendency to treat furthering a child's autonomy and ensuring her protection as opposing aims. Doing so places parents and other adults in the position of protector and does not recognize the child as an agent who can also help to ensure her own well-being. Recognizing that protection and autonomy are not strict opposites allows the claim that furthering a child's autonomy, while acknowledging her current competence to decide for herself, likely increases her ability to protect herself. Just as one's ability to say yes is compromised by his inability to say no, to be able to refuse consent a child must have potential consent to give. To say what is not okay children must have some idea of what is okay (which is not to say that any level of sexual activity will actually be okay). Not only that, but when a child appreciates her body, and knows her own desires, needs and abilities she is in a much better position to refuse activities that she knows she does not want. In other words, increasing teen sexual agency will allow young people to feel in control of their choices and improve their ability to say no and protect their own rights. Janet Holland and Rachael Thomson concur, reporting that a number of women they interviewed were able to negotiate safer sex with their partners when they came to value their own pleasure, which did not depend on having intercourse with penetration (Holland and Thomson 1998: 72–74).

At the same time, understanding autonomy relationally makes it easier to reconcile the need to respect children's autonomy with their need for adult and parental input and protection. To be autonomous a child doesn't have to make decisions in isolation. The interpersonal skills, self-regard, ongoing social support, information and input on sexual values that a child needs to make autonomous decisions develop with and because of her interactions with others. As many feminist theorists have argued, the same is true of adults.

14.6 Conclusion

We have reviewed two prevailing discourses of child sexuality, argued for the need to further investigate the status of (semi)autonomous sexual choice by minors given their potential competence but also potential bad decisions, and pointed to two gaps in conversations about child sexuality in relation to present goods and autonomy versus protection. Our hope is that this brief foray will spark broader philosophical conversations about childhood sexuality.

In particular we suggest that the following questions deserve further investigation: What is the relevant difference between competent minors and adults that would allow the latter and not the former to make high risk decisions about sexuality? What kinds of bad sexual choices, if any, is it alright to allow minors to make? Is sexuality a *good* of childhood? If so, in what way? How does the development of agency in childhood contribute to opportunities for well-being linked to sexuality? What are the connections between respecting a child's autonomy and ensuring her protection? How might thinking of autonomy as relational and recognizing the potential for semi-autonomy alter our response to childhood sexual exploration? What constitutes childhood sexual well-being, and how can we best support it? We have raised and sketched the beginnings of answers to these questions but there is more work to be done.

We believe that "child + sexuality = okay" is important for both the present and future well-being of our children. But we also know that not all forms of sexual experience will support a child's well-being. Until adults stop focusing solely on sex education, abuse, contraception and consent we will be unable to answer the questions raised above. And in that case we will be unable to fully support the children we love, as they are now and as they will be.

References

Archard, D. (1998). *Sexual consent*. Boulder: Westview Press.
BBC News Online. (2005). Is sex education good enough in schools? In *Have your say stories*. http://news.bbc.co.uk/1/hi/talking_point/4574991.stm. Accessed 30 July 2013.
Brennan, S. (2002). Children's choices or children's interests: Which do their rights protect? In C. Macleod & D. Archard (Eds.), *The moral and political status of children: New essays* (pp. 53–69). New York: Oxford University Press.
Brennan, S. (forthcoming). The goods of childhood, children's rights, and the role of parents as advocates and interpreters. In F. Baylis & C. McLeod (Eds.), *Family-making: Contemporary ethical challenges*. New York: Oxford University Press.
Brennan, S., & Noggle, R. (1997). The moral status of children: Children's rights, parent's rights, and family justice. *Social Theory Practice, 23*(1), 1–26.
Bronski, M. (2002). Review of harmful to minors. *Z Magazine 15*(6). http://www.zmag.org/ZMag/articles/jun02bronski.html
Brown, M. (2011). Sex-ed classes and the rape of our children's innocence. In *Townhall columnists*. http://townhall.com/columnists/michaelbrown/2011/12/01/sex_education_and_the_assault_on_childrens_innocence. Accessed 31 July 2013.
Center for Genetics and Society. (2012). Eugenics in California: A legacy of the past? In *Berkeley Law School panel presentation*. http://www.youtube.com/watch?v=BrF1Q0G4g5o. Accessed 2 Aug 2013.
Christman, J. (2009). Autonomy in moral and political philosophy. In *Stanford encyclopedia of philosophy*. http://plato.stanford.edu/entries/autonomy-moral/. Accessed 31 July 2013.
Coleman, J., & Roker, D. (1998). Introduction. In J. Coleman & D. Roker (Eds.), *Teenage sexuality: Health, risk, and education* (pp. 1–20). Amsterdam: Harwood Academic Publishers.
Collins, P. H. (1999). Mammies, matriarchs, and other controlling images. In J. Sterba Kourany & R. Tong (Eds.), *Feminist philosophies*. NJ: Upper Saddle River.
Corrina, H. (2003). 10 of the best things you can do for your sexual self (at any age). http://www.scarleteen.com/article/body/10_of_the_best_things_you_can_do_for_your_sexual_self_at_any_age. Accessed 26 July 2013.
Coyle, A. (1998). Developing lesbian and gay identity in adolescence. In J. Coleman & D. Roker (Eds.), *Teenage sexuality: Health, risk, and education* (pp. 163–188). Amsterdam: Harwood Academic Publishers.
Downs, C., & Whittle, S. (2000). Seeking a gendered adolescence: Legal and ethical problems of puberty suppression among adolescents with gender dysphoria. In E. Heinze (Ed.), *Of innocence and autonomy* (pp. 195–224). London: Ashgate Publishing.
Ekman Ladd, R. (1996). *Children's rights re-visioned: Philosophical readings*. Belmont: Wadsworth Publishing Company.
Ferguson, F. (2003). The afterlife of the romantic child. *South Atlantic Quarterly, 102*(1), 215–234.
Fields, J. (2005). Children having children: Race, innocence, and sexuality education. *Social Problems, 52*(4), 549–571.
Fox News. (2011). Parenting tips linked by federal site describe children as "sexual beings." In *Politics home*. http://www.foxnews.com/politics/2011/08/24/parenting-tips-linked-by-federal-site-describe-children-as-sexual-beings/. Accessed 31 July 2013.
Friedrich, W. N. (2003). Studies of sexuality of nonabused children. In J. Bancroft (Ed.), *Sexual development in childhood* (pp. 107–120). Bloomington: Indiana University Press.
Hanson, E. (2004). Knowing children: Desire and interpretation in the exorcist. In S. Bruhm & N. Hurley (Eds.), *Curiouser: On the queerness of children* (pp. 107–138). Minneapolis: University of Minnesota Press.
Holland, J., & Thomson, R. (1998). Sexual relationships, negotiation and decision making. In J. Coleman & D. Roker (Eds.), *Teenage sexuality: Health, risk, and education* (pp. 59–80). Amsterdam: Harwood Academic Publishers.

Ince, J. (2004). *The politics of lust*. Vancouver: Pivotal Press.
Irvine, J. M. (2002). *Talk about sex: The battles over sex education in the United States*. Berkeley: University of California Press.
Johnson, C. G. (2013). Female inmates sterilized in California prisons without approval. In *Center for investigative reporting*. http://cironline.org/reports/female-inmates-sterilized-california-prisons-without-approval-4917. Accessed 2 Aug 2013.
Kincaid, J. R. (1998). *Erotic innocence: The culture of child molesting*. Durham: Duke University Press.
Knowles, J. (2002). *Masturbation – From stigma to sexual health*. Katharine Dexter McCormick Library for Planned Parenthood Federation of America Inc. http://www.plannedparenthood.org/pp2/portal/files/portal/medicalinfo/sexualhealth/white-020904-masturbation.xml
Krepel, T. (2011). Right-wing noise machine repeats misguided attack on Obama admin. over sex ed. In *Media matters for America blog*. http://mediamatters.org/blog/2011/08/23/right-wing-noise-machine-repeats-misguided-atta/182512. Accessed 31 July 2013.
Larsson, I. (2001). *Children and sexuality: "Normal" sexual behaviour and experiences in childhood*. Doctoral thesis, Linköping University Department of Molecular and Clinical Medicine, Child and Adolescent Psychiatry.
Levine, J. (2002). *Harmful to minors: The perils of protecting children from sex*. Minneapolis: University of Minnesota Press.
McCreery, P. (2004). Innocent pleasures? Children and sexual politics. *GLQ: Journal of Lesbian Gay Studies, 10*(4), 617–630.
McKay, A., & Bissell, M. (2010). Sexual health education in the schools: Questions & answers, 3rd edition. In *Sex information and education council of Canada*. http://www.sieccan.org/pdf/she_q&a_3rd.pdf. Accessed 31 July 2013.
Meeker, M. (2004). *Epidemic: How teen sex is killing our kids*. Washington, DC: LifeLine Press.
Meeker, M. (2005). Doctor addresses sex risks for teens: Excerpt from "*Epidemic: Raising great teens in a toxic sexual culture*." MSNBC News Online http://www.msnbc.msn.com/id/6867511/. Accessed 30 July 2013.
Monk, D. (2000). Health and education: Conflicting programmes for sex education. In E. Heinze (Ed.), *Of innocence and autonomy* (pp. 179–194). London: Ashgate Publishing.
Moore, S., & Rosenthal, D. (1998). Adolescent sexual behaviour. In J. Coleman & D. Roker (Eds.), *Teenage sexuality: Health, risk, and education* (pp. 35–58). Amsterdam: Harwood Academic Publishers.
Ohi, K. (2004). Narrating the child's queerness in what Maisie knew. In S. Bruhm & N. Hurley (Eds.), *Curiouser: On the queerness of children* (pp. 81–106). Minneapolis: University of Minnesota Press.
Packer, C. (2000). Sex education: Children's right, parent's choice or state obligation? In E. Heinze (Ed.), *Of innocence and autonomy* (pp. 163–178). London: Ashgate Publishing.
Piper, C. (2000). Historical constructions of childhood innocence: Removing sexuality. In E. Heinze (Ed.), *Of innocence and autonomy* (pp. 26–46). London: Ashgate Publishing.
Postman, N. (1982). *The disappearance of childhood*. New York: Delacorte Press.
Potter, R. H., & Potter, L. A. (2001). The internet, cyberporn, and sexual exploitation of children: Media moral panics and urban myths for middle-class parents? *Sexuality Culture, 5*(3), 31–48.
Princeton Survey Research Associates International. (2004). *NBC/People: National survey of young teens sexual attitudes and behaviors*.http://msnbcmedia.msn.com/i/msnbc/Sections/TVNews/Dateline%20NBC/NBCTeenTopline.pdf. Accessed 30 July 2013.
Rees, J., Mellanby, A., & Tripp, J. (1998). Peer led sex education in the classroom. In J. Coleman & D. Roker (Eds.), *Teenage sexuality: Health, risk, and education* (pp. 137–162). Amsterdam: Harwood Academic Publishers.
Rodman, H., Lewis, S. H., & Griffith, S. B. (1984). *The sexual rights of adolescents: Parental competence, vulnerability, and parental control*. New York: Columbia University Press.
Ross, T. (2013). Fears over 11-year-olds sending sex texts. In *The telegraph*. Published 14 February 2013.

Rotermann, M. (2008). Trends in teen sexual behaviour and condom use. Component of Statistics Canada Catalogue no. 82-003-X Health Reports. http://www.statcan.gc.ca/pub/82-003-x/2008003/article/10664-eng.pdf. Accessed 30 July 2013.

Stainton Rogers, R., & Stainton Rogers, W. (1992). *Stories of childhood: Shifting agendas of child concern.* Toronto: University of Toronto Press.

The Guardian. (2011). A child's innocence is precious. That's why it must be protected. In *The observer.* http://www.theguardian.com/commentisfree/2011/oct/02/observer-editorial-parenting-children. Accessed 31 July 2013.

The Oprah Winfrey Show. (2002). *Dr. Phil on alarming sexual behavior among children.* http://www.oprah.com/tows/pastshows/tows_2002/tows_past_20020507_b.jhtml. Accessed 31 July 2013.

Tolman, D. L. (2002). *Dilemmas of desire: Teenage girls talk about sexuality.* Cambridge, MA: Harvard University Press.

Chapter 15
The Grounds and Limits of Parents' Cultural Prerogatives: The Case of Circumcision

Jurgen De Wispelaere and Daniel Weinstock

In June 2012, a German court in Cologne outlawed the circumcision for non-medical reasons of male children, when a young Muslim boy suffered complications after having undergone the procedure. The court judged that in the absence of consent, circumcision constitutes an assault on the physical integrity of children, one that cannot be justified by any offsetting benefit. The court opined that though males capable of giving consent should not be prevented from having their foreskins surgically removed in order to mark their belonging to a religious community that requires circumcision as a condition of membership, children are incapable of giving that consent. In the view of the judges, while parental consent is acceptable for surgical procedures for which there is a medical rationale, it cannot override the state's very great interest and responsibility in protecting children from this kind of physical assault. Consent for this kind of procedure should be limited to agents who are capable of providing consent for themselves.[1]

Unsurprisingly, given the history of German-Jewish relations, the decision created a political firestorm, and by the end of the year, the German *Bundestag* had introduced legislation that reaffirmed the permissibility of such elective circumcisions, on condition that they be carried out in medically appropriate ways, and that parents be provided with information about the possible complications arising from circumcision.

---

[1] For an account of the German case, see Heimbach-Steins (2013).

J. De Wispelaere
Institute for Health and Social Policy, McGill University, 3644 Peel Street, Montreal, QC H3A 1 W9, Canada
e-mail: jurgen.dewispelaere@gmail.com

D. Weinstock (✉)
Faculty of Law, McGill University, 3644 Peel Street, Montreal, QC H3A 1 W9, Canada
e-mail: daniel.weinstock2@mcgill.ca

This controversy has reignited debate around the permissibility of circumcision.[2] It also points to a broader ethical and political question, which has to do with the nature of the prerogative that ought to be granted by the state to parents to raise their children as they see fit, and in particular, to raise them in accordance with the tenets of a religion, even when in so doing they impose what would (but for their religious identification) represent setbacks to their interests. We will be exploring the question of the permissibility of circumcision in the context of this broader set of questions. In particular, we are interested in the question of the degree and ways in which parents should be allowed by the state to make decisions for their children which, though they may serve the cause of facilitating the integration of these children into their cultural or religious communities, may not be in the interest of children. To anticipate, we will argue that there are both prudential and ethical reasons to provide parents with the leeway to subject their children to a surgical procedure that, though it is not medically required, does not impose serious harms, and is perceived as essential to the identification of the child to the religious group to which parents belong.

We will proceed as follows. First, we will argue that a legitimate parental prerogative exists to achieve intimacy with their children through the sharing of cultural scripts. Second, we will argue that a principal ethical criterion that must be satisfied by such scripts is that they do not deny children the right to a reasonably open future. Scripts through which parents seek to achieve the "goods of intimacy" with their children should also satisfy other moral criteria. In particular, they should not be demeaning either to those that are subjected to them, or to those who are affected by them in other ways. We argue that male circumcision can be construed as part of such a script, and that it satisfies the criteria just laid out, much more than do practices that are unproblematically accepted as falling well within the parental prerogative. We will conclude by arguing that there are prudential reasons not to prohibit circumcision, which have to do with the opportunity to regulate the potentially more harmful aspects of the practice that outright prohibition would have us forego. We end by arguing that such prudential considerations cannot be extended, as some have argued they should, to the case of female "circumcision", as that practice fails to satisfy the criteria for *prima facie* moral permissibility that in our view are satisfied in the case of male circumcision.

We will in what follows be operating under the assumption that male circumcision is not medically necessary, and that it may have some moderately harmful long-term consequences. Though the medical debate continues apace, as a quick perusal of the medical literature makes clear, we will be operating, for the sake of argument, on the assumption that it is better, all things considered, for children not to be circumcised, but that the harms associated with circumcision are not severe.[3] Clearly, the plausi-

---

[2] The *Journal of Medical Ethics* has recently devoted an entire issue to the medical, ethical, and legal dimensions of the question. See *Journal of Medical Ethics*, vol. 39, no. 7 (2013).

[3] For a sample of recent papers that reveal just how broad disagreement is among medical researchers as to the balance of potential harms and benefits associated with male circumcision, see Short (2004); AAPTF (2012); Lang (2013); Svoboda (2013). Opponents of the practice argue that there

bility of the position we will be defending here depends upon certain empirical hypotheses to do with the fairly moderate nature of the harm caused to children who undergo the procedure. Were that harm to prove to be greater, the normative grounds that we adduce to defend the permissibility of the practice would be defeated. Were the harm to prove negligible, or were there to turn out to be on-balance *benefits* associated with the practice, then the controversy over permissibility would presumably not arise.

15.1 A Case for Parental Prerogatives

It is only fairly recently that political philosophers have begun to pay attention to the family. Though John Rawls believed that the family was an institution within the basic structure, and that the bestowal of advantages and disadvantages conferred by the family upon children risked making the ideal of equality of opportunity unrealizable, he also depicted the "Original Position" in his original version of that part of his theory as bringing together "heads of households". While the positioning of the family within the basic structure might lead one to believe that there existed Rawlsian reasons to view what happens within the family as a subject of concern for theories of justice and for social and political institutions, the assumption that heads of households negotiate within the Original Position on behalf of their family members suggests a more privatistic conception of the family. Now, within the Rawlsian edifice, these two positions are easily reconciled by the idea that injustices that occur within the family as a result of the operation of the natural mechanisms of affection and partiality can be compensated by other institutions within the basic structure. (In Rawls' view, justice must characterize the basic structure as a whole, rather than particular institutions within the basic structure, taken one by one). But his musings about the family and its compatibility with the goal of equality of opportunity opens up an area of ethical investigation that others have begun to explore.[4]

Now whatever the case as far as Rawls was concerned, it seems clear that until quite recently political philosophers have opted for the privatistic side of the complex Rawlsian picture. To the extent that that picture has been disturbed somewhat, it has been under the pressure of the feminist critique, rather than because of a concern

---

are risks associated with the practice that cannot be entirely eliminated, that it causes significant pain and discomfort, and that it can lead to later sexual dysfunction. Defenders of the right of parents to have their male children circumcised hold that risks and harms are minimal. Circumcision has, finally, been associated with significantly lower rates of HIV transmission in sub-Saharan Africa.

[4] Rawls' discussion of the family in *Theory of Justice* occurs in various places, including p. 74, and p. 511, where he moots the idea that the family might have to be abolished to realize fair equality of opportunity (Rawls 1971). Among theorists who very early took up the challenge of thinking about the family in the context of a largely Rawlsian theory of social justice, see Fishkin (1984). See also Munoz-Darde (1998). Rawls dropped that simplifying assumption within the theory as a result of the critique that was addressed to him by the liberal feminist critique of Okin (1989).

with the intergenerational dimension of family life. Thus, though few philosophers if any would have gone as far as to represent children as being the *property* of their parents, the question of what parents owe their children *as a matter of justice*, and the related question of how the state ought to regulate family life in order to contribute to just intergenerational relations within the family, has received fairly short shrift.

A natural, but ultimately overly simplistic way in which to represent justice within the family is on the basis of the claim that families are from a moral point of view, and from a policy point of view as well, institutions whose sole function is to realize children's interests. Talk of "parental rights" is according to this conception of the family ultimately a shorthand for parental obligations. Parents are trustees to whom certain prerogatives are granted on the assumption that they will make use of their decision-making authority in order to promote the interests of their children. According to this account of the family, parents are essentially trustees, who have no interests in the way that family life transpires that are not reducible to the interests of their children (or to the extent that they do have independent interests, these are viewed as paling in significance relative to the interests of children).

Though it would be implausible to deny that the interests of children loom large in the overall justification of the family, and represent an important criterion that state agencies appropriately apply to the assessment of the functioning of families, we believe that the most adequate theory of the family is a pluralist one. Specifically, we believe that parents also have very important interests in family life, and that these interests are not always in natural harmony with the interests of children. There are plural goods at stake in the life of the family, and this plurality leads to potential conflicts that call for just adjudication.[5]

That parents have such interests is attested to massively by the very great lengths to which many people who cannot have children through unassisted sexual reproduction go through in order to acquire children to parent, either through assisted reproduction technologies, with their attendant costs and physical burdens, or through adoption, with its considerable costs and bureaucratic aggravations.[6] Clearly, people would not go to the lengths of having children simply in order to take up the role of trustee with respect to them.

But should the state give any weight to the desire that parents have to realize their own values and projects through family life, and specifically through the parenting relationship? We follow several theorists who have begun to theorize the political philosophy of families, and who hold that the regulation of family life through family policy should be sensitive at least in some measure of the legitimate interests of parents.[7] This is so for both prudential and for more fully moral reasons. If, as seems obvious, the ability to parent is a crucial and unsubstitutable component of the conception of the good of those adults who choose to parent, then the state

---

[5] This point is developed at greater length in Weinstock (2013).
[6] Cf. De Wispelaere and Daniels (2014).
[7] We are indebted in particular to Brighouse and Swift (2006).

should all things equal facilitate the realization of that good. But prudentially, it could very well be that the realization of the interests of children within the family requires that parental interests be seen to as well. Indeed, it does not seem outlandish to suppose that many parents will perform their role of trustee with diligence to the extent that they can also realize some fundamental aspect of their conceptions of the good through family life. Though this is an empirical hypothesis rather than a conceptual truth, it is possible that children have an interest in being parented by parents who feel that the efforts they deploy in parenting are in the service of values that are not solely those that a mere trustee would be sensitive to.

But what *are* the legitimate, irreducible interests that parents have in the parenting relationship? In an influential account, Adam Swift and Harry Brighouse have argued that there is a certain kind of intimacy that can only be realized through the kind of relationship that obtains in the parenting relationship. "Intimacy" in this account is a shorthand for a wide range of more specific goods: a kind of affection that can only be realized through the parent-child relationship, an intensity of concern that is also unlike any other, and so on.[8]

The principal claim we want to add to the account that Swift and Brighouse have developed is that *intimacy is paradigmatically mediated through cultural scripts*.[9] By this we mean that one of the principal ways in which intimacy is realized in family life is through the introduction of children into narratives, rituals, practices that are central to the identity of parents, and which represent what might be called the "currency of intimacy". Intimacy does not arise simply through parents and children being located side by side. It emerges through families extending cultural scripts intergenerationally through the induction of children into them.

Now, these cultural scripts can be multiple. They can take the form of the sharing by parents of artistic forms and practices that have meant a lot to them. It can involve sharing one's partisanship for a particular sport, or for a particular sports team. It can take very idiosyncratic forms, as for example in the sharing by a parent with a child of a particularly cherished place. But it has very often taken the form of the desire by parents that their children share a particular cultural or religious identity with them, and that they partake in the rituals and practices that are central to that identity.

An apparent difficulty with this aspect of the parent-child relationship is the fact that in many cases, the rites and practices into which parents bring their children up are only in the interest of children *in the context of that relationship*. It is not the case, in other words, that children have an interest in x, but rather that they have an interest in x given the centrality of x to their parents' pre-existing identity. One of us has explored this apparent paradox in the context of language acquisition.[10] Considered in isolation of the significant relationships into which they are brought up, children have an interest in learning whatever language or languages will

---

[8] Brighouse and Swift (2009).
[9] This idea was suggested to us in a paper presented by Colin Macleod to a conference at the University of Western Ontario in June 2013.
[10] Weinstock (2011).

maximize their communicative reach. Were a simple trustee to teach them, say, Welsh, that would arguably constitute a harm relative to the child's interest in as open a future as possible. But when Welsh identity is central to the parents' identity, when the narratives that constitute the self-understanding of the Welsh identity are used in family life as ingredients of the stories that parents tell their children, the teaching of a language with such limited communicational reach takes on an entirely different significance from an ethical point of view. Welsh becomes a privileged medium through which the (culturally mediated) goods of intimacy are realized.

Now, clearly, there are limits to the degree to which the interests of children can be determined by the cultural scripts on the basis of which parents establish intimate relationships with their children. Racist, sexist, and homophobic cultural scripts are clearly to be excluded. But the kinds of limits that I am interested in exploring are the ones through which the state attempts to ensure that children's "right to an open future" is respected to as great a degree as possible.

15.2 The Right to an Open Future

Joel Feinberg's notion that children have a right to an "open" future has attracted a lot of attention since it was first put forward in the context of a critique of the *Yoder* decision of the American Supreme Court.[11] As has been pointed out by many commentators,[12] there is something both absurd and unattractive about the notion, when interpreted in its most extreme form. Indeed, as Claudia Mills has pointed out, there is only a limited amount of time within which children can through the stewardship of their parents explore more than a handful of options. At the limit, the vision of child-rearing that Feinberg's paper might seem to point toward is a recipe for paralysis rather than agency. As Eamonn Callan has pointed out, agency requires not simply revising one's conception of the good, or changing memberships and allegiances, on a whim. Rather, it means knowing what it is to *have* a conception of the good, to explore its resources, run up against its contradictions, see the world through the perspective that it affords.[13]

But the "right to an open future" does not necessarily mean maximizing the range of options that a child can choose to exercise by prescinding from inculcating any conception of the good and associated set of practices in him. Rather, and more sensibly, it can mean ensuring that while the child is being raised within a determinate conception of the good (a particular religious tradition, for example) the conditions are nonetheless in place that might allow him to exit that conception and consider taking on a new one. To express the point in terms of a familiar distinction among theories of individual autonomy, what is required is not that an individual be reared according to a substantive conception of autonomy (according to which

---

[11] Feinberg (1980).
[12] E.g., Mills (2003).
[13] Callan (1997).

the "good life" consists in large measure in not identifying too closely with any particular conception of the good or any particular community), but rather that they possess procedural autonomy (that is, the ability to reflect upon one's commitments, and withdraw from them if they are no longer viewed as attractive).[14]

If the parental interest in achieving culturally mediated intimate relations with one's children is to be compatible with the interest of children in the acquisition of the tools required in order to allow them to realize their right to an open future, then it will have to avoid what might be termed "indoctrination". Indoctrination occurs when children are raised within a cultural script that is presented as uniquely capable of realizing values in their lives, and that accordingly involves the denigration of rival conceptions, and when it fails to provide them with critical tools with which to question the practices that they have been raised in.

The state has a role in ensuring that the right of children to an open future in the sense that has been put forward here is realized. It can do so, for example through its control of the educational agenda, by preventing parents who are so inclined from creating a totalizing educational environment for children, one in which they are subjected to indoctrination as understood here from all of the institutions into which they are raised – family, places of worship, and schools. Though the state cannot without running roughshod over the right to freedom of assembly intervene in the life of the family – or in that of churches, mosques, synagogues, and the like –, it can legitimately limit the educational reach of parents by requiring schools to provide children with alternative perspectives, and with the cognitive tools that they require in order for their right to an open future to be more than simply formal.[15]

The fundamental interest of children in securing the conditions for the right to an open future is most seriously threatened by attempts at limiting the child's cognitive and imaginative horizons through indoctrination. An implication of this is that when parents raise children in ways that may not be in the child's best interest, when that interest is considered in isolation from the interest that the child has in common with its parents to a certain kind of intimate parent-child relation, but that nonetheless secure the child's interest in possessing both a right to an open future and the wherewithal to exercise it, the state appropriately steps aside. It does so because the kind of relationship that is made possible in this manner is valuable, but also for the prudential reason that parents will most likely be better parents if they feel that they are more than just their children's trustees.

15.3 Parental Prerogatives and Male Circumcision

If the arguments of the foregoing two sections are plausible, it follows that parents should be granted a certain prerogative within which they can pursue culturally mediated intimate relations with their children, even when the activities through

---

[14] The canonical formulation of the distinction is in Dworkin (1986).
[15] Cf Clayton (2006).

which such relationships are forged and pursued might be considered not to be in the interest of the children outside the relationship in question.

How does the rite of circumcision fit into this picture? As is well known, circumcision is considered to be an integral part of what it means to be a Jew or a Muslim. Circumcision is a visible mark of the induction of the male child into a community that is presumed central to the identity of parents.

Now, some commentators have claimed that circumcision is incompatible with the child's right to an open future, because it is an irreversible physical mark of that membership. Were an individual to reconsider his membership in the community upon arriving at the age of consent, there is nothing that could be done to undo this mark.[16]

The first thing to note in responding to this concern is that circumcision is still widely practiced among non-Jewish and non-Muslim men in many parts of the world. Moreover, the practice is unlikely to disappear any time soon, as it is still widely believed that circumcision carries with it some medical benefit. (To repeat, we are assuming for sake of argument that the practice is moderately contra-indicated. But the empirical evidence continues to be a matter of controversy among medical researchers). Thus, unlike other forms of ritual markings, circumcision does not uniquely designate belonging to a particular religious or ethno-cultural group. It bears reminding, moreover, that unlike markings of the face practiced by certain groups, circumcision is visible only in the most intimate of contexts.

Given the fact that circumcision does not identify males who have undergone the procedure as members of a particular religious group, the idea that it makes it impossible for them to reconsider and to reject membership when they reach the age of consent is implausible. As we have suggested, moreover, educational and child-rearing practices that aim to indoctrinate are much more prejudicial to the child's capacity to disassociate from the groups and rituals that its parents introduced it to than are ritual markings, especially when they do not mark uniquely.

Perhaps what lies at the basis of the concern with the permanent nature of circumcision is not so much that it cannot be reversed, but that it was not consented to in the first place. According to some, an individual's religious identity should be theirs to choose when they reach the age of consent. If an individual chooses upon reaching that stage that he wants to affirm his membership in a religion that requires circumcision of its male members, then there should be no objection forthcoming from the state of from anyone else to their procuring one. The problem lies when such an irreversible act is imposed upon a child when they are still incapable of providing meaningful consent.[17]

To prevent parents from taking any steps to inculcate the rituals, practices and beliefs of their religious culture upon their children until such a time as children are capable of providing a consent in our view imposes too great a constraint on the parental prerogative. As we have suggested, there are certain goods that are inherent

---

[16] Darby (2013).
[17] Svoboda et al. (2001).

to the familial bond that are made possible by parents sharing their cultures with their children. Intimacy, as we have argued, is not an unmediated dimension of human relationships. One achieves intimacy by sharing worthwhile practices with other individuals, and in the case of the parent-child relationship, those practices are often intertwined with the culture, tradition, and religion.

One could imagine an opponent of this view accepting the claim that intimacy is by its nature culturally mediated, but who would argue that in order not to deny the child's right to an open future cultural forms that, as it were, lie further from the core of a person's identity than religious culture does ought to be chosen by parents in order to serve this intimacy-facilitating function. This claim would misunderstand however the way in which intimacy is achieved through the inculcation of children into cultural "scripts". Indeed, the argument we are advancing is that intimacy is only achieved when the rituals and practices one introduces one's children to are perceived by parents as important, as repositories of central values, and as enacting traditions that connect parents and children to a temporally more extended narrative. What's more, there is likely very little discretion in the case of particular parents as to what kinds of cultural forms will have the requisite level of meaningfulness for them. For some parents, sharing their love of a particular sport might have the required level of centrality, but this will be a function less of choice as to which kind of cultural forms achieves the required level of intimacy while prejudging central components of the child's identity as little as possible, and more of what practices just happen to have become central to parents themselves as a result of the manner in which *they* have been raised, and the way in which they have led their lives.

A final claim that might be made to opponents of a parental prerogative that would allow parents to circumcise their male children for religious or cultural reasons would be to return to the idea of harm. We are assuming for the sake of argument within the context of this paper that the harm experienced by children as a result of circumcision is minimal or moderate. But opponents of the practice could claim that *any* harm visited upon children by their parents should be prohibited.

The initial plausibility of this claim is lessened when one realizes that parents often willingly place their children in harm's way in the pursuit of activities that we standardly think of as falling well within the bounds of permissible parental prerogative. Well before they are able to consent meaningfully, many children are placed in competitive sporting activities, many of which are accompanied by significant risks of short and long-term physical harm. Girls who train seriously as gymnasts must maintain a weight that often interferes with regular menstruation. They also suffer from eating disorders at a rate far greater than occurs in the general population. In Canada, young boys are put at risk of concussive head injuries, that often have severe long-term consequences, in competitive hockey leagues. Recent studies have indicated that concussion-like symptoms may arise from the practice of "heading" a soccer ball. Soccer is played by literally millions of children around the world. Though there are measures that can – and should—be taken to lessen the risks of harm associated with sports, there are limits to what can be done to eliminate the risks associated with sports entirely.

Now, opponents of the permissibility of circumcision would counter by saying that there is an obvious difference between sports and circumcision, which is that sports confer a benefit. Sports conduce to overall good health, and team sports arguably have a positive impact on the socialization of children. Thus, it is unlikely that most people would respond to the risk associated with sport by requiring of parents that they prescind from placing their kids in sporting activities until they are able to provide their fully informed consent.

In the light of these predictable benefits, most people would in the face of this evidence probably stop short of requiring of parents that they prescind from placing their children in *any* sports that bear some kind of risk of injury or harm. They would insist that preventive measures be taken to ensure that those risks are kept to a minimum, and that the most grievous risks are eliminated. But they would probably agree that where sport is concerned responsible parenting requires the minimization of risk rather than its elimination.

Properly regulated by appropriate medical oversight and guidelines, it is quite likely that the harms associated with circumcision are far less grave than those that parents subject their children to when they sign them up for sports. Should the conclusion not then be that in the face of predictable harm, the appropriate policy response is not prohibition, but rather regulation?

The obvious response is that circumcision, unlike sport, does not confer any benefit. (Indeed, we have stipulated that it does not, even though the empirical literature on this point is still mixed). That response would be overly hasty, however. For circumcision, to the extent that it is taken to signify the accession of a child into the religious community, can be seen as a condition for the realization of the "goods of intimacy" that are inherent in parents and children participating together in the rites and practices of a religious tradition that is central to the identity of parents, and which, in virtue of that fact, is for religious parents a privileged locus of culturally mediated intimacy. Thus, though circumcised boys derive no *medical* benefit from circumcision, the claim being made here is that they derive benefit from being in virtue of circumcision brought into a relationship with their parents that procures certain "goods of intimacy".

A final way in which the disanalogy might be maintained between the (unconsented-to) harms of sports and those that arise from circumcision is to claim that unlike what is the case in sports, the benefits associated with the harms of circumcision are only benefits because of a decision made by parents to make the harm a condition of the corresponding goods. Were parents to decide that circumcision was not required in order to procure the culturally mediated goods of intimacy, then those goods could be realized, as it were, risk-free. It is by way of comparison difficult to imagine how even a carefully regulated sport could confer benefits without associated risks.

A number of rejoinders to this point can be made. It actually would be possible to design sporting activities that conferred as much cardiovascular and muscular benefit as sports currently practiced do, with almost no risk attached. We could imagine competitive sports, especially sports in which there is significant contact between players, and between players and projectiles, being banned, in favour of extremely low-risk sports. This suggestion would undoubtedly be resisted, and we hypothesize that a good part of the resistance would stem not from an objective assessment by parents of the relative risks and benefits of different sports, but rather from the cultural centrality of certain sports rather than others in the intergenerational lives of families and communities into which one is introducing one's child.

The second observation to make is that the idea that circumcision is an optional aspect of religion is to misunderstand the manner in which many believers stand to their religious obligations. They do not take them as matters of choice, but rather as meaning-conferring parameters within which to lead their lives. This is not to say that religions do not change in terms of what believers take to be central and peripheral to their religious obligations and identities. Thus, despite the centrality of circumcision to the vast majority of the world's Jews and Muslims, only 40 % of Swedish Jews undergo the procedure. Female circumcision, about which we will be saying more in the final section of this paper, was successfully rooted out in many communities when it was discovered by sociologists that the principal reason for which the anatomically devastating practice was still being carried out had to do with the perception by all members that they had to circumcise their daughters because others were as well, and because in the absence of the procedure their daughters would be considered unmarriageable. The structure of a collective action problem was thus uncovered, and a solution found, in the form of "abandonment ceremonies" whereby entire communities agreed to abandon the practice as a currency of eligibility for marriage.[18]

The point is not to deny that change happens in this area. But change occurs when practices such as circumcision lose their significance for members of the community. And this loss of significance is not likely to occur as a result of legal prohibition of the practice. On the contrary, prohibition may if anything strengthen the resolve of those who might come to feel embattled and persecuted by the prohibition. Ayelet Shachar has for example warned of the dangers of "reactive culturalism" in the face of restrictions of religious practices.[19] Though the German government moved quickly to counteract the decision of the Cologne Court in the case that touched off the controversy in Germany in 2012, the reaction of the Jewish and Muslim communities to news of the prohibition gives us reason to think that the prohibition would have been met by resistance, rather than by compliance.

15.4 Prohibition or Regulation? The Seattle Compromise

That legal prohibition would not have eradicated the practice, but rather driven it as it were "underground", gives us further reason to hold that from the point of view of the state, regulation, rather than prohibition, is the prudentially best policy. The case of male circumcision is indeed one in which a policy of harm reduction seems

---

[18] Mackie (1996).
[19] Shachar (2001).

advisable.[20] The natural habitat of such policies is one in which, first, a practice that obtains within a segment of society is the object of reasonable disagreement not likely to be resolved through discussion or deliberation, and in which, second, even those who are opposed to it realize that attempts at prohibition are likely to backfire because they exceed the carrying capacity of law-enforcement agencies, for epistemic or cost-effectiveness reasons. That is, the practice may simply be difficult to detect, or else the resources that would need to be deployed for effective detection and enforcement would be disproportionate to the good that would be achieved through effective prohibition. In such cases, that include policy areas such as drugs, gambling, sex work, euthanasia and assisted suicide, and a host of others, moral debate can in effect be bracketed, and a focus on the effectiveness of prohibition and of various modes of regulation can be adopted as an appropriate lens through which to determine the best policy response to a practice which in an unregulated form could give rise to significant harms.

In the case of circumcision the concern is of course that the legal prohibition of male circumcision would not diminish the incidence of the practice considerably, but would simply prevent the state from exercising regulatory oversight over it. The German legislative response to the Court's attempt at prohibition provides us with a sense of the kinds of regulations it seems appropriate to impose upon male circumcision. According to the law that was drafted in December 2012, the practice can only be carried out in a medically appropriate setting. Up until the age of 6 months, non-medical personnel can however carry out circumcisions, complications that might arise after that age being seen as requiring the intervention of trained medical personnel. The law also imposes the requirement that parents only be able to consent to the practice on behalf of their sons if they are provided with full medical information about it, including information about possible complications and long-term physiological consequences.[21] In a context in which the practice was rendered illegal but not effectively prohibited, harms resulting from what would in effect be an entirely deregulated practice of circumcision would likely be much worse than they would be under an appropriate set of regulations.

There are thus prudential reasons not to prohibit circumcision, even for those who do not accept the moral argument that has been put forward here in favour of including it within the range of parents' legitimate prerogative.

The argument we have been developing in the case of male circumcision is however, on inspection, not a pure case of the harm reduction approach. A "pure" harm reduction strategy prescinds from any moral judgment. Its aim is not to censor nor to attempt to eradicate or even to lessen the occurrence of a practice, but rather to minimize the harmful consequences that tend to accompany it. Our approach is to be distinguished from pure harm reduction in that we do not think that it should

---

[20] Ben-Yami (2013).

[21] Studies indicate however that information about the potential deleterious effects of circumcision do not significantly deter parents from requesting that the procedure be carried out. See for example Binner et al. (2002).

be applied to practices that offend against the principles that we have invoked in our discussion of male circumcision.

To see this more clearly, consider the case of female "circumcision". On a number of occasions in the past decade or so, Somali immigrants to Western countries, first Italy, and then the United States, approached medical practitioners in local clinics to ask them to practice genital scarring of their girls, in lieu of the much more extensive mutilation of girls' sexual organs carried out in many communities in the countries from which they have arrived, mutilation that often involved the removal of the clitoris and of the labia minora. The scarring of the hood of the clitoris that was proposed by representatives of the Somali communities was comparatively minor from an anatomical point of view, and would in particular not involve the removal of any tissue, nor would it preclude women being able to enjoy sex. It would moreover be carried out in sterile, medically appropriate settings. The alternative in both these communities would have been for girls to continue to be subjected to a much more painful and anatomically devastating form of female genital cutting, in non-medical settings, with the attendant risks of sepsis. This proposal came to be known as the "Seattle compromise", as it had initially been proposed to the Harborview Medical Center located in that city.[22]

In both the Italian and American clinics in which the compromise was proposed, medical practitioners who dealt on a regular basis with members of the Somali communities in question agreed to the compromise. They were clearly motivated at the very least by the kind of harm reduction rationale that we have presented as providing independent support for the moral grounds which in our view allows male circumcision as part of the parents' legitimate range of prerogative. In both cases, however, social and political pressures to refuse the compromise were such that regulatory bodies exercising oversight over the practitioners required that the practice be halted, even at the cost of placing young girls back in the hands of untrained ritual cutters operating in unsanitary conditions.[23]

Who was right in this case? To the extent that the physical harm imposed on girls as a result of the Seattle compromise is no greater, and may actually be less, than that which results from the much more broadly accepted practice of male circumcision, it would seem that our analysis should apply to that practice as well.[24] Where the medical contra-indication is moderate rather than grave, why should we not view it as falling within the range of what parents can decide for their children? Are our very different responses to the two kinds of cases a reflection of discriminatory attitudes that we may harbor toward the groups that engage in female cutting, who are viewed with greater suspicion than the much more familiar groups that engage in male circumcision?[25]

There does seem to us to be a morally salient difference between the two cases, however, even if we accept for the sake of argument that a medicalized version of

---

[22] For an account of the basic facts of the case see Lambelet Coleman (1998).
[23] See AAPCB (2010).
[24] Cf. Shell-Duncan (2001).
[25] On this issue see Davis (2010); Tamir (2006); Gaelotti (2007).

genital scarring might be as medically innocuous as male circumcision. In ways that are not present in the case of male circumcision, female genital cutting has to do with the control of women's sexual and reproductive lives. It seems intrinsically connected to the wish that seems to be felt by families in communities in which the practice is widespread to make daughter eligible for marriage. It suggests that only where women are rendered unable to experience pleasure in sexual relations can this condition be satisfied. Clearly, the meaning attached to the practice, even in the more moderate form suggested in the "Seattle compromise", is incompatible with the norm of gender equality. (What's more, even if it was possible to carry out an analogous procedure on males, it would instantiate an unattractive view of human sexual relations).

Now, some might argue that there are in fact a number of meanings associated with the practice of female genital "circumcision", some of which betoken precisely the kind of group membership that we have claimed as a ground to accept circumcision in the case of males.[26] But the abandonment ceremonies recounted by Gerry Mackie seem premised on the fact that the morally objectionable meanings are those that attach most robustly to the practice.[27] Indeed, they were carried out on the basis of the hypothesis formulated by Mackie that the persistence of the practice had the structure of a collective action problem, born from the desire of members of communities that engage in the practice to trade in the currency of marriageability, whatever that currency might be. The success of the abandonment ceremonies indicated that community members were not wedded to the particular currency of female genital cutting. But it also indicates that the meaning that most spontaneously attached to the practice had to do with a desire to control women's lives as sexual beings. Were other meanings robustly attached to the practice, the agreement not to consider it a condition of eligibility for marriage would not have lead to widespread abandonment of the practice that the "convention" account pioneered by Mackie predicted that it would. To the extent that one of the restrictions that we have imposed upon the cultural mediations through which familial intimacy is achieved included the requirement that such mediations not be premised upon values inimical to liberal democracies, there is reason to prohibit the practice even in its more moderate, "Seattle compromise" form, since it reflects the same set of values as the more thoroughgoing form of genital cutting.

Another way of putting the point is that the question of whether or not a practice of genital cutting should be tolerated as part of parental prerogative cannot be determined by anatomical facts alone. The meanings that attach to those facts must also be considered. Though the Seattle compromise establishes anatomical equivalence between male and female circumcisions, it does not establish moral or symbolic equivalence.

---

[26] On the other meanings that female genital cutting has at various times been taken to have, see Kopelman (1994).

[27] Mackie (1996).

15.5 Conclusion

To summarize the argument: the interest in certain kinds of intimate relations with their children are culturally mediated through a range of practices, rituals, communities, beliefs, etc., that constitute the scripts through which "the goods of intimacy" are realized. In some cases, these cultural scripts require parents acting in ways toward their children that might be seen deleterious to their children's interests, but for the intimate relationships within which they occur. What matters is not that children be completely shielded from such practices, which would occur on a trustee model in which parents always acted according to the child's best interest, where that best interest would be defined independently of the familial relationship. Rather, the state's role is to ensure that children are not subjected to excessive harm, that the cultural practices through which the familial relations and the goods of intimacy are not themselves predicated upon values that are contrary to the basic normative commitments of a liberal democracy, and that children are shielded from practices of indoctrination that aim at making it difficult for children to revisit their communal attachments when they reach the age of consent. Male circumcision appears to us when seen in the light of this framework to fall within the range of permissible actions that parents can impose upon their children. We have assumed for the sake of the present argument that the medical contra-indication, if any, is not an emphatic one, and the nature of the physical mark that circumcision represents is less deleterious to the child's being able to revisit his attachments in later life than are other, non-physical attempts at indoctrination that parents may be inclined to visit upon their children, and which the state must attempt to counteract, most notably through the education system.

References

American Academy of Pediatrics Committee on Bioethics (AAPCB). (2010). Policy statement: Ritual genital cutting of female minors. *Pediatrics, 125*(5), 1088–1093.
American Academy of Pediatrics, Task Force on Circumcision (AAPTF). (2012). Technical report: Male circumcision. *130*(3), 756–785.
Ben-Yami, H. (2013). Circumcision: What should be done? *The Journal of Medical Ethics, 39*, 459–462.
Binner, S. L., et al. (2002). Effects of parental education on decision-making about neonatal circumcision. *Southern Medical Journal, 95*(4), 457–461.
Brighouse, H., & Swift, A. (2006). Parents' rights and the value of the family. *Ethics, 117*, 80–106.
Brighouse, H., & Swift, A. (2009). Legitimate parental partiality. *Philosophy and Public Affairs, 37*(1), 43–80.
Callan, E. (1997). *Creating citizens*. Oxford: Oxford University Press.
Clayton, M. (2006). *Justice and legitimacy in upbringing*. Oxford: Oxford University Press.
Darby, R. L. (2013). The child's right to an open future: Is the principle applicable to non-therapeutic circumcision? *The Journal of Medical Ethics, 39*, 463–468.
Davis, D. (2010). Cultural bias in responses to male and female genital surgeries. *The American Journal of Bioethics, 3*(2), W1–W9.

De Wispelaere, J., & Weinstock, D. (2014). Privileging adoption over sexual reproduction? A state-centered perspective. In R. Vernon, S. Hannan, & S. Brennan (Eds.), *Permissible progeny*. Oxford: Oxford University Press.

Dworkin, G. (1986). *The theory and practice of autonomy*. Cambridge: Cambridge University Press.

Feinberg, J. (1980). The child's right to an open future. In A. Aiken & H. Laffollette (Eds.), *Whose child? Parental authority and state power*. Totowa: Rowman and Littlefield.

Fishkin, J. (1984). *Justice, equal opportunity, and the family*. New Haven: Yale University Press.

Gaelotti, A. E. (2007). Relativism, universalism, and applied ethics: The case of female circumcision. *Constellations, 14*(1), 91–111.

Heimbach-Steins, M. (2013). Religious freedom and the German circumcision debate. *EUI working papers*, RSCAS 18.

Kopelman, L. M. (1994). Female circumcision/genital mutilation and ethical relativism. *Second Opinion, 20*(2), 55–71.

Lambelet Coleman, D. (1998). The Seattle compromise: Multicultural sensitivity and Americanization. *Duke Law Journal, 47*(4), 717–783.

Lang, D. P. (2013). Circumcision, sexual dysfunction and the child's best interest: Why the anatomical details matter. *The Journal of Medical Ethics, 39*, 429–431.

Mackie, G. (1996). Ending footbinding and infibulation: A convention account. *American Sociological Review, 61*(6), 999–1017.

Mills, C. (2003). The child's right to an open future? *The Journal of Social Philosophy, 34*(3), 499–509.

Munoz-Darde, V. (1998). Rawls, justice in the family, and justice of the family. *The Philosophical Quarterly, 48*(192), 335–352.

Okin, S. (1989). *Justice, gender, and the family*. New York: Basic Books.

Rawls, J. (1971). *A theory of justice*. Cambridge, MA: Harvard University Press.

Shachar, A. (2001). *Multicultural jurisdictions*. Cambridge: Cambridge University Press.

Shell-Duncan, B. (2001). The medicalization of female circumcision: Harm reduction or promotion of a dangerous practice. *Social Science and Medicine, 52*, 1013–1028. col.

Short, R. V. (2004). Male circumcision, a scientific perspective. *The Journal of Medical Ethics, 30*, 241.

Svoboda, J. S. (2013). Circumcision of male infants as a human rights violation. *The Journal of Medical Ethics, 39*, 469–474.

Svoboda, J. S., Van Howe, R. S., & Dwyer, J. G. (2001). Informed consent for neonatal circumcision: An ethical and legal conundrum. *Journal of Contemporary Health Law Policy, 17*, 61–133.

Tamir, Y. (2006). Hands off clitoridectomy. *The Boston review*. Accessed 26 Nov 2013.

Weinstock, D. (2011). Do the interests of children pose a limit on cultural rights? In E. Rude-Antoine & M. et Pievic (Eds.), *Éthique et famille*. Paris: L'Harmattan.

Weinstock, D. (2013). La famille comme institution politique. In D. Robichaud, D. et Anctil, & P. Turmel (Eds.), *Penser les institutions*. Sainte-Foy: Les presses de l'Université Laval.

CPSIA information can be obtained
at www.ICGtesting.com
Printed in the USA
LVOW13*1745080418
572701LV00009B/932/P

9 789401 792516